Accidental Cure 3:

AI vs Ancient Intelligence

A Medical Acupuncture Series

Simon Yu, MD

Accidental Cure 3:

AI vs. Ancient Intelligence

A Medical Acupuncture Series

1st Edition

No part of this book may be reproduced or transmitted in any form by any means, graphic, electronic, or mechanical, including photocopying, recording, taping, or by any information storage retrieval system, without the written permission of the publisher.

All Rights reserved © 2025 by Simon Yu, MD

This book is written for informational purposes and not intended as medical advice. The views in this book are those of the author, who has not been paid or sponsored by any institution for the content within.

Prevention and Healing, Inc.

For information, contact:

10908 Schuetz Road
St. Louis, Missouri 63146

www.preventionandhealing.com

ISBN 979-8-9935009-0-4

Dedication

For all my patients struggling and willing to try the unknown territory of integrative energy medicine and dentistry.

Many patients recovered but many did not respond despite my and their best efforts, but their experiences are not forgotten.

Their successes and failures are included here, in storytelling form, throughout my book: *Accidental Cure 3*.

Acknowledgments

Special thanks to:

Laura Henze Russell for helping me edit and organize my writing into a book, and editing my articles, e-letter, and website.

Shawn Cornell for his gifted graphic art on my cover and in the figures and illustrations throughout the book.

My staff who have supported me, take care of patients, and provided me with valuable feedback from our work with patients.

My colleagues who come to learn, share information, spread the word, and put up with my sense of adventure and humor.

Special thanks to those who read, reviewed, and enriched my book: Dr. med. Helmut Retzek for thoughtful additions, Dr. med. Atel Hemat for writing comprehensive FAQs, Scott Forsgren for careful review and edits, and Dr. Tim Guilford, Dr. Murat Isci, Dr. Kelly Blodgett, DDS, and Dr. Michael Karlfeldt for their thoughts. Any errors are mine.

This book would not be possible without my wife Kate's unconditional support.

Also by Simon Yu, MD

Accidental Cure: Extraordinary Medicine for Extraordinary Patients

AcciDental Blow Up in Medicine: Battle Plan for Your Life

Reviews & Recommendations

"In the last decade, few physicians have bridged the worlds of conventional and complementary medicine as effectively—and as boldly—as Dr. Simon Yu, internist from St. Louis, Missouri. What sets his approach apart is its simplicity, speed, and accuracy. His AMA method provides a reproducible, independent testing system."

Helmut Retzek, Dr. med, Vöcklabruck, Austria

"When I finally met Dr. Yu, everything fell in place. He had developed what I was searching for: a diagnostic and therapeutic tool that helps uncover hidden causes for the many weird and therapy-resistant symptoms that my patients were suffering from."

Atel Hemat, Dr. med., Cologne, Germany

"When I graduated from medical school, the commencement speaker explained that a medical license was a license to learn. Simon Yu is an example of using his medical license as a license to learn."

Tim Guilford, MD, Your Energy Systems, LLC

"For any dentist who considers themselves to be "Biological" or "Holistic" in nature, incorporating energy assessments into daily care is a must!"

Kelly Blodgett, DMD, NMD, Blodgett Dental Care, Portland, OR

"In his third life-altering book, *Accidental Cure 3*, Dr. Simon Yu again challenges conventional dogma and looks outside the medically accepted box to find solutions that truly empower patients to find their road back to vibrant health. His brilliance as a medical doctor, paired with his bravery as a human being, is a magical formula that often results in cures that may not be so accidental after all."

Scott Forsgren, FDN-P, HHP, Better Health Guy

"Dr. Simon Yu's work has revolutionized how we view chronic illness and unresolved health issues. His parasite protocol has become an instrumental part of my clinical toolkit. The stories in *Accidental Cure 3* reflect what I've seen in practice—remarkable recoveries once hidden infections are addressed. Dr. Yu's Acupuncture Meridian Assessment is not just diagnostic; it's a roadmap to restoration."

Michael Karlfeldt, ND, PhD, Founder, The Karlfeldt Center

"This book is essential reading for physicians, dentists, and healers of any background who are ready to engage with medicine's emerging frontier—not through guesswork, but through a structured, tested, and patient-centered system that listens to what the body already knows."

Murat Isci, MD, Istanbul, Turkey

Forward

In the last decade, few physicians have bridged the worlds of conventional and complementary medicine as effectively—and as boldly—as Dr. Simon Yu, internist from St. Louis, Missouri.

Dr. Yu's groundbreaking work fuses bioenergetic testing techniques with mainstream pharmacological treatments in a way that is both radically efficient and clinically astonishing. His method, known as Acupuncture Meridian Assessment (AMA), is a streamlined and far more accessible evolution of the traditional electroacupuncture according to Voll (EAV). In just minutes, he can energetically assess a patient and develop a treatment protocol, often using conventional antiparasitic, antibacterial, antiviral, and antifungal medications—yet with unconventional precision and success.

This rapid diagnostic approach is not theoretical. I have personally witnessed the remarkable demand for Dr. Yu's expertise at medical conferences, where entire groups of physicians line up, sometimes into the night, eager to be tested by him. At Europe's largest integrative medicine conference in Baden-Baden, I saw more than two dozen doctors follow him back to his hotel at 10 p.m.—where he continued testing into the early morning hours.

Dr. Yu's journey began during his time in the U.S. Army Reserve Medical Corps, where he served for 25 years and retired as a full Colonel. On a humanitarian mission to Bolivia, he treated over 10,000 people with antiparasitic medications—witnessing astonishing improvements in a wide range of chronic symptoms. These experiences shaped his clinical philosophy and eventually led to the fusion of energetic diagnostics with evidence-based pharmaceuticals.

What sets Dr. Yu's approach apart is its simplicity, speed, and accuracy. His AMA method provides a reproducible, independent testing system—comparable in principle to other bioenergetic testing methods—but clearly faster, more precise, and more intuitive in practice. I can state this confidently, having been trained in all these modalities.

A particularly striking case Dr. Yu once shared with me in London concerned a woman suffering from chronic fatigue, brain fog, neuropathic symptoms, and irritable bowel syndrome. After a course of antiparasitic therapy, her condition improved dramatically. So much so, in fact, that she gave the same medication to her autistic son—who then experienced a surprising and profound improvement in his symptoms. These are not isolated results, but part of a growing body of clinical observations.

Equally essential to Dr. Yu's method—and often overlooked in standard medical practice—is his systematic focus on hidden dental infections, cavitations, and focal interference fields in the mouth. These silent disruptions of the body's energy system can sabotage even the best medical treatment plans. Dental foci, if unrecognized, may prevent healing and perpetuate chronic disease. Dr. Yu trains practitioners to identify and correct these blockages with the same precision he applies to parasitic, microbial, and energetic issues. In this, he has made an invaluable contribution to modern integrative diagnostics.

I first encountered Dr. Yu in 2016 at a cancer hyperthermia conference in Munich, where he presented a series of patients—some with conditions as severe as amyotrophic lateral sclerosis—showing extraordinary improvements. He presented before-and-after meridian measurement graphs, clearly documenting not only energetic normalization but tangible clinical recovery. These were not anecdotes—they were documented transformations.

Since then, my wife and I have travelled multiple times to train directly under Dr. Yu in St. Louis. We have now organized and attended eight additional AMA training seminars in Europe. As we move toward retirement, we are glad to see that Dr. Atel Hemat in Cologne and Düsseldorf is continuing Dr. Yu's legacy with great fidelity—step by step, method by method. He is well on his way to becoming Dr. Yu's leading European successor.

Dr. Simon Yu's influence pervades not only our clinical practice but also my writings, lectures, and large integrative medicine platform, www.ganzemedizin.at. His work exemplifies what it means to be a true physician-healer: using whatever means necessary to help the patient—not constrained by rigid protocols but guided by results and deep insight.

Following his previous books—*Accidental Cure* and *AcciDental Blow Up in Medicine*—this new volume, *Accidental Cure 3*, adds an even richer layer of case studies and clinical wisdom. It is not only timely but essential reading for anyone who takes healing seriously.

Dr. med. Helmut Retzek
Vöcklabruck, Austria
www.ganzemedizin.at/en

Onward

In 2018, Dr. Helmut Retzek and his wife and assistant, Lenna Retzek, from Austria introduced me to Dr. Yu. Since then, I have successfully applied AMA for diagnostic and therapeutic purposes. I have witnessed firsthand the transformative power of a holistic treatment approach that combines dental work, parasite cleansing, balancing nutritional deficiencies, removing environmental toxins, avoiding intolerant foods, and addressing emotional traumas.

I trained as an internist in Germany, specializing in emergency medicine. While conventional medicine excels in treating acute and life-threatening conditions, it often falls short when addressing chronic illnesses. From the very start of my medical education, I sought complementary approaches to better serve chronically ill patients.

Over the years, I have attended numerous seminars on homeopathy, basic acupuncture, environmental medicine, nutritional medicine, and repurposed drug therapies. My goal has always been to explore diagnostic and therapeutic tools that are holistic, practical, and beneficial for my patients, as well as my family and friends.

When I finally met Dr. Yu, everything fell in place. He had developed what I was searching for: a diagnostic and therapeutic tool that helps uncover hidden causes for the many weird and therapy-resistant symptoms that my patients were suffering from: AMA = Acupuncture Meridian Assessment. Although I already had attended basic EAV classes before, Dr. Yu's AMA was opening a whole new dimension to energetic testing.

I was fascinated by Dr. Yu's approach, which combined AMA with prescription parasite medications, antifungal treatments, and chelating agents. Inspired after my first seminar, I purchased a Vistron EAV device from Kindling and began practicing. It took time to achieve consistent and reliable results, but each training session deepened my understanding and proficiency in AMA.

To date, I have attended seven AMA seminars in St. Louis and Europe, including two advanced training sessions, and organized an AMA seminar in Germany with Dr. Yu.

I am grateful to my friends and mentors, Dr. Helmut Retzek and Ms. Lenna Retzek. They have generously shared their vast knowledge and experience with me without expecting anything in return. Their selflessness is truly inspiring.

I would like to express my gratitude to Dr. Yu, his wife Kate Yu, and his whole team for their unwavering support in helping me learn the method, for selflessly sharing their knowledge, and for their warm-hearted support during my stay in their clinic and during the seminars.

Atel Hemat, Dr. med.
Cologne, Germany
www.dratelhemat.com/en/

Inward

For centuries dentistry has been performed in a very mechanical fashion following a "drill it and fill it" mentality. Little to no consideration has been given to the inherent energetic shifts that occur to the body when its native structures are altered in the mouth. Even to this day dental schools continue to teach from a purely mechanical perspective.

As a dentist whose goal is to optimize the health of my patients, it came to my attention about 20 years into my practice life that all living things are an embodiment of energy. I also discovered that energy can be measured by various means of energetic assessment. The version that resonated most with me is called "Acupuncture Meridian Assessment" and was developed by Dr. Simon Yu. It is an efficient and streamlined version of the original "EAV" (Electroacupuncture According to Voll) technique.

Since incorporating Acupuncture Meridian Assessment into my practice, my team and I have been able to verify when the body's energy is balanced. This has tremendous practical application when removing infection from people's jaws, ensuring that materials are well tolerated, or that a person's bite is balanced. For any dentist who considers themselves to be "Biological" or "Holistic" in nature, incorporating energy assessments into daily care is a must! I encourage all healthcare professionals to learn Acupuncture Meridian Assessment so that we are better able to listen to what the energy of our patients is trying to tell us.

Kelly Blodgett, DMD, NMD, IBDM
Blodgett Dental Care, Portland, OR
www.blodgettdentalcare.com

Outward

I first met Simon Yu, MD, almost 15 years ago at a medical conference hosted by Dietrich Klinghardt, MD. Given my prior exposure to Dr. Klinghardt's powerful Autonomic Response Testing work, I was immediately drawn to Dr. Yu's explorations into the energetic realm and in the creation of his Acupuncture Meridian Assessment (AMA) system; now also referred to as AI or Acupuncture Intelligence.

Shortly after, I attended Dr. Yu's International Alternative Medicine Conference in St. Louis to learn more about his work. On the same trip, I scheduled my first appointment with Dr. Yu to be evaluated using his AMA system; with the goal of further progressing my own healing from years of Lyme disease, mold illness, Chronic Fatigue Syndrome/ME, and Fibromyalgia.

Dr. Yu immediately detected two dental cavitations, parasites, and heavy metals in our first visit. In later visits, he also found a fungal overgrowth and an issue with my bite. Addressing the factors that he identified using AMA further assisted me in unlayering the hidden contributors to my longstanding health challenges.

I later attended his AMA Practitioner Training to learn more about his life's work and had the somewhat stressful opportunity to test Dr. Yu using AMA while I was blind-folded and at the head of the class in front of many brilliant minds. Fortunately, he was a great teacher, and I rose to the challenge.

What makes Dr. Yu's work so profound is that he often finds the roadblocks to health that everyone else is missing; or those where available testing is unable to adequately detect an issue. Addressing the core, often unexplored barriers to health, such as dental infections and parasites, can allow the body to regain homeostasis.

Then, you combine his brilliance with his bravery which makes a powerful combination. He is an outside-the-box thinker and does not limit his approach to what others may consider the standard of care. The standard of care should be caring about patients, but that's not how modern medicine often works.

I remember asking Dr. Yu once how he got away with using his AMA testing device and prescribing antiparasitics in the military. His response was, "I was the colonel. Who was going to tell me I couldn't do it?"

Dr. Yu is one of the bravest practitioners and human beings I have encountered on my own health journey. I applaud him for doing what is right for patients and for having the bravery to go against conventional wisdom. His patients greatly benefit from both his brilliant mind and his brave soul.

Many have suggested that when his patients get better that it was just an accident, but how many accidents does it take for the realization that it was "No Accidental Cure" to emerge?

My life is better today as a result of crossing paths with Dr. Yu! The world needs more brave healers like him.

Scott Forsgren, FDN-P, HHP
Patient, Health Coach, and Creator
www.betterhealthguy.com

Preface

In December 2023, I gave a talk, "Infections, Inflammation, and the Unknown" to a group of physicians in Berlin, Germany. My focus was a new understanding of the role of dental issues, parasites, and fungi in infectious diseases and chronic illnesses. What hides within our patients and ourselves, impacting health and disease - long before we can detect them by conventional exams and lab tests - if we are even looking for them? Key questions: Can we treat dental infections before they become visible on x-rays or cone beam scans? Can we address parasites and fungi when reliable tests to detect these covert infections are lacking?

En route to Berlin, my wife Kate and I made a stop in Istanbul, Turkey, to visit the Göbekli Tepe. This recently unearthed archaeological site dates back nearly 11,600 years, predating the last ice age and the time of Abraham in Biblical chronology. Despite being in the early stages of excavation, we observed monumental stone carvings depicting animals aligned with astronomical constellations.

This site represents an advanced civilization whose existence was previously unknown. The deliberate burial of this monumental work to preserve it underground remains a mystery. This discovery will undoubtedly transform our understanding of human history, necessitating a rewrite of the era predating the early Sumerian civilization; effectively doubling our historical timeline, or more.

Similarly, can we unearth ancient knowledge from the era predating Ayurvedic medicine, Traditional Chinese Medicine, and Acupuncture? There is much ancient wisdom yet to be discovered.

This book explores the known and unknown as I perceive it, sense it, and beyond. It covers how to use ancient, authentic, acupuncture intelligence to help detect and treat underlying problems and restore health and vitality.

In my first ten years of practice, I rose to medical director at a midwestern HMO. I became frustrated with the limits of prescribing medications to treat symptoms vs. detecting and reversing underlying causes of disease. I embarked on a journey to learn more, building on my medical school training, clinical practice, and service in the US Army Reserves Medical Corps, from which I retired after 25 years as a full colonel.

I also studied acupuncture at Helms Medical Institute, then housed at Stanford University Medical School, learned German Biological Medicine at conferences in Europe, learned about dentistry from my biological dentist mentor Doug Cook, DDS, and have investigated and trialed many other modalities, from insulin potentiation and stem cell therapies to Frequency Specific Microcurrent and brain neuromodulation therapies.

Promise vs. Pitfalls of AI for Medicine

Let's fast forward to today's Artificial Intelligence (AI). AI has revolutionized the world, including the field of medicine.

A patient of mine attended the inaugural IBM Watson Hackathon in Brooklyn, NY, eager to explore the potential of AI in diagnosing, guiding treatment, and curing complex chronic diseases. She was disappointed to find that Watson's AI was limited to peer-reviewed medical journals. It focused on diagnosing and treating symptoms of named diseases via pharmaceuticals based on established research, overlooking recent innovations, preliminary results, and case studies.

In Berlin, I gave a lecture and demonstration on Acupuncture Meridian Assessment (AMA) for a complex chronic disease patient. The physicians were intrigued by how I could treat parasite problems when laboratory tests for parasites are notoriously unreliable. This was based on my experience with the US Army military mission in Bolivia, as described in my first book, *Accidental Cure*.

Your mysterious chronic disease may come with a fancy medical diagnosis in Latin. However, a cure is possible when we ignore the name of the diagnosis and rediscover a better understanding of ancient forgotten knowledge in the acupuncture meridian system.

Increasingly, genetic mutations, viral infections, especially post-COVID syndrome, or unresolved emotions such as PTSD are blamed as the cause of patients' problems. What if these are not the true underlying problems but instead, they reflect the impacts of unrecognized dental infections, parasite-fungal infections, environmental toxins, and nutritional imbalances?

My Approach to the Parallel Universe of AI

Artificial Intelligence (AI) is applied to the domain of medicine: electronic written universe of medical literature and published research, images and scans, and guidelines and orthodoxy to suggest diagnoses and potential treatments to consider.

In contrast, Acupuncture Intelligence is applied to the domain of the whole body - physical, physiological, and emotional - of each patient. It reflects what our bodies, brains, organs, systems, and cells signal, or tell us, encoded in the bioenergetic frequencies resonating within each patient. It assesses how the patient will respond to various treatments, and how to sequence them, starting with the biggest problem first.

This book is my attempt to weave together AI applied to the domain of the whole body - the ancient acupuncture intelligence contained in the living body's meridian system - to explain why and how to detect, treat, and effectively rebalance these systems.

Let's rediscover and explore Acupuncture Intelligence, in which your whole body is the domain. The body's subtle energy fields can communicate Ancient, Applied, Authentic, Accurate, and Advanced Intelligence, if we learn how to read the meridian frequencies like musical scales and interpret them.

We can test medications against the underlying problems revealed by electrical disturbances, finding ones that restore meridian balances by utilizing the body's internal intelligence network to guide effective treatment. We can apply an expanding universe of therapies, supportive treatments, and tools to help patients recover, rebuild, and enjoy healthy and vibrant lives.

No Accidental Cure

When I wrote my first book in 2010 after 10 years of practicing AMA, I didn't want to claim too much, so I called it, *Accidental Cure*. My second book, *AcciDental Blow Up in Medicine*, carried the theme forward. Based on my experiences and those of others practicing AMA, I am naming this book, (It Ain't No) *Accidental Cure 3*.

Disclaimer

I do not claim to cure my patients and never promise a cure. Healing and recovery are something the patient undertakes – physically, emotionally, and spiritually. My work is to remove obstacles to healing – to identify and address the hidden invaders – so that the biological terrain improves, making it easier to heal.

I am not an oncologist, and I do not treat cancer. However, I do see cancer patients and help treat their underlying problems. They come to see me for a second opinion and to look for nutritional support and immune-enhancing therapy. I leave chemotherapy to their oncologists.

I am not a parasitologist. However, I see patients who have parasite problems, and I have developed experience in treating them since my tour as a US Army Reserve medical officer in Bolivia in 2001. We treated thousands of patients with antiparasitics and saw them report resolving a host of other medical problems. Parasites are not simply a Third World problem or an issue for people with animals or pets. Parasites and fungi often co-occur. Heavy metals and toxins can help fuel their growth and complicate treatment.

I am not a dentist. However, I understand the integral connections between oral and whole-body health. I often refer people to a biological dentist or oral surgeon as part of their healing journey. My initial patient exam includes looking for dental-related medical problems. I also test patients' teeth and jaws energetically to unmask problems that may not show on x-ray to assess their systemic impacts on health.

Within the framework of biocybernetics, the tools of Acupuncture Meridian Assessment can be applied to detect and help guide treatment of root underlying causes of cancer and chronic diseases.

Table of Contents

Forward 7
Onward 10
Inward 12
Outward 13
Preface 15
Introduction 29
Part 1 Rediscovering the Domain of the Body 31
Chapter 1 Awakening the Healer Within You 32
   From EAV to AMA: by Dr. med. Helmut Retzek 41
Chapter 2 Utilizing Acupuncture Intelligence to Uncover Hidden Issues 48
   Medical Acupuncture on Dental-Oral Cavity Meridian: Dental as a Missing Link for Medical Failures 51
      Case Study: Man with Squamous Cell Cancer 53
Chapter 3 My Protocol for Radical Healing 58
Part 2 Medical Acupuncture on the Meridian System 64
   Introduction 65
Chapter 4 Large Intestine, Lung, Stomach, and Spleen/Pancreas Meridians 66
   Medical Acupuncture on Large Intestine Meridian: Ancient Romans and US Army Target Demons 67
      Large Intestine Meridian and Related Teeth 69
   Medical Acupuncture on Lung Meridian: Pulmonary Hypertension, Covid-19, Lyme, more 70
      Lung Meridian and Related Teeth 75
   Medical Acupuncture on Stomach Meridian: Global Whining and Fearmongering to Global Healing - Rebellious Stomach for Nobel Prize 76
      Stomach Meridian and Related Teeth 79

Medical Acupuncture on Spleen/Pancreas Meridian: Case
Studies of Military Officers 81
    First Case Study: Military Colonel 81
    Second Case Study: Retired Brigade General 83
    Spleen/Pancreas Meridian and Related Teeth 84

Chapter 5 Gallbladder, Liver, Triple Warmer, and
Circulation/Pericardium Meridians... 86
    Medical Acupuncture on Gallbladder Meridian: Therapeutic
    Illusion on IBS and Autism... 87
        Gallbladder Meridian and Related Teeth 91
    Medical Acupuncture on Liver Meridian: Deworming in the
    Nile Forgotten Art of Preventive Medicine 92
        Liver Meridian and Related Teeth... 96
    Medical Acupuncture on Triple Warmer Meridian: Adrenal,
    Thyroid, Lyme, Breast Cancer, Chronic Fatigue Syndrome,
    CFS/ME, and Dental.. 98
        Case Study: 60-year-old Physician with Lyme 99
        Triple Warmer Meridian and Related Teeth 105
    Medical Acupuncture on Circulation/ Pericardium Meridian:
    Questioning the Scientific Merits of Old and New Medicine
    106
        Circulation/Pericardium Meridian and Related Teeth..........110

Chapter 6 Heart, Small Intestine, Kidney, and Bladder Meridians
....112
    Medical Acupuncture on Heart Meridian: Portals of Entry for
    Squirrels and Dragon 112
        Heart Meridian and Related Teeth 117
    Medical Acupuncture on Small Intestine Meridian: From
    Allergy and Autoimmune to Immune Deficiency....................118
        Small Intestine Meridian and Related Teeth 122
    Medical Acupuncture on Kidney Meridian: Acute and
    Chronic Kidney Disease Saved by Dentists?........................... 123
        Kidney Meridian and Related Teeth 126

Medical Acupuncture on Bladder Meridian: Two Prostate
  Cancer Patients.. 128
    Bladder Meridian and Related Teeth................................. 131
Part 3 Lesser-Known Medical Acupuncture Meridians............... 133
Chapter 7 Joint/Cartilage, Skin, and Nerve Degeneration Meridians
.... 134
  Medical Acupuncture on Joint/Cartilage Meridian: Untangle
  Rheumatism, Breast Cancer, and Dental Problems 135
  Medical Acupuncture on Skin Meridian: Better Than
  Biologics for Eczema, Psoriasis, and More? 138
  Medical Acupuncture on Nerve Degeneration Meridian: ALS,
  MS, Parkinson's Disease on the Rise! 141
Part 4 Dental: Portal to Hell or Health? 146
Chapter 8 Deadly Dental Trap 147
  Live Longer One Less Tooth at a Time: The Secret of
  Antiaging, Cancer, Lyme and Wellness Depends on Dental
  148
  Autoimmune Disease and Missing Links: A Cure for…
  Misdiagnosis? Dr. Johann Lechner's Dental Research on
  RANTES 152
  Toothless in St. Louis, God Forbid – Toothless in Vienna:
  Fairy Death Tale from Berlin 157
  Dental Parasites, Fungal and Bacterial Infections: Dreaded
  Periodontal Surgery is like Oral What?! 161
    Parasites, Fungi, and Bacteria in Periodontal Infections 163
    Physician Perspective: Tim Guilford, MD 170
  Antiparasitic and Antifungal Medications for Targeting
  Cancer Cells Literature Review and Case Studies.................. 172
  Bite, Breathing, Brainstem (BBB), and More: Better Bite,
  Better Life 174
  Guidelines for Treating Dental Infections............................. 178
Part 5 Cancer: Infection, Inflammation, and Mitochondrial
Dysregulation... 181

Chapter 9 Cancer: Who is Afraid of Cancer? 182
  Metabolic Therapy for Cancer: Theory and Practice - Keys to Longevity 182
  The Holy Grail of Antiaging is in your hands: Biohacking Wnt signaling pathway to beat cancer 191
    Patient Story: Prostate Cancer Treatment 196
  Leukemia and Lymphoma: Simple Solution A Possibility? ... 199
    Patient Story: Mantle Cell Lymphoma 203
  Glioblastoma Multiforme (GBM) Case Studies: Biological Dentistry in Oncology Care 205
    Case Study: A 46-Year-Old Canadian Patient with Glioblastoma Multiforme (GBM) 209
    Patient Story: We are thankful her mass is resolved 212

Part 6 Pathogens Hijacking the Genome and Other Unexpected Encounters 214

Chapter 10 Russian Genetic Roulette, Epigenetic Reprogramming, and Other Topics 215
  Ehlers-Danlos Syndrome (EDS) and More: Pathogens Biohacking and Reprogramming the Epigenome? 216
    Patient Story: Pain Free after Ankylosing Spondylitis 220
  Accidental Cure for Macular Degeneration: Vision Loss Affects 37 Million Americans 222
  Excerpt: Lyme and Post-Lyme Syndrome: Forensic Case Study from New York 225
  Palladium, not Polonium! Am I Dead? 227
  Toxoplasmosis Parasite Deceiving Medicine: Reversing Unsuspected Mental Illness? 232
  Three Million Dollar Kentucky Woman's Case: Adrenal Burnout, Lyme, Seizures and More 237
  Excerpt: RNA Based Nutrigenomic Therapy: New Treatment for Autism and Neurodegenerative Disease 240

Part 7 COVID and Post-COVID Syndrome 242

Chapter 11 COVID and Post-COVID Syndrome 243

COVID-19: Hidden Coinfections and Chain Reactions
Parasitic Infectious Relationships within Us 244
COVID-19, FUO and UFO Phenomenon: Ivermectin to Treat
Fever of Unknown Origin? 247
Ivermectin Deficiency Syndrome, Part 2: Staying Out of the
COVID-19 Graveyard 252
Parasites Follow the Money: Disease Follows the Money 255
Physician Perspective: Murat Isci, MD 258
Part 8 How to Reboot Your Brain 260
Chapter 12 Brain, Bioresonance, Neuromodulation, Cyber, and
More 261
Cognitive Decline to Dementia & Alzheimer's Disease:
Unsuspected Parasite-Dental-Oral Infections 262
Brain Neuromodulation Therapy from Cyprus: Transcranial
Direct Current Stimulation 269
Five Seconds Saves Ten Years of Suffering: Quantum
Random Non-Sense AI 273
Part 9 Biohacking Basics to Advanced Therapies 279
Chapter 13 Blending AMA, AI, and Biohacking for Health 280
Color Me Red, Color Me Blue: Red Light and Methylene
Blue Therapy May Save Your Life 281
Excerpt: Parasite Treatment Hacked by an MIT Engineer:
Think Small, Dream Big for Pandemic 288
Patient Story: Chronic Illness from Parasites 290
Excerpt: Insulin Potentiation Therapy (IPT) for All Chronic
Disease: Can Old Cranky Physicians Try New Approaches?
.... 290
Excerpt: EBOO – Ozone Dialysis Therapy for Veterans,
Firefighters, Farmers and Others Exposed to Toxins 292
Part 10 Biology of Belief 294
Chapter 14 Looking Back, Looking Ahead 295
Bruce Lipton's Biology of Belief and Epigenetics: Quantum
Entanglement of Parasites? 295

Unresolved Feelings and Their Target Organs 301
    Patient Story: Dr. Yu Saved my Life 303
Igor, my Bad Patient: Deworming as a New Uncertain Preventive Medicine 304
    Patient Story: Understanding Dr. Yu's Approach 307
Emotional Response to Stress, and Your Response? Mark Twain's Way of Looking at Things 308
Placebo Effects on the Brain's Inner Pharmacy: Quantum Uncertainty of Matching Reality with Expectation 313
Seventh Sense for Your Health 317
Unscientific Basis of Anti-Aging Program: Power of N-of-1 320
    Conclusion: Knowledge for Healing Comes from Within 324

Part 11 Everything You Want to Know About Acupuncture Meridian Assessment 326

Chapter 15 Frequently Asked Questions 327
  1. General Questions 327
  2. Parasite Treatment 336
  3. Dental Treatment 346
  4. Allergy-Immunology Meridian Disturbance: Mycotoxins, Toxic Metals, and Environmental Toxins 354
  5. Accompanying Treatments 356
  6. FAQs for Practitioners 359

Appendix: Patient Resources on my Website 366
About the Author 370
Endnotes 373
Bibliography 380
Index 386

List of Figures

Figure 1: Microcurrent as Musical Frequency 35
Figure 2: Chart of Patient's AMA Evaluation 36
Figure 3: Key to Meridians on AMA Chart 37
Figure 4: AMA Chart Compared to Musical Notes, Scale 38
Figure 5: Hand Control Measurement Points (14) 38
Figure 6: Foot Control Measurement Points (11) 39
Figure 7: The Biocybernetic Loop 47
Figure 8: Dental–Organ Meridian Chart (Maxillary) 49
Figure 9: Dental–Organ Meridian Chart (Mandible) 50
Figure 10: Unsuspected Dental/Medical Complex Problems 52
Figure 11: Translation of Medical History to Musical Scale 53
Figure 12: AMA Chart for Man with Cancer 54
Figure 13: DNA Connexions for Man with Cancer 55
Figure 14: Medical and Dental Disconnection 56
Figure 15: Multiple Factors Contributing to Lyme & Cancer 57
Figure 16: Large Intestine Meridian, Connection to Dental 69
Figure 17: Initial AMA Testing for 67-Year-Old Woman 72
Figure 18: Second AMA Testing for 67-Year-Old Woman
(Enhanced Interrogation Technique) 73
Figure 19: Lung Meridian, Connection to Dental 75
Figure 20: Stomach Meridian, Connection to Dental 80
Figure 21: Symptoms and Diagnoses: Military Officer 82
Figure 22: Initial AMA Testing for Military Officer: 82
Figure 23: Spleen/Pancreas Meridian, Connection to Dental 85
Figure 24: Gallbladder Meridian, Connection to Dental 91
Figure 25: Life Cycle of Schistosomiasis 94
Figure 26: Parasites speak many languages 95
Figure 27: Liver Meridian, Connection to Dental 97
Figure 28: IGeneX Lab Results for Lyme Blot IgM, IgG 100
Figure 29: DNA Connexions Lab Results: Oral and Lyme 102
Figure 30: Triple Warmer Meridian, Connection to Dental 106
Figure 31: Circulation/Pericardium, Connection to Dental 111

Figure 32: Störtebecker Diagram 115
Figure 33: Heart Meridian, Connection to Dental 117
Figure 34: Initial AMA Testing for Oregon Woman: Four
Meridians Out of Balance 120
Figure 35: Initial AMA Testing for Missouri Woman: Four
Meridians Out of Balance... 121
Figure 36: Small Intestine Meridian, Dental Connection 122
Figure 37: Initial AMA Reading: Impact of Tooth Injury on
Kidney, Dental and Allergy.. 124
Figure 38: AMA Reading After Extraction: Impact of
Tooth Injury on Kidney, Dental and Allergy................................ 125
Figure 39: Kidney Meridian, Connection to Dental 127
Figure 40: Bladder Meridian, Connection to Dental 132
Figure 41: Thermogram of Woman with Dental Infection 137
Figure 42: 68-year-old with ALS 143
Figure 43: AMA, Non-Small Cell Lung Cancer Patient 149
Figure 44: Inflammation, Infections and Immune Dysregulation
.... 153
Figure 45: Jawbone Osteonecrosis and Inflammatory Cytokine
RANTES 156
Figure 46: Case 1 Physician with Dental Infections 168
Figure 47: Case 2 Man with ALS and Dental Infections 168
Figure 48: AMA Before and After Test Plate with
Tinidazole/Ivermectin... 180
Figure 49: Multiple Causes of Mitochondrial Damage 184
Figure 50: Wnt Signaling Pathway 194
Figure 51: Medications Targeting Cancer Cells 194
Figure 52: Initial AMA Evaluation 200
Figure 53: Post-Treatment AMA Evaluation 202
Figure 54: Three Glioblastoma Multiforme Patients 207
Figure 55: Initial AMA Readings for Three Glioblastoma
Multiforme Patients 207

Figure 56: Panoramic X-rays for Three Glioblastoma Multiforme Patients 208
Figure 57: MRI of Recurrent Tumor, Pre-Visit, April 2023 209
Figure 58: MRI of Recurrent Tumor, Post-Treatment, May 2024 210
Figure 59: Pre- and Post-Treatment AMA for Canadian Patient . 211
Figure 60: DNA Connexions Result of Dental Biopsy 219
Figure 61: Symptoms Associated with Mercury 229
Figure 62: Symptoms Associated with Lead 230
Figure 63: Initial AMA Evaluation: 9 of 40 Meridians Out of Balance 238
Figure 64: Second AMA with "Enhanced Interrogation" Technique: 22 of 40 Meridians Out of Balance 239
Figure 65: Evolutionary Tree of Universal Ancestors 244
Figure 66: Parasitic Infectious Relationships: 245
Figure 67: Seasonal COVID Activity 247
Figure 68: Risk Factors for Alzheimer's and Neurodegeneration 264
Figure 69: AMA Evaluation of Retired Air Force Pilot 278
Figure 70: Color Spectrum, Wavelength, Notes, Pitch 282
Figure 71: Color Spectrum, Wavelength and Chakras 283
Figure 72: Universal Ancestors: RNA, DNA – Evolution via Cooperation vs. Competition 298
Figure 73: Multiple Signs of Parasite Infections 299
Figure 74: Unresolved Emotions and Target Organs 302

Introduction

This book is written in storytelling format to explain and illustrate the use of Acupuncture Meridian Assessment (AMA) in all 12 of the classical meridian systems, and additional more recent ones discovered by Dr. Reinhold Voll, which I find useful in my practice. It includes new articles and updates on the major challenges facing patients today. It is organized into 11 parts:

>Part 1 Rediscovering the Domain of the Body

>Part 2 Medical Acupuncture on the Meridian System

>Part 3 Lesser-Known Medical Acupuncture Meridians

>Part 4 Dental: Portal to Hell or Health?

>Part 5 Cancer: Infection, Inflammation, and Mitochondrial Dysregulation

>Part 6 Pathogens Hijacking the Genome and Other Unexpected Encounters

>Part 7 COVID and Post-COVID Syndrome

>Part 8 How to Reboot Your Brain

>Part 9 Biohacking Basics to Advanced Therapies

>Part 10 Biology of Belief

>Part 11 Everything You Want to Know About Acupuncture Meridian Assessment

Figures and illustrations are by the gifted artist Shawn Cornell. AMA charts from patient cases are produced by MORA equipment and software. The illustrations of meridians are from Traditional Chinese Medicine. Tables and slides are from my PowerPoint presentations at my Acupuncture Meridian Assessment (AMA)

Training Seminars for physicians and dentists, many conference presentations, and monthly seminars. All my articles are on my website, preventionandhealing.com.

Any mistakes are my own. All successes belong to my patients.

Part 1
Rediscovering the Domain of the Body

Chapter 1 Awakening the Healer Within You

It's time to recognize the human body as a domain from which we can learn, using an updated yet age-old form of AI – Acupuncture Intelligence. This 5,000-year-old disruptive technology can awaken the healing power within you - whether you're a physician, a dentist, or a patient - through the meridians via a life force known as Chi. Consider your body as a fine musical instrument, like a violin. The steps to begin to play and master this instrument include inspecting the violin, playing, tuning, practicing, learning, and practicing more.

Acupuncture Meridian Assessment (AMA)

Our bodies operate in several different energy realms, including bioelectrical and magnetic systems, as well as the familiar biomechanical and biochemical systems. Einstein's theory of relativity, Heisenberg and Schrodinger's quantum theory of uncertainty opened a new dimension of wave-particle theory, the duality of energy and matter, and the nature and behavior of matter and energy on the atomic and subatomic levels. Humans and all living and non-living things are both matter and energy.

In truth, energy animates life. You might be surprised to learn that pathways of electrical impulses – meridians – run throughout your body, each with a specific frequency. These meridians connect specific organs, sensory organs, joints, teeth, and tissues with points located next to the skin, called acupuncture points. Each meridian has an energy frequency that indicates healthy functioning, like a violin string when it is in tune. When the frequency is thrown off, it goes out of tune and does not work as well, indicating disease and dysfunction.

All Living Organisms Possess Complex Electromagnetic Fields

The new breakthroughs in medicine will come from understanding the biophysics and biocybernetics of cells and organs, not only from the Human Genome Project. Here's what scientists know about the biocybernetics of cells and organs:

- All living organisms possess complex electromagnetic fields and an invisible body.

- Biophotons trigger all biochemical reactions in the living cell.

- Electromagnetic fields disappear completely with death.

Franz Morell, MD from Germany, said, "The oscillation (frequency) of the universe is the cause of the phenomenon called LIFE." These oscillations bring both health and disease. Without electromagnetic oscillations, life is probably inconceivable. Oscillations have four dimensions: length, width, height, and time. Self-healing requires an active cancellation of pathological oscillations and a rebalancing of a disturbed equilibrium.

I highly recommend reading *The Biology of Belief*, by Bruce H. Lipton, PhD. He is a revolutionary thinker in the field of New Biology, stating: "All living organisms are as much energy as matter." Trained as a cell biologist, he learned how the environment, more than the gene itself, signals cells and governs their fate with respect to health and disease. "It's not the cell, it's the membrane – the true brain that controls cellular life." Or to put it more simply, "It's the environment, stupid." He adds, "We need to step back and incorporate the discoveries of quantum physics into biomedicine so that we can create a new, safer system of medicine that is attuned to the laws of nature." [1]

For those interested in reading more in this area, consider:

Dr. Robert O. Becker, *The Body Electric: Electromagnetism and The Foundation of Life*,
Dr. Richard Gerber, *A Practical Guide to Vibrational Medicine*,
Dr. Jerry L. Tennant, *Healing is Voltage: The Handbook*,
Claude Swanson, *Life Force, The Scientific Basis: Volume 2 of the Synchronized Universe*,
James L. Oschman, *Energy Medicine: The Scientific Basis*, and
Dr. Carolyn McMakin, *The Resonance Effect*.

Here are some interesting points that connect the oscillations in biocybernetics with acupuncture meridians:

> • Information exchange within a living organism can only be transmitted by oscillations that move at the speed of light (Popp).
>
> • We are living in the matrix of a biocybernetic system.
>
> • The oscillations of the organs are present on the acupuncture points in a bunched and concentrated form.

The frequency spectrum of an organ is conducted via the meridians and can be detected at the acupuncture points. Nearly the whole oscillation spectrum of the body exists in the palms of the hands and the soles of the feet.

Mapping the Invisible Body of the Biocybernetic Matrix

To my amazement, we already have an "invisible body map of the biocybernetic matrix" in the acupuncture meridian system taught in Traditional Chinese Medicine (TCM) and the chakra system taught in Ayurvedic medicine. Acupuncture Meridian Assessment (AMA), also known as Electroacupuncture According to Voll (EAV), is one of the most effective ways to learn about the biocybernetic system. It provides a physical means to measure invisible energy functions unknown to Western medicine.

Understanding the biological terrain and measuring the biocybernetic regulation of the body allows us to detect hidden dental infections, parasites, allergies, heavy metals, and toxins in the body. This opens up a treatment plan that seems almost impossible in the context of current medical science. This aspect of my practice may seem magical to new patients and highly suspicious to my medical colleagues in academia or clinical practice. For me, the biocybernetic medicine component of my practice is fascinating, fun, and rewarding. Best of all, it never gets boring. It provides an invaluable forensic tool to help identify and counteract the asymmetric threats causing cancers and chronic illnesses.

Reading AMA on a Digital Scale

Here is a brief overview of AMA, which I have described in my previous books. In AMA, we measure subtle microcurrent frequencies in the body along the meridian pathways. See Figure 1. On a scale of 0 to 100, 50 is considered ideal, the normal range is 45 to 55, and the range of the actual scale is 0 to 600,000 ohms (ohm is a unit of electrical resistance).

Figure 1: Microcurrent as Musical Frequency

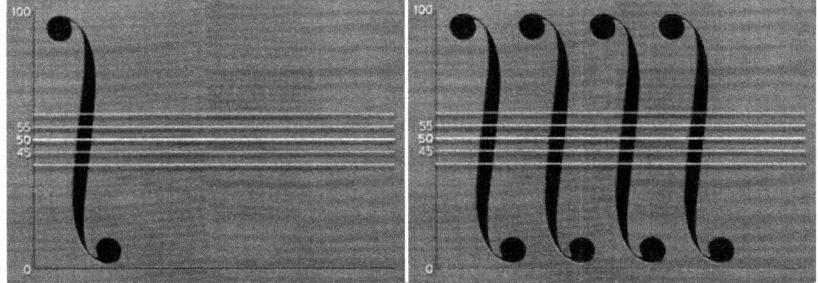

In terms of music, "consonance" is when two or more tones complement each other to produce a sound that is pleasant to the ear. Consonant intervals include the major/minor third, the perfect fourth, the perfect fifth, and unison/octave. "Dissonance" is when two or more tones clash and create a harsh, unpleasant sound.

Patients come to me with a multitude of complaints, often with a history of many consultations with specialists, lab tests, and other diagnostic tests. What do I do? I use Acupuncture Intelligence to read the domain of the body, tell me where and what things are wrong, and how to fix them. This approach allows me to address the root causes of their health issues, rather than just treating their symptoms.

As illustrated in the program I use for recording patients' AMA readings, middle bars represent the normal range of 45-55, low bars (under 45) indicate chronic conditions, and high bars (over 55) signify recent inflammatory responses. I measure 10 points each on the right and left hand, and on the right and left foot, respectively, totaling 40. Here is an example in Figure 2.

Figure 2: Chart of Patient's AMA Evaluation

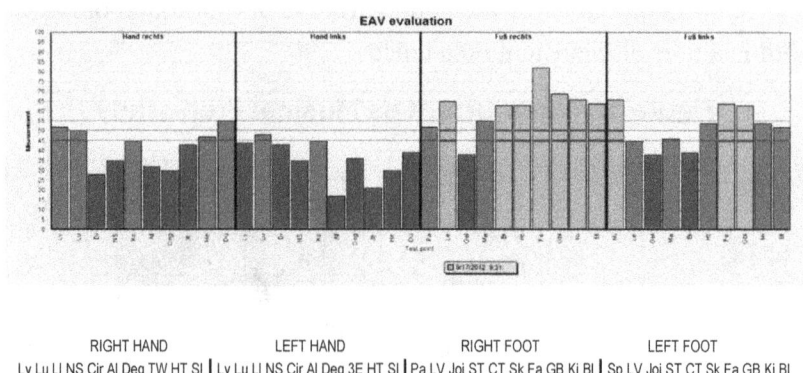

In this patient's case, sixteen meridians show chronically low values, ten are in an acute high inflammatory state, and fourteen are within normal range. This patient presents a series of issues to address. I typically start with the most significant—the lowest value—first. Figure 3 gives the key to the Meridian Chart.

Figure 3: Key to Meridians on AMA Chart

Right Hand: Lymph (Ly), Lung (Lu), Large Intestine (LI), Nervous System (NS), Circulation (Cir), Allergy (All), Degeneration (Deg), Triple Warmer (3E), Heart (HT), Small Intestine (SI)

Left Hand: Lymph (Ly), Lung (Lu), Large Intestine (LI), Nervous System (NS), Circulation (Cir), Allergy (All), Degeneration (Deg), Triple Warmer (3E), Heart (HT), Small Intestine (SI)

Right Foot: Pancreas (Pa), Liver (LV), Joints (Joi), Stomach (ST), Connective Tissue (CT), Skin (Sk), Fat (Fa), Gallbladder (GB), Kidney (Ki), Bladder (Bl)

Left Foot: Spleen (Sp), Liver (LV), Joints (Joi), Stomach (ST), Connective Tissue (CT), Skin (Sk), Fat (Fa), Gallbladder (GB), Kidney (Ki), Bladder (Bl)

Note: Symbols vary on the AMA charts based on language of the program (e.g. English, German, etc.)

RIGHT HAND	LEFT HAND	RIGHT FOOT	LEFT FOOT
Ly Lu LI NS Cir Al Deg TW HT SI	Ly Lu LI NS Cir Al Deg 3E HT SI	Pa LV Joi ST CT Sk Fa GB Ki Bl	Sp LV Joi ST CT Sk Fa GB Ki Bl

AMA Readings, Like Music: Harmony or Disorder

AMA readings can be compared to musical notes on a scale. Some are harmonious, while others are discordant and disordered, reflecting pathology along the acupuncture meridian pathways, as illustrated in Figure 4.

Figure 4: AMA Chart Compared to Musical Notes, Scale

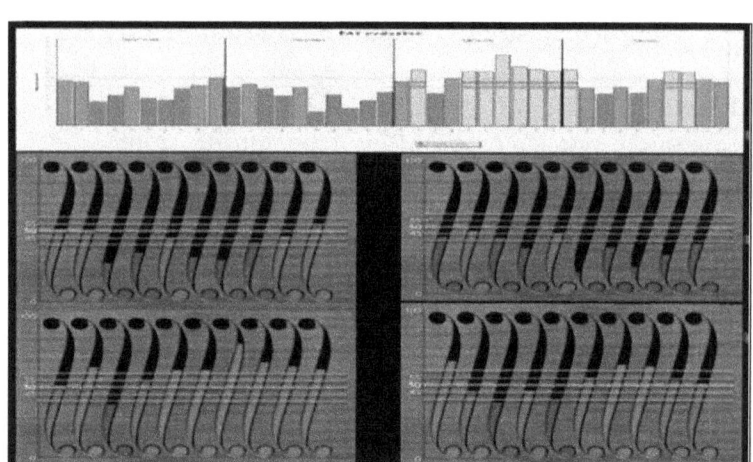

Measuring Acupuncture Intelligence

Acupuncture Intelligence is measured through meridian control measurement points on the hands and feet. There are 14 acupuncture meridian control measurement points (CMPs) on the hands: Lymph, Lung, Dental, Large Intestine, Nerve, Circulation, Allergy (two are marked on the chart), Organ, Adrenal, Triple Warmer, Breast, Heart, and Small Intestine; see Figure 5.

Figure 5: Hand Control Measurement Points (14)

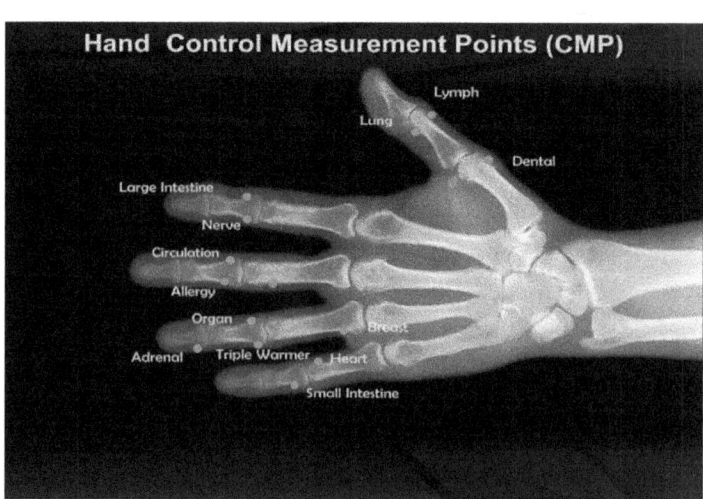

There are 11 acupuncture meridian control measurement points (CMPs) on the feet: Pancreas (right foot)/Spleen (left foot), Liver, Joints, Stomach, Connective Tissue, Skin, Fat, Gallbladder, Kidney, Bladder, and Prostate/Uterus; see Figure 6.

Note that there are 40 points in the main meridian system, but I check some additional points as indicated.

Figure 6: Foot Control Measurement Points (11)

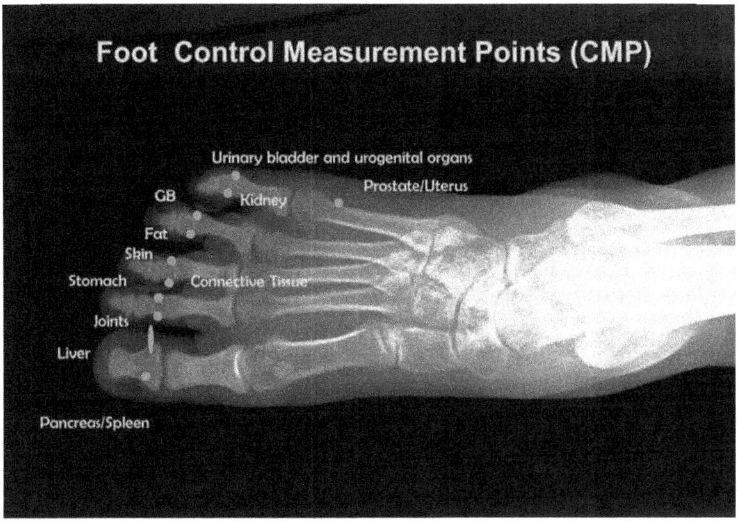

The heart of this book includes the articles in my Medical Acupuncture series. My primary goal is to explain why it is crucial to understand which meridians are out of balance, and what combinations and sequence of medications and therapies will help rebalance them. "Acupuncture Intelligence" guides the development, monitoring, and adjustments of each patient's treatment plan.

I will present clinical case examples to aid physicians, dentists, and patients in exploring new healing possibilities. I will also include guidance, tips, and advice from physicians and dentists I have trained who share their experiences in applying AMA – Acupuncture Intelligence – in their practices.

The book includes several of my favorite articles I have written in the years since I published the second book in my series, *AcciDental Blow Up in Medicine*. You can find all the 250 plus articles I have written to date on the articles/blog page on my website, preventionandhealing.com. You can also search them by category, or by keyword, or key phrase.

Dr. Atel Hemat of Cologne, Germany, who has attended many of my AMA and Advanced AMA Training Seminars, and organized AMA Training Seminars in Europe, has prepared an excellent Frequently Asked Questions (FAQs) for Patients and for Practitioners. It is included in Chapter 15 as an excellent reference and resource.

This book on Medical Acupuncture is my interpretation based on Electroacupuncture According to Voll from Germany and my internal medicine practice, and my military experience. I will share an excellent overview by Dr. med. Helmut Retzek of Austria. It is time to embrace holistic medicine based on science and energy medicine: Ancient Intelligence or Acupuncture Intelligence, AI^3.

From EAV to AMA: by Dr. med. Helmut Retzek

The rest of this chapter contains an excellent overview of EAV and AMA written by Dr. med. Helmut Retzek of Austria.

History

Electroacupuncture According to Voll (EAV) was developed in the 1950s by German physician Dr. Reinhold Voll, in collaboration with engineer Fritz Werner. The method combines the principles of Traditional Chinese Medicine (TCM) with Western electrodiagnostic techniques, measuring electrical conductivity at acupuncture-related skin points. Dr. Voll observed that certain points showed distinct electrical characteristics in the presence of organ dysfunction or chronic disease, offering a novel diagnostic tool that bridged Eastern and Western concepts of medicine.

Technical Background

EAV works by applying a low-voltage DC current (typically 1–1.5 volts) to the skin through a handheld electrode, measuring electrodermal conductance at specific acupuncture and meridian endpoints, mostly located on the hands and feet. A healthy point generally measures around 50 on a scale from 0 to 100. Deviations indicate energetic disturbances, which may correspond to subclinical organ dysfunction, infections, toxic load, or other pathological influences.

EAV also allows testing the resonance of various substances—originally mostly homeopathic remedies, herbal medicines, and nutritional supplements—by observing whether they normalize abnormal meridian readings.

Research Overview

EAV has been investigated in several observational and experimental studies, though its full recognition in academic medicine remains limited. However, within biological, integrative, and environmental medicine, it has gained widespread use and clinical support.

Selected Studies

1. Schimmel H. (1983): Developed the VEGA test, refining Voll's method for allergy and toxin screening
2. Galle & Stauner (1998): Studied EAV application in chronic pain and functional disorders
3. Moser et al. (2000): Demonstrated reproducibility of electrodermal measurements in double-blind settings
4. Zhang et al. (2005): Reported EAV-based detection of heavy metal toxicity

Motivation for Innovation by Dr. Simon Yu

Dr. Simon Yu, a board-certified internist and former U.S. Army medical officer, recognized the diagnostic power of EAV but also its practical limitations: the need to measure hundreds of points, the reliance on complementary test substances, and the complexity of interpretation. Drawing from over 30 years of clinical experience, Dr. Yu developed a more focused and reproducible system called Acupuncture Meridian Assessment (AMA).

Technical Advancements

AMA reduces the testing process to 40 core meridian endpoints located on the extremities. These were carefully selected to represent all major organ systems and offer a fast, yet sensitive way to detect hidden dysfunctions. The method dramatically reduces testing time and increases consistency between practitioners.

Benefits of AMA include:

- Faster testing (approx. 10–15 minutes)
- High clinical relevance and reproducibility
- Improved clarity and therapeutic precision

- Greater accessibility for physicians and dentists unfamiliar with traditional EAV

Integration of Allopathic Test Substances

Unlike traditional EAV, which focused on homeopathic or naturopathic substances, AMA primarily uses conventional pharmaceutical agents for resonance testing. These include:

- Antibiotics (e.g., doxycycline, metronidazole, tinidazole)
- Antiparasitic agents (e.g., albendazole, ivermectin, praziquantel)
- Antifungals, and occasionally antivirals

When a meridian point shows pathological values that normalize in the presence of a specific medication, this indicates a resonance—suggesting a hidden infection or toxicity responsive to that substance. This approach directly links diagnosis to a treatment path, significantly enhancing therapeutic outcomes.

Hidden Dental Infections and Jawbone Pathologies

One of the most crucial and unique contributions of Dr. Yu's work is the consistent identification of hidden dental infections, especially those associated with root canals, jawbone cavitations, and failed extractions. These dental foci often escape detection on conventional X-rays but can lead to systemic chronic illness:

- Neuroinflammation
- Neurological symptoms (e.g., brain fog, fatigue, balance disorders)
- Chronic pain syndromes
- Cancer-promoting immune activation

Dr. Yu routinely finds that previously root-canaled or cavitated teeth harbor 70–100+ pathogenic species, identified through genetic analysis of extracted material. This is exacerbated by the absence of venous valves in the head and neck region, allowing oral pathogens to reach the brain when the patient is lying down—potentially contributing to neurodegenerative or autoimmune disorders.

Of particular importance is the cytokine RANTES (CCL5), which is frequently found in very high concentrations in jawbone lesions and is strongly linked to tumor growth and immune dysregulation. These findings correlate consistently with abnormal meridian readings in AMA.

AMA as the Only Reliable Diagnostic Tool

According to Dr. Yu, AMA is often the only method capable of detecting these covert dental burdens, especially when conventional imaging (X-rays, CBCT) appears normal. The dental meridians—particularly associated with molars and wisdom teeth—often reveal energetic disturbances long before structural changes are visible.

Dr. Yu emphasizes:

- Persistent health issues cannot resolve unless these silent infections are surgically addressed
- He often refers patients repeatedly to biological dentists or oral surgeons for precise surgical correction
- Without this step, in his clinical experience, full recovery is rarely possible

This makes the dental component of AMA not just an optional enhancement, but a core pillar of the system—especially in chronic illness, neurological disorders, and treatment-resistant conditions.

Biocybernetics: The Invisible Operating System of Life

In my world of medical acupuncture and energetic diagnostics, biocybernetics is not just a word from physics textbooks or engineering labs. It is the *hidden language of life*, the invisible operating system through which your body communicates, compensates, and—when permitted—***heals***.

If you ask most physicians about biocybernetics, they may shrug, unfamiliar with its implications for medicine. But ask the body—it knows. It is already speaking in cybernetic code: oscillations, frequencies, resonance, resistance, and coherence.

Biocybernetics, at its core, is the study of control and communication in living systems. But unlike the clinical sterility of traditional cybernetics, *biological* cybernetics recognizes that living tissues are not just passive recipients of biochemical commands—they are dynamic, self-regulating, intelligent fields of energy and information.

I like to think of the acupuncture meridian system as an ancient map of this cybernetic intelligence. When we use Acupuncture Meridian Assessment (AMA) to measure microcurrent frequencies across the meridians, we are tapping into the body's regulatory software—its energetic feedback loops, self-repair mechanisms, and intercellular messages that move at the speed of light.

This is not metaphor. Scientists like Albert Popp have shown that biophotons—ultra-weak light emissions from cells—are involved in cellular communication. When someone dies, those light emissions vanish. No electromagnetic field, no life. The oscillations cease.

In my practice, these oscillations—their balance, distortion, or absence—tell me what the patient's labs and scans cannot. A meridian that is dissonant reflects a biocybernetic breakdown—a disruption in the communication pathways between organ systems, the gut, the brain, and the subtle field we call *Chi*. It might be caused by parasites, a hidden dental infection, unresolved emotional trauma, or toxic metals. But once I read the disturbance, I can ask the body how to fix it.

"The oscillation of the universe is the cause of the phenomenon called life," said Franz Morell, the German pioneer who understood this decades ago. Life is not a random collection of molecules—it is a harmonized dance of electrical impulses, magnetic fields, and vibrational intelligence. That's biocybernetics.

This system cannot be understood through the Human Genome Project alone. Genes are the hardware. Biocybernetics is the software. The instructions. The real-time diagnostics and corrections occurring below your awareness but well within your body's innate intelligence.

In this way, Acupuncture Intelligence (AI^2) becomes a kind of bio-forensic tool. AMA allows me to read the meridians like a conductor tuning the instruments of a grand orchestra. I don't diagnose in Latin or treat based on pharmaceutical algorithms—I listen. I measure. I decode.

When a meridian is out of tune, we adjust it—sometimes with a medication, sometimes with a homeopathic, sometimes with light or frequency, and often with dental intervention. The result is not a mechanical repair. It is a rebalancing of the biocybernetic matrix. And when the matrix rebalances, healing becomes not just possible—it becomes inevitable.

Biocybernetics, then, is not an abstract theory. It is a living truth. It is the connective tissue between quantum medicine and practical healing. Between Traditional Chinese Medicine and modern energetic diagnostics. Between the unseen and the undeniable.

It is the bridge between chaos and coherence. See Figure 7 for a simple diagram.

If you know how to read it, it will guide you to the hidden causes—and the unexpected cures.

Figure 7: The Biocybernetic Loop

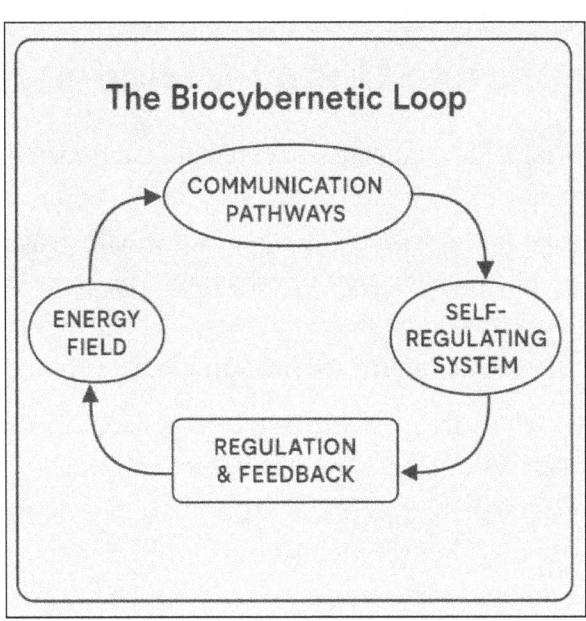

Conclusion

Acupuncture Meridian Assessment (AMA), as developed by Dr. Simon Yu, represents a paradigm shift in energetic medicine—streamlining and upgrading EAV to serve as a practical, reproducible, and clinically potent diagnostic and therapeutic tool. Its integration of conventional pharmaceuticals, focus on root causes like dental infections, and energetic-organic correlations make it one of the most advanced diagnostic models in modern integrative medicine.

Through AMA, Dr. Yu bridges the gap between bioenergetic diagnostics and evidence-based clinical action, offering hope for patients with complex, unresolved illnesses—and setting a new standard in the field of biological medicine.

My thanks and appreciation to Dr. Retzek for this excellent overview. His website and blog are at www.ganzemedizin.at/en/.

Chapter 2 Utilizing Acupuncture Intelligence to Uncover Hidden Issues

The most formidable challenges in evaluating chronically ill patients who present with undiagnosed medical conditions stem from concealed dental issues. I frequently attribute dental problems as the reason why patients aren't improving. This missing link, which I call a Medical and Dental (MAD) disconnection, often triggers chronic and complex medical problems.

While dental issues are a leading overlooked factor in chronic illness and a driver of meridian imbalances, hidden parasite/fungal infections are equally neglected. Together and in synergy, these "known unknowns" impact internal organs, the gut, the microbiome, organs, the circulatory, immune, and nervous systems, and the brain.

Applying Acupuncture Intelligence to the domain of the whole body, teeth, and dental cavity can aid in detecting and guiding treatment on a comprehensive, holistic, integrative basis – a necessity for recovery and health.

Before delving into each of the main meridian systems, I will begin with dental. It is both overlooked and fundamental. Each tooth is connected to a different meridian. See the Tooth-Organ Meridian Chart, in Figure 8 and Figure 9, on the next two pages.

If we can accurately identify and address dental problems using Acupuncture Intelligence and eradicate hidden parasite/fungal infections, we can decode the domain of the body and learn how to restore its harmony and health. I use AMA to determine which problems to treat first - the correct sequence is crucial to lasting success - and to test medications for their effectiveness in each patient. Welcome to the journey and continue to practice.

Figure 8: Tooth–Organ Meridian Chart (Maxillary-Upper)

	R								L							
Upper Teeth	1	2	3	4	5	6	7	8	9	10	11	12	13	14	15	16
Sense Organs	Inner Ear	Maxillary Sinus	Maxillary Sinus	Ethmoid Cells	Eye	Eye	Frontal Sinus	Frontal Sinus	Frontal Sinus	Frontal Sinus	Eye	Eye	Ethmoid Cells	Maxillary Sinus	Maxillary Sinus	Inner Ear
Joints (upper)	Shoulder, Elbow	Jaws	Jaws	Shoulder, Elbow			Back of Knee	Back of Knee	Back of Knee	Back of Knee			Shoulder, Elbow	Jaws	Jaws	Shoulder, Elbow
Joints (mid)					Hip	Hip	Sacrococcyx	Sacrococcyx	Sacrococcyx	Sacrococcyx	Hip	Hip				
Joints (lower)	Hand, Ulnar; Foot, Plantar; Toes, Sacroiliac Joint	Front of Knee	Front of Knee	Hand, Radial; Foot, Big Toe		Foot	Foot			Foot	Foot		Hand, Radial; Foot, Big Toe	Front of Knee	Front of Knee	Hand, Ulnar; Foot, Plantar; Toes, Sacroiliac Joint
Spinal Segments	C8 T1 T5 T6 T7 S1 S2 S3	T11 T12 L1	T11 T12 L1	C5 C6 C7 T2 T3 T4 L4 L5	T8 T9 T10	T8 T9 T10	L2 L3 S4 S5 Coccyx	L2 L3 S4 S5 Coccyx	L2 L3 S4 S5 Coccyx	L2 L3 S4 S5 Coccyx	T8 T9 T10	T8 T9 T10	C5 C6 C7 T2 T3 T4 L4 L5	T11 T12 L1	T11 T12 L1	C8 T1 T5 T6 T7 S1 S2 S3
Vertebrae	C7 T1 T5 T6 S1 S2	T11 T12 L1	T11 T12 L1	C5 C6 C7 T2 T3 T4 L4 L5	T9 T10	T9 T10	L2 L3 S3 S4 S5 Coccyx	L2 L3 S3 S4 S5 Coccyx	L2 L3 S3 S4 S5 Coccyx	L2 L3 S3 S4 S5 Coccyx	T9 T10	T9 T10	C5 C6 C7 T2 T3 T4 L4 L5	T11 T12 L1	T11 T12 L1	C7 T1 T5 T6 S1 S2
Organs	Heart-R	Pancreas	Pancreas	Lung-R	Liver-R	Liver-R	Kidney-R	Kidney-R	Kidney-L	Kidney-L	Liver-L	Liver-L	Lung-L	Spleen	Spleen	Heart-L
Organs (paired)	Duodenum	Stomach-R	Stomach-R	Large Intestine-R	Gallbladder	Gallbladder	Bladder-R, Urogenital Area	Bladder-R, Urogenital Area	Bladder-L, Urogenital Area	Bladder-L, Urogenital Area	Bile Ducts-L	Bile Ducts-L	Large Intestine-L	Stomach-L	Stomach-L	Jejunum, Ileum-L
Endocrine Organs	Pituitary, Ant. Lobe	Parathyroid	Thyroid	Thymus	Pituitary, Post Lobe	Pituitary, Post Lobe	Pineal Gland	Pineal Gland	Pineal Gland	Pineal Gland	Pituitary, Post Lobe	Pituitary, Post Lobe	Thymus	Thyroid	Parathyroid	Pituitary, Ant. Lobe
Others	CNS Psyche	Mammary Gland-R													Mammary Gland-L	CNS Psyche

Figure 9: Tooth–Organ Meridian Chart (Mandible-Lower)

Lower Teeth	R	32	31	30	29	28	27	26	25	24	23	22	21	20	19	18	L	17
Others		Energy Metabolism																Energy Metabolism
Endocrine Glands Tissue System		Peripheral Nerves	Arteries	Veins	Lymph Vessels	Gonad (Testes or Ovary)		Adrenal Gland				Gonad (Testes or Ovary)	Mammary Gland-L	Lymph Vessels	Veins	Arteries		Peripheral Nervous System
												Mammary Gland-R						
Organs		Ileum-R	Large Intestine-R		Stomach-R Pylorus	Gall-bladder		Bladder-R Urogenital Area			Bladder-L Urogenital Area	Bile Ducts -L	Stomach-L		Large Intestine-L			Jejunum Ileum-L
		Ileoceal Region																
Vertebrae		Heart-R	Lung-R	C5 C6 C7 T2 T3 T4 L4 L5	Pancreas	T11 T12 L1	Liver-R	L2 L3 S3 S4 S5 Coccyx			L2 L3 S3 S4 S5 Coccyx	Liver-L	Spleen	T11 T12 L1	Lung-L	C5 C6 C7 T2 T3 T4 L4 L5		Heart-L
		C7 T1 T5 T6 S1 S2					T9 T10					T9 T10						C7 T1 T5 T6 S1 S2
Spinal Segments		C8 T1 T5 T6 T7 S1 S2 S3		C5 C6 C7 T2 T3 T4 L4 L5	T11 T12 L1	T8 T9 T10		L2 L3 S4 S5 Coccyx			L2 L3 S4 S5 Coccyx	T8 T9 T10	T11 T12 L1		C5 C6 C7 T2 T3 T4 L4 L5			C8 T1 T5 T6 T7 S1 S2 S3
Joints		Shoulder and Elbow	Hand, Radial Foot Big Toe		Front of Knee	Jaws	Hip	Sacrococcyx			Sacrococcyx	Hip		Jaws	Front of Knee			Shoulder and Elbow
		Hand, Ulnar Foot, Plantar Toes, Sacro-iliac Joint						Foot			Foot					Hand, Radial Foot Big Toe		Hand, Ulnar Foot, Plantar Toes, Sacro-iliac Joint
Sense Organs		Ear	Ethmoid Cells		Maxillary Sinus	Eye		Frotal Sinus			Frotal Sinus	Eye	Maxillary Sinus		Ethmoid Cells			Ear

Medical Acupuncture on Dental-Oral Cavity Meridian:
Dental as a Missing Link for Medical Failures

Do you want to live a longer, healthier life free from chronic aches, pain, or chronic illness? Your oral cavity, gum and dental status can provide an ample "mouthful of evidence" about your health status. Your physician has likely overlooked the dental-oral connection to your health. Medical doctors rely on dentists to care for your teeth, and common procedures can worsen your health over time. I have witnessed medical and dental disconnections for the last 30 years thanks to my mentor, biological dentist Doug Cook, DDS, a pioneer in the field of Energy Medicine in Dentistry. I wrote the Forward to his book, *Rescued By My Dentist*.[2]

Hidden dental problems may be as bad or worse for your health than obesity, hypertension, and diabetes as a preexisting medical condition. Yet, medical professionals are often blindsided by dental problems as a preexisting condition and source of inflammation and chronic disease.

Modern dentistry, with its current Newtonian-based mechanical model focused on physical function and cosmetics, may inadvertently create a larger medical problem. The future of dentistry will understand and embrace Energy Medicine, a part of holistic, integrative biological medicine. Acupuncture meridians are an integral part of energy, the basic language of Nature; energy medicine is essential to understanding health and disease.

There isn't a clearly defined dental-oral cavity meridian according to Classical Acupuncture literature. More recently, German medical doctor, homeopath, and acupuncturist Reinhold Voll described the lymphatic system of the jaw (dental-oral cavity), which overlaps with the classical Lung meridian. The Dental meridian represents the upper lymphatic system of the throat, tonsils, sinus, and oral cavity.

> **Medical professionals are often blindsided by dental problems as a preexisting condition and source of inflammation and chronic disease.**

One of my severe asthma patients, who did not respond to standard and alternative care, did respond to the extraction of a root canal-treated tooth (which had a normal dental X-ray). It corresponded to the Lung on the Tooth-Organ Meridian Chart, see Figures 8 and 9. For more information, refer to my books, *Accidental Cure*, and *AcciDental Blow Up in Medicine*, and the color version of the Chart on my website, preventionandhealing.com/resources.[3]

Acupuncture Meridian Assessment (AMA) can translate the medical history, physiology, and biochemistry of individual patients to a frequency (think musical) scale based on meridians: a 5,000-year-old technology. Some common unsuspected Dental/Medical Complex Problems are listed in Figure 10.

Figure 10: Unsuspected Dental/Medical Complex Problems

Amalgams	Bonding Materials
Root Canals	Metal Allergies
Galvanic Currents (the mouth battery)	Composite Materials
	High Speed Drill
Cavitations	Biological Dentistry?
TMJ	Proprioception
Airway	Parasites and Bruxism
Implants	Pleomorphism of Bacteria
Heavy Metals	and Protozoa

What have I learned over the years? Dental is a commonly overlooked cause of many health problems. Think "dental" when the latest medical therapy fails.

How do I explain the meridian system at medical conferences? Figure 11 is from a presentation I gave in Boston, "Dental as a Missing Link for Medical Failures: Lyme, Cancer, Neurological Disorders and More." See the normal range for AMA readings superimposed on the scale. My lecture focused on evidence-based case studies that connected the dots of Medical and Dental (MAD) disconnection: lymphatic drainage to the brain, breast, thyroid, etc. and using Acupuncture Meridian Assessment as a guiding tool.

Figure 11: Translation of Medical History to Musical Scale

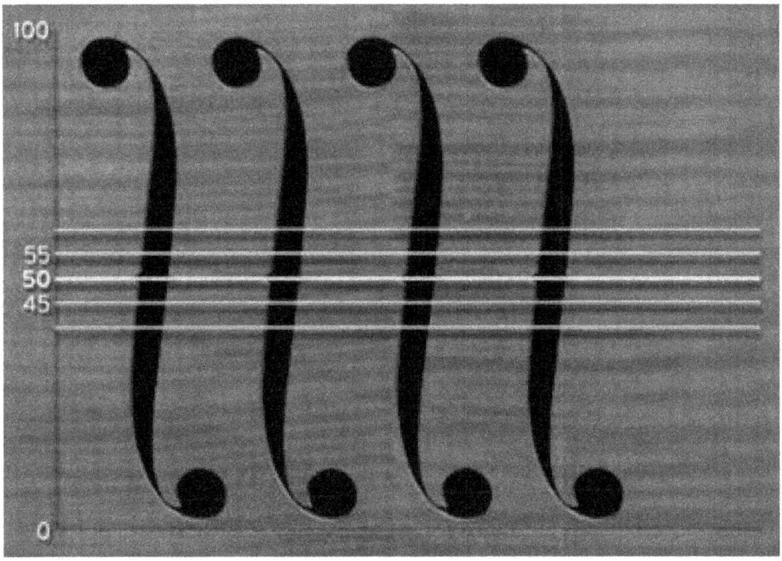

Case Study: Man with Squamous Cell Cancer

Here is a case study of a man with a long history of ulcerative colitis who also had persistent chronic pus draining from his thumb. His chronically infected thumb eventually turned into squamous cell carcinoma, and it was recommended for amputation. He came to see me, and his initial AMA evaluation indicated he needed parasite medications for his ulcerative colitis.

After intense parasite cleansing and detoxification, his tumor shrank so rapidly I did not believe it was possible. His next 40-point AMA evaluation showed only his dental/lymph meridian out of balance (Figure 12), represented by the lower bar on the left side of the chart below. His biological dentist was reluctant to extract it as it appeared normal on cone beam and X-ray.

Figure 12: AMA Chart for Man with Cancer

Case: 52-year-old with Ulcerative Colitis & Squamous cell cancer of right thumb

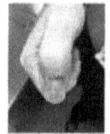

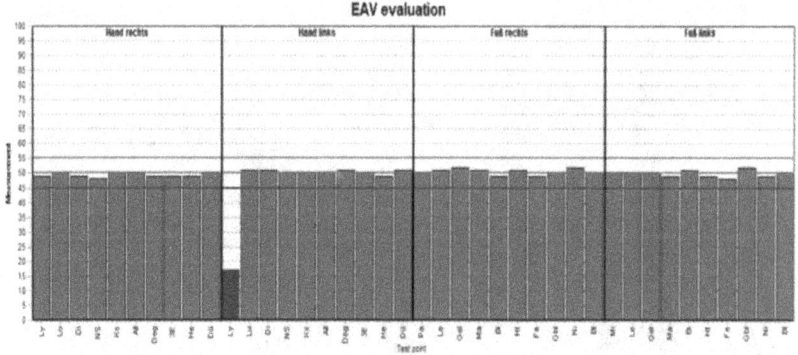

He finally extracted the tooth, but his cancer had advanced, and it was too late. It took over 1½ years to convince his biological dentist to remove his infected tooth. A Dental DNA test (Figure 13) revealed many different microorganisms hidden in his seemingly normal healthy-looking tooth. I learned that even CBCTs can be misleading.

This case underscored for me that AMA frequency readings based on ancient meridian systems provide a new perspective on human energy fields. It made a deep and lasting impression on me. I refer to it often, and it is why I want biological dentists to learn about energy medicine and incorporate it in their practice.

Figure 13: DNA Connexions for Man with Cancer

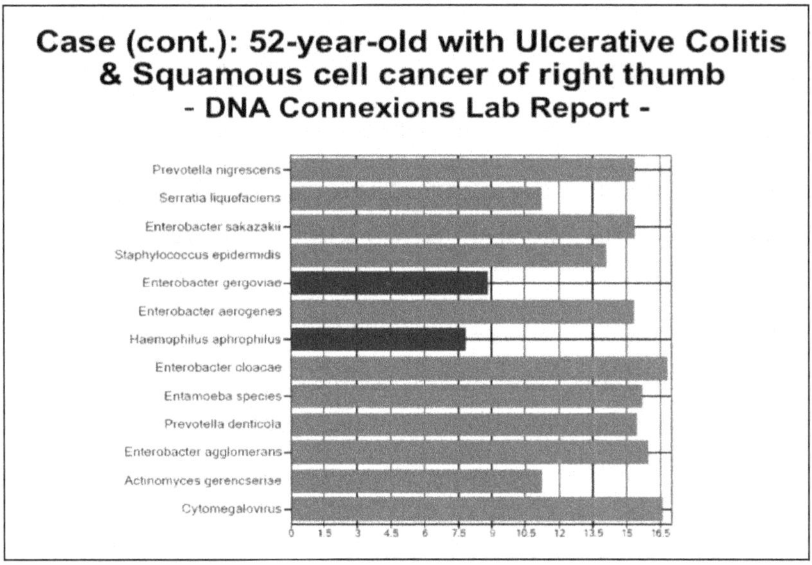

Case (cont.): 52-year-old with Ulcerative Colitis & Squamous cell cancer of right thumb
- DNA Connexions Lab Report -

- Prevotella nigrescens
- Serratia liquefaciens
- Enterobacter sakazakii
- Staphylococcus epidermidis
- Enterobacter gergoviae
- Enterobacter aerogenes
- Haemophilus aphrophilus
- Enterobacter cloacae
- Entamoeba species
- Prevotella denticola
- Enterobacter agglomerans
- Actinomyces gerencseriae
- Cytomegalovirus

The Dental DNA test indicated 13 different infectious microorganisms in his extracted tooth. They were evidently a factor in his squamous cell cancer and its progression.

Sir William Osler, the founder of Johns Hopkins, stated that the "Mouth is the Mirror of all Disease." Dr. Norman Doidge discussed the power of the tongue and the brainstem's ability to create new brain cells and new neural connections in, *The Brain That Changes Itself*.[4] The oral cavity represents about 46 percent of the brain's sensory cortex and motor cortex area.

I have corresponded with a Canadian dentist, Dr. George Paul Greenacre, DDS of Ottawa, who says there are five major brains: 1) Central Brain, 2) Mouth Brain, 3) Gut Brain, 4) Spinal Brain, and 5) Breath Brain. He underscores the importance of the Mouth-Brain and Gut-Brain connection. These are regulated by the Trigeminal nerve and the Vagus nerve as an integral part of our Central Brain.

When a patient does not respond to standard medical care, it is time to consider dental, parasites, and fungal issues! Medical Acupuncture on the Dental-Oral Cavity Meridian will guide you beyond a dental X-ray or CBCT scan. Some of the key points of Medical and Dental (MAD) disconnection are listed below.

> **Dental is a commonly overlooked cause of many health problems. Think "dental" when the latest medical therapy fails.**

In Figure 14, the left column represents medical-related factors, and the right column represents dental-related and overlapping problems. Applying this information with patients takes some time: learn the science, tools and techniques, practice AMA, connect the dots, and prioritize and treat in the proper sequence.

Figure 14: Medical and Dental Disconnection

Dental as a Missing Link for Medical Failure Take Home Points	
Parasites	Dental Parasites
Nutrition and Diet	Dental Infections
Vaccinations	Root Canals
Environmental Toxins	Galvanic Metal Currents
EMF	Cavitations/Endotoxins
Heavy Metals	Amalgams
Medications	TMJ
Chemical Stresses	Airway/Sleep Apnea
Surgery Scars	Implants
Allergy/Immunology	Dental Material Allergy

As shown in Figure 15, multiple factors can contribute to Lyme, Post-Lyme, cancer, neurological disorders, and more. The same principle applies to COVID, post-COVID activation of Epstein-

Barr Virus (EBV), Bartonella, Mycoplasma, chronic disease, and cancer: reactivation of underlying problems.

Figure 15: Multiple Factors Contributing to Lyme & Cancer

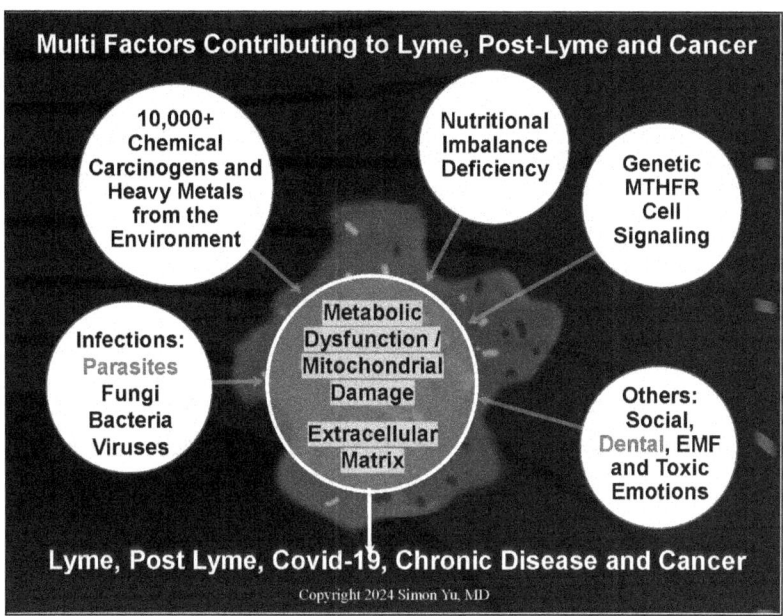

I have written many articles on Medical and Dental disconnection. Go to the Articles page on my website and search on "dental." When it comes to dental problems, I tell my patients to expect the unexpected. This is also sound advice for physicians and dentists.

> **When it comes to dental problems, I tell my patients to expect the unexpected. This is also sound advice for physicians and dentists.**

Chapter 3 My Protocol for Radical Healing

Patients, physicians, and dentists often want to understand exactly what I do, why I do it, and how I diagnose and treat in the way I do. I have done my best to explain my condensed protocol in my first two books. Let's try to explain it in a different format here. You may consider this a manual for unrestricted, unlimited, radical healing tailored to you, and only you, an N-of-1 approach. It's a given fact that not everyone responds to my unconventional therapies, and I accept this and strive to understand my limitations.

Step 1: Take a medical history before evaluating for Acupuncture Meridian Assessment (AMA). Every patient has their unique background of events, often including diagnosis, treatment, and misadventures within the modern medical system. Although I document all their medical diagnoses, I try not to be biased by their suspected diagnoses as a reliable source of information. They may have had over ten medical diagnoses based on their symptoms and test results, but that did not contribute to their recovery.

Sometimes, a patient gets overwhelmed with providing too many details of every event, procedure, lab test, and each diagnosis that happened to them. This can add more confusion than being helpful. If I cannot get a good grasp of why they came to see me within twenty minutes, I may abruptly stop them from talking further. I tell them, stop talking, and I will evaluate you and commence designing a battle plan based on Acupuncture Meridian Assessment (AMA). Another way of saying this is that I will inspect the violin, play the violin, and tune the violin that is You. I prefer not to compare our body to a fine machine but rather to a fine, delicate musical instrument. For your information, I do not play the violin. As a youngster, I spent my energy and time avoiding my violin lessons rather than practicing the violin.

> **Although I document all their medical diagnoses, I try not to be biased by their suspected diagnoses as a reliable source of information.**

Step 2: Assess and evaluate 40 main acupuncture meridians to find out how many meridians, to what degree, and in what sequence are out of balance or out of tune. This is crucial information for me to read the meridians like a musical scale, looking for "pattern recognition" based on the teaching of acupuncture and EAV. Does the medical history and diagnosis match my AMA evaluation? Each medical acupuncture article in my series will give you a glimpse or snapshot of the acupuncture meridian, its function, a case study or example, and how all these meridians interact.

> **Assess and evaluate 40 main acupuncture meridians to find out how many meridians, to what degree, and in what sequence are out of balance or out of tune.**

Step 3: If my initial assessment does not correspond with their symptoms or diagnosis, I will do a second evaluation, repeat 40-point measurement for advanced AMA after flashing colored light to the eyes at 8 hertz. I initially nicknamed this technique, Operation Open Sesame or Advanced Interrogation Techniques, to explore the body and meridians at a deeper level. Our body will always compensate and try to restore our bodily function. The body absorbs light and creates a phase-contrast, and I can see and hear the difference in the meridian assessment before and after the light therapy.

A good example: A patient comes with a multitude of medical diagnoses and multiple medications to correct their symptoms with the standard treatment according to the diagnosis. He or she may be on psychiatric medications for anxiety/depression, insomnia, chronic pain, ADD/ADHD, etc. with many medications, and the initial 40 points AMA will be almost normal. This does not make sense, so I do advanced AMA using light therapy to unmask hidden problems revealed through the meridian system. The name of the medical diagnosis is not as important as rebalancing the meridians in the right sequence. If I can balance and maintain the meridians using medication testing, often our body will correct itself. You may call it healing from within: Spontaneous Healing, Radical Healing, or Accidental Cure.

> **The name of the medical diagnosis is not as important as rebalancing the meridians in the right sequence.**

Step 4: Despite using the Operation Open Sesame technique to detect hidden layers of the problem, some patients still do not reveal deeply embedded problems. Their medical history may not match with the meridian assessment. For instance, cancer patients who have been on chemo, radiation, steroids, and taking parasite medications on their own, like fenbendazole, ivermectin, and albendazole, may present such a case. After much trial and error, I have used different acupuncture needles to target certain sensitive areas, such as the conception and governing vessels, revealing another deeper layer of the problem. This process can continue with each visit. I call it my "Enhanced Interrogation Technique."

> **After much trial and error, I have used different acupuncture needles to target certain sensitive areas, such as the conception and governing vessels, revealing another deeper layer of the problem.**

Step 5: Once I've established which areas are overlooked by their medical doctors - usually parasites/fungal, environmental toxins, and dental/oral cavity related - I commence the treatment plan. This starts with intestinal cleansing, which means using cleansing herbs to get the bowel to move at least one or two times a day.

Then, I start parasite/fungal medications that can last a few weeks to many months depending on the degree of the infection.

> **Once I've established which areas are overlooked by their medical doctors - usually parasites/fungal, environmental toxins, and dental/oral cavity related - I commence the treatment plan.**

Step 6: Hair Tissue Mineral Analysis (HTMA) from Analytical Research Lab, food allergy IgG delayed response test from Genova Lab, and Blood Type tests are recommended for all patients, and typically done at the first visit. Hair tissue mineral composition, calcium, magnesium, sodium, and potassium level, and the ratio of these minerals provide a unique metabolic pattern for individual patients—fast, slow, and mixed oxidizer. It also checks trace elements and screens for toxic metals. Metabolic type testing gives you information about what proportion of protein, fat, and carbohydrates are needed. Food allergy tests and blood type diet provide individualized, personalized dietary guidelines.

> **Hair Tissue Mineral Analysis from Analytical Research Lab, food allergy IgG delayed response test from Genova Lab, and Blood Type tests are recommended for all patients, and typically done at the first visit.**

Step 7: I may do additional tests depending on the AMA evaluation. A DMPS heavy metal provocation test measuring 20 toxic metals, and tests for fungal mycotoxins and/or environmental toxins, are recommended if indicated based on AMA.

> **I may do additional tests depending on the AMA evaluation.**

Step 8: The second visit is about one month later. I review the lab test results and repeat the 40-point meridian assessments to see how my patient is responding to treatment, looking for both changes in physical symptoms and changes in the meridians. As a rule, improvements in the meridian assessment come first before noticing physical improvements. There is a lag time from energetic improvement to manifest into physical improvement.

> **I review the lab test results and repeat the 40-point meridian assessments to see how my patient is responding to treatment, looking for both changes in physical symptoms and changes in the meridians.**

Step 9: I may readjust the medications, start the nutritional program based on the above tests results, and begin a detox program or chelation therapy based on the initial lab findings.

Step 10: Dental procedures like removal of the amalgams are usually addressed on the second or third visit. If I suspect a patient has active dental infections like root canals or cavitation (jaw infection), *I may recommend extracting root canals or cleaning up the cavitation as soon as possible depending on dental care availability. This is a very sensitive subject and often patients drop out.* Even if they see a dentist, their dentist may not agree with my assessment if the dental X-ray does not reveal any sign of infection, or it might be too costly to get the dental work done. *The cost for American dentistry can be shocking to many patients.*

> **Dental procedures like removal of the amalgams are usually addressed on the second or third visit.**

Step 11: Two months later, there will be a third visit. At that point, I expect to see significant physical improvements, and balancing of most of the meridians except dental related or environmental toxin related problems, which still need to be addressed. Of course, not everyone responds as I projected, and may need reevaluation with more advanced AMA evaluation which I nicknamed, Enhanced Interrogation Technique (EIT), described later in this book. These are my typical evaluation and treatment plans for complex, chronically ill patients who do not have life-threatening conditions like ALS or advanced cancer.

> **I expect to see significant physical improvements, and balancing of most of the meridians except dental related or environmental toxin related problems, which still need to be addressed.**

Step 12: For the most serious patients with advanced cancer, the tempo of evaluation and the treatment will be faster and different than for typical patients. I do not treat cancer. I treat the whole body. I try to work with oncologists who are open to my medical philosophy of holistic medicine and support the patients if they are going through chemotherapy or radiation therapy. More IV infusion therapy and expedited dental work is needed. Expect to stay near the clinic for a few days to a few weeks at a time. The magnitude and the importance of dental work cannot be overemphasized as you will see in my article, "Live Longer One Less Tooth at a Time."

Summary

In summary, this is a quick overview of what to expect when you come to see me, and how to get to know me. The most important first step is mapping out the 40-point meridian assessment which I call, "inspecting the violin," developing a treatment plan based on it, and monitoring your progress in balancing the meridians.

The Medical Acupuncture Meridian series which follows in Part 2 explains how the main 12 meridians operate and interact with each other in maintaining the Chi or Life Force. Part 3 includes the lesser-known meridians. Part 4 focuses on the dental/oral/lymph meridian. The dental AMA evaluation is one of the most crucial parts of the evaluation and treatment plan; implementing its recommendations is the biggest barrier for patients to address.

Part 2
Medical Acupuncture on the Meridian System

Introduction

Acupuncture Meridian Assessment (AMA) measures the subtle energy flow, Chi, which encompasses the physical, emotional, and spiritual spectrum of life force. I use AMA as a tool to determine the sequence of treatment and to test the effectiveness of medications for each patient. Balancing the forty main meridians can lead to spontaneous, accidental, placebo, or even miracle healing, regardless of one's religious or spiritual beliefs.

In my lectures on Spiritual Wellness, I often begin with the provocative statement, "What if doctors don't heal and God doesn't forgive?" While most patients intuitively understand that healing comes from within, not from the doctor, they often struggle with the concept that "God does not forgive." By the end of the lecture, I clarify that "God does not forgive because God has nothing to forgive. God embraces all and does not judge, therefore, there is nothing to forgive. It is humans who judge others and need to learn forgiveness."

> **Balancing the forty main meridians can lead to spontaneous, accidental, placebo, or even miracle healing, regardless of one's religious or spiritual beliefs.**

Forgiveness is a crucial part of the healing process, especially for chronically ill patients who do not respond to conventional, alternative, or integrative medical care. I have written about this in many of my previous articles and will continue to explore how unresolved emotional conflicts can manifest as disturbances in the meridian system throughout this series on medical acupuncture. Now, let's delve into how I apply Medical Acupuncture Meridian Assessment. Welcome to the journey.

Chapter 4 Large Intestine, Lung, Stomach, and Spleen/Pancreas Meridians

Why is the Large Intestine meridian a critical gateway to understanding the enigmatic world of parasites? This meridian was my initial breakthrough in comprehending parasites and their interconnections with the rest of the body's domain.

When I returned from a US Army mission in Bolivia in 2001, I was already measuring meridians using the German EAV system based on Dr. Voll's work. Instead of using typical herbs for parasites like black walnut, wormwood, and clove oil (the classic Hulda Clark formula), which had moderate success for various intestinal problems, I experimented with mebendazole or pyrantel pamoate. These were prescription parasite medications that we used in the US Army missions.

The results were surprising. Not only did GI symptoms improve, but many patients also reported that their asthma, bronchitis, bronchiectasis, or pneumonia responded quickly. Chronic fatigue and fibromyalgia improved, ADD/ADHD symptoms lessened, some autistic children responded positively, an MS brain lesion disappeared, and cancer became more manageable.

Initially, I thought it was pure coincidence, but a pattern emerged. Parasite medications were the quickest way to rebalance all meridian systems, except for dental and allergy-immunology.

Here begins my series of medical acupuncture articles, which include clinical case descriptions, in the next several chapters. They are organized by paired meridians, which together form a complete cycle of interrelated meridian systems.

Medical Acupuncture on Large Intestine Meridian: Ancient Romans and US Army Target Demons

Imagine divinity, humanity, and demons in the context of homeopathy, herbs, and pharmaceuticals. What if I propose that parasites are akin to demons? Parasites are deceptive, malevolent, elusive entities. They drain your energy, hijack your mind, and overpower your will. If we replace the term "parasites" with "demons" we can view the history of mankind and medicine from a unique perspective.

My firsthand experience with prescribed parasite medications came in 2001, during my deployment to Bolivia as a US Army Reserve medical officer. Our medical team extensively used the most affordable parasite medications provided by the US Army for about 10,000 Bolivian native Indians. These medicines were pyrantel pamoate and mebendazole.

When treating patients with IBS-like intestinal symptoms, detected based on disturbances on the large intestine meridian, some of my patients reported not only an improvement in their IBS symptoms but also a disappearance of their asthma, resolution of eczema or psoriasis, no recurrence of pneumonia, improvement in chronic fatigue and fibromyalgia, improvement in anxiety/depression, disappearance of fever of unknown origin, resolution of migraine headaches for the first time in many years, disappearance of brain lesions on MRIs in MS patients, and sometimes shrinkage of tumors, among other medical conditions.

I wasn't treating these conditions directly, but rather addressing parasites based on disturbances in the large intestine meridian. This information was not part of my medical school or Internal Medicine training. My treatment approach was informed by 30 years of medical practice and my experience with the US Army.

Parasites are pervasive yet challenging to detect with modern medical science. Relying solely on standard stool or blood tests to detect parasites is gravely insufficient. We need to embrace and understand the concepts of subtle Energy Fields, Matrix, Prana, and Meridians, as described in ancient civilizations.

In *The Process of Healing,* H. Van Gelder, DO, ND, suggests that homeopathy has been known for thousands of years in India, according to the ancient Indian science of Ayur Veda (Sanskrit for Knowledge of Life). The narrative suggests that Pythagoras, an Ionian Greek philosopher, studied Ayur Veda in India. Paracelsus, a mystical scientist of the Middle Ages, experimented based on Pythagoras's manuscripts. Samuel Hahnemann then based his theory of Homeopathy on Paracelsus's works.[5]

If Van Gelder's assertions are correct, the ancient Indian Ayurveda might be the precursor to modern Homeopathy. According to Van Gelder, the Ayurveda outlines three types of medicine for healing:

- **Divine** – Homeopathy
- **Human** – Herbs
- **Demonic** – Drugs

In this context, "drugs" are reserved for "demonic" entities, which I interpret as parasites. I've had moderate success with homeopathic and natural herbal parasite remedies. However, when I used the correct combinations of prescribed parasite medications in the right sequence (alongside resolving hidden dental problems), there were dramatic responses to many unexpected medical conditions that seemed impossible to cure. I am convinced that deeply embedded parasites can manifest in various forms of acute and chronic illnesses. Unlike antibiotics, parasite medications do not merely cover symptoms and suppress conditions.

While I oppose the use of medications to merely mask symptoms, as often promoted by pharmaceutical companies, I believe that parasite medications have been underutilized due to the deceptive, shadowy, and 'demonic' nature of parasites. Pharma, recognizing the demand for parasite medications, has been aggressively raising prices, becoming monetary parasites in the process.

Large Intestine Meridian and Related Teeth

The Large Intestine (LI) Meridian, which is paired with the Lung Meridian, plays a crucial role in our body. The LI is the last part of the digestive system; it is also called the large bowel and includes the colon. It absorbs water and electrolytes, produces and absorbs vitamins, and forms feces for elimination.

Ancient Acupuncture Intelligence reveals many interconnections along the Large Intestine meridian. Today's AI further illuminates these interconnections. Note the same teeth are associated with the large intestine and lung meridians; see the Tooth-Organ Meridian Chart. These organs and meridians are associated with upper bicuspids #4, 5 and #12, 13, and lower molars #18, 19 and #30, 31. See Figure 16.

Figure 16: Large Intestine Meridian, Connection to Dental

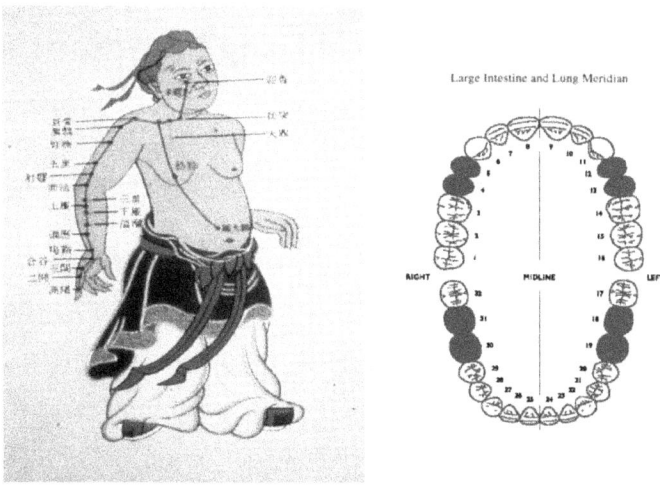

The Large Intestine functions and regulates with the Lung Meridian. What do these interconnections mean? Imbalances in any part of the meridian are often associated with problems elsewhere in that system, as seen in the Tooth-Organ Meridian Chart, which shows teeth, sensory organs, joints, spinal segments, vertebrae, organs, endocrine organs and tissues, and more.

In Traditional Chinese Medicine (TCM), organs and meridians are also associated with feelings. The Large Intestine is associated with being overcritical, controlling, dogmatic, and uptight. Fixing the underlying problems and rebalancing or restoring healthy meridians can help resolve these negative feelings.

It's worth noting that unresolved emotions, such as being a "control freak," are often associated with the large intestine and its meridian. This connection between emotional states and physical health is a fascinating aspect of holistic medicine.

I've observed when the LI meridian is balanced with parasite medications, it often clears a variety of bronchial and asthma-like conditions, including post-Covid syndrome.

Medical Acupuncture on Lung Meridian:
Pulmonary Hypertension, Covid-19, Lyme, more

Pulmonary hypertension, a type of high blood pressure that affects the arteries in the lungs and right side of the heart, can be caused by unrecognized dental infections and parasites. This is a bold statement: can it be substantiated with evidence from case studies?

Could asthma, COPD, post-COVID syndrome (Long COVID), Lyme, pulmonary hypertension, pneumonia, and lung cancer share an overlooked common denominator? In addition to smoking, allergies, molds, environmental chemicals, and viral and bacterial infections (which are common risk factors) could we be missing something? Overlapping parasite and dental infections may trigger medically unexplained symptoms (MUS), including pulmonary hypertension. This is my mantra, or broken record: Accidental Cure by treating unrecognized hidden dental and parasite infections. I have seen it many times.

I once treated a retired 67-year-old microbiologist from Ohio who had a history of pulmonary hypertension, shortness of breath, wheezing, coughing, thick mucus production, and vibrating sensations in her chest and lungs. She also had Lyme, hypothyroidism, hypertension, and suspected parasite problems, which manifested as fatigue, leg edema (swelling), skin sores all over her body, and incontinence.

She brought forensic evidence of parasites: microscopic pictures of skin lesions, a wet mount slide from sputum, parasite eggs in stool, and larva in a blood smear. Her doctors had tried different combinations of parasite medications: albendazole, fenbendazole, mebendazole, and doxycycline, but she was not responding. She was not suffering from delusions of parasitosis; she had forensic evidence of parasites.

After not responding to treatments with numerous parasite medications, the question arises: how and where do we start? As a rule, if parasites are not killed with sufficient duration and high-dose medications, they will continue their reproductive lifecycles, morph (some are pleomorphic), and hide deeper into tissues.

She had already undergone extensive blood tests, which were positive for many viral infections, but the rest of her blood tests were unremarkable. More blood tests would not be helpful for her treatment plan.

When I checked her 40 acupuncture points using Acupuncture Meridian Assessment, 13 out of 40 meridians were out of balance.

See Figure 17 below, which measures 40 meridians from the hand and foot on the right and left side. A reading of 45 to 55 on a scale of 100 is considered within the normal range; while low (under 45) is out of balance (scale 0 - 600,000 ohms).

Figure 17: Initial AMA Testing for 67-Year-Old Woman

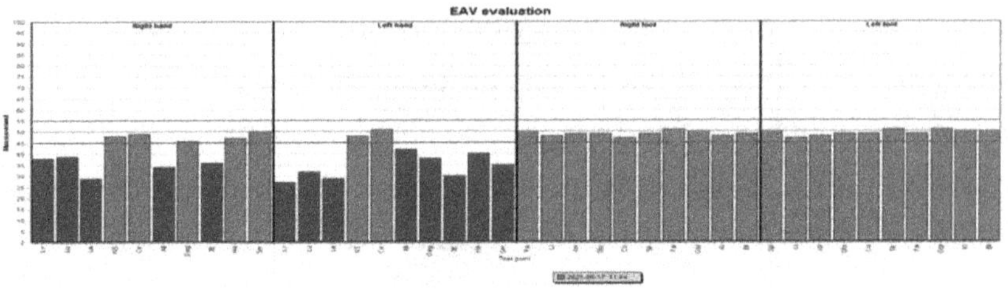

My first evaluation indicated that her primary problems were coming from the large intestine and lung meridians, a primary suspect for persistent parasite problems that had not been fully treated; she also had disturbances showing in allergy-immunology, dental, hormonal, heart, and small intestine meridians.

Advanced Enhanced Interrogation Technique

On her second evaluation the same day – which I sometimes do for patients with complex issues to unmask deeper-level problems - I used six acupuncture needles on her head.

I call this my "Advanced Enhanced Interrogation Technique." It unmasked 12 additional problems for a total of 25 out of 40 meridians out of balance: Liver, Gallbladder, Stomach, Skin meridians, among others. See Figure 18.

This indicates that most of her previous medications were not in the right combinations, with too small doses and too short duration. They were not potent enough to kill the parasites, so they went hiding in deeper layers of organs – almost like a cloaking device – and were still causing damage.

Figure 18: Second AMA Testing for 67-Year-Old Woman (Enhanced Interrogation Technique)

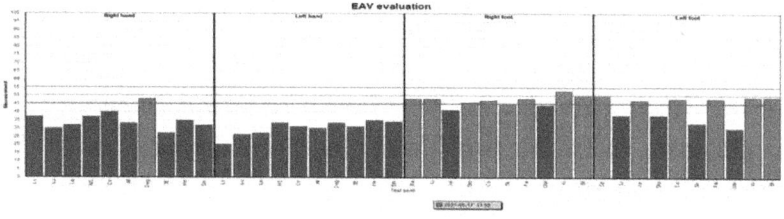

Based on her enhanced AMA reading and previous history, I selected high doses of ivermectin, pyrantel pamoate, praziquantel, tinidazole, doxycycline, and nystatin for 30 days and also gave her homeopathic liver, kidney, allergy, gallbladder, dental, and lymph support remedies as a first step in targeting parasite, dental, and fungal infections.

I told her that this was a shotgun approach to get hyperinfection under control before we can do more fine-tuning: that often requires dental operations and ruling out environmental toxins. I can predict, based on statistical probability, and expect her response after a 30-day course of medications to indicate better balancing of her meridians in response to the medications.

The real test begins when the patient returns for reevaluation. The odds are in her favor for a positive response when most of her 40 meridians are balanced. However, this is just the beginning of the healing process.

Fine Tuning the Treatment Process

Fine-tuning involves treatment with rotating parasite/fungal medications to break the lifecycle, dental work as indicated by further AMA testing and other diagnostics, and detoxification of environmental toxins and heavy metals. These steps must be executed in the correct sequence.

Recovery is gradual and may take over a year; dental work is always an unknown factor beyond my control, in the hands of the dentist. Holistic biological dentists and oral surgeons are a part of my medical team.

> **Fine-tuning involves treatment with rotating parasite/ fungal meds to break the lifecycle; dental work as indicated by further AMA testing and other diagnostics; as well as detoxification of environmental toxins and heavy metals.**

According to the NIH National Heart, Lung, and Blood Institute (NHLBI), pulmonary hypertension is also known as pulmonary arterial hypertension (PAH). The increased pressure in the blood vessels of the lungs means that your heart must work harder to pump blood into the lungs. This can cause symptoms such as shortness of breath, chest pain, and lightheadedness.

Dental Infections: Overlooked Cause of Heart Disease

In the US, the most common cause of pulmonary hypertension is heart disease. From my perspective, hidden dental infections are the most overlooked factor underlying heart problems - not high cholesterol.

> **From my perspective, hidden dental infections are the most overlooked factor underlying heart problems - not high cholesterol.**

Other conditions that can cause pulmonary hypertension include sickle cell disease, pulmonary embolism, a type of venous blood clot, and chronic obstructive pulmonary disease (COPD). If left untreated, the increased pressure can damage your heart. This may lead to serious or life-threatening complications, such as heart failure or irregular heart rhythms.

Lung Meridian and Related Teeth

As noted earlier, the Lung and Large Intestine are intimately connected as paired meridians. The lungs are responsible for respiration, bringing oxygen into your body and transferring it into the bloodstream, and removing and expelling carbon dioxide. The Lung meridian governs the inspiration of Chi from air and expulsion of impure Chi from the body.

My initial observation about these paired meridians was that opening the Large Intestine meridian with parasite medications often alleviated various lung-related bronchial symptoms and asthma-like medical conditions, including post-COVID syndrome.

Today's AI further illuminates these interconnections. Note the same teeth are associated with the lung intestine and large intestine meridians; see the Tooth-Organ Meridian Chart. These organs and meridians are associated with upper bicuspids #4, 5 and #12, 13, and lower molars #18, 19 and #30, 31. See Figure 19.

Figure 19: Lung Meridian, Connection to Dental

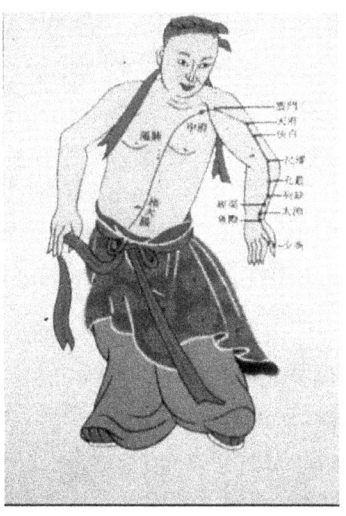
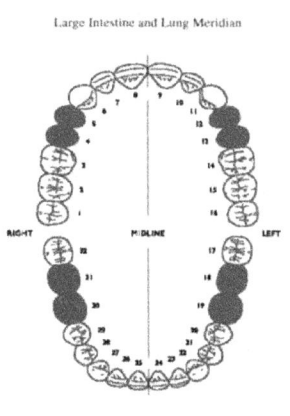

The Lung Meridian controls respiration, the throat, nose, and skin, and is paired with the Large Intestine Meridian. Imbalances in any part of the meridian are often associated with problems elsewhere in that system, as seen in the Tooth-Organ Meridian Chart, which shows teeth, sense organs, joints, spinal segments, vertebrae, organs, endocrine organs and tissues, and more.

In Traditional Chinese Medicine (TCM), organs and meridians are also associated with feelings. The lung meridian is associated with grief and sadness. Unresolved emotional conflict from chronic grief, sadness, longing, or loss of zest in life may manifest in an imbalance of the lung meridian. Fixing the underlying problems and rebalancing or restoring healthy meridians can help resolve these negative feelings.

Regardless of diagnosis with asthma, COVID-19, Post COVID syndrome, Lyme, Pulmonary Hypertension, lung cancer, and other medically unexplained symptoms (MUS), look for hidden unrecognized parasites and dental infections as part of the solution.

Medical Acupuncture on Stomach Meridian:
Global Whining and Fearmongering to Global Healing - Rebellious Stomach for Nobel Prize

Historically, medical consensus attributed stress and lifestyle factors as the primary causes of peptic ulcer disease. However, this theory was challenged by Australian Dr. Barry Marshall and pathologist Robin Warren.

In a daring act of self-experimentation, Marshall ingested a cocktail of *H. pylori*, inducing the disease, and then used antibiotics to cure it. Their groundbreaking discovery in 1982 revealed that the gram-negative bacteria H. pylori was responsible for more than 90 percent of duodenal ulcers and up to 80 percent of gastric ulcers.

Infection is the Root Cause of Inflammation

This revelation sparked a paradigm shift in medical thinking: infection, not stress or lifestyle, is the root cause of inflammation, ulcers, gastro-esophageal reflux, and esophageal/stomach cancers. The unexpected finding that *H. pylori* caused gastritis and peptic ulcers earned him the 2005 Nobel Prize in Physiology.[6] This achievement disrupted the established medical community and paved the way towards Global Healing.

> **This revelation sparked a paradigm shift in medical thinking: infection, not stress or lifestyle, is the root cause of inflammation, ulcers, gastro-esophageal reflux, and esophageal/stomach cancers.**

If you're experiencing severe acid reflux, burping, nausea, gas, indigestion, gastritis, or peptic ulcer disease, it may indicate an imbalance in your Stomach meridian. Ancient acupuncture texts metaphorically describe these symptoms as a rebellious stomach or global whining. The Stomach meridian, one of the most complex, regulates not only digestion but also your brain, central nervous system, and neuromuscular system down to your toes.

Acid reflux and indigestion often respond to apple cider vinegar, hydrochloric acid, and over-the-counter digestive enzymes. For a more detailed explanation, refer to my article, "Acid Reflux and Rebellious Stomach: Killing the Messenger for Profit." More advanced cases with abdominal pain, bloating, gastritis, and ulcer may respond to doxycycline/tinidazole to cover H. pylori and microscopic GI parasites, along with adding bile products and pancreatic enzymes.

The selection of medications is based on Acupuncture Meridian Assessment, and the origin of the problem is often not in the stomach, but usually in the pancreas, gallbladder, liver, or small intestine. Many patients also have hidden dental infections, unique individual parasites/fungal problems, and/or environmental toxins. The root of the problem is often not in the stomach, but in the pancreas, gallbladder, liver, or small intestine.

Stomach/Esophageal Cancer: A Lethal Disease with Multiple Risk Factors

Stomach and esophageal cancer are often aggressive and lethal diseases. *H. pylori* infection is one of many risk factors. Although *H. pylori* is common, most people colonized with it never develop esophageal or stomach cancer. For instance, Indians rarely develop gastric cancer compared to the Japanese. This disparity may be due to differences in diets, parasites, and bacterial infections between these populations, which may interact differently and help counteract bacterial infections. We must also consider the impact of stress, lifestyle, smoking, alcohol, drugs, environmental toxins, and pollution.

I recently lost a patient to stage 4 esophageal cancer. This patient also had parasites, fungi, and bacterial infections, and had been exposed to massive amounts of xylene petrochemical products while working on a road crew many years ago. Despite a 20+ year history of acid reflux and diabetes, and being unable to swallow food, he did not respond to natural remedies, antiparasitics, or antifungal medications while undergoing radiation and chemotherapy. His advanced stage made any response unlikely. His high xylene level was surprising, as he had been promoted to supervisor and had not been directly exposed to or used any petrochemical products for many years.

Driving Forces for Mitochondrial Dysfunction

The ancient understanding of the Rebellious Stomach led to the discovery of *H. pylori* and the Nobel Prize awarded to Dr. Marshall and Warren. This major paradigm shift in medical history is just beginning. Parasites, fungi, and bacterial infections, along with environmental toxins, dental/medical complex, and EMF, are driving forces for inflammation and metabolic derangement down to mitochondrial dysfunction.

These factors may manifest in a myriad of medical diagnoses such as autism, asthma, cancer, chronic fatigue syndrome, chronic pain, fibromyalgia, Lyme, and migraine headache, to neurodegenerative conditions like MS, Parkinson's disease, and ALS, and every known chronic complex illness.

Responding to every physical symptom and medical diagnosis is akin to responding to Global Whining. We face a Global COVID-19 Pandemic and Global Warming, but without an effective early Global Warning System – whether for climate change or patients' medical problems – we can only face troubling and unpredictable outcomes. Now is the time to focus on learning, understanding, preventing, and correcting the underlying problems and move from Global Whining and Global Fearmongering to Global Healing.

Stomach Meridian and Related Teeth

The Stomach and Spleen/Pancreas meridians are paired meridians. The stomach moves things downward: it gets food from the esophagus, mixes it with digestive enzymes and gastric acid, begins breaking it down, and stores it until it is ready to move into the small intestine.

The Stomach meridian, one of the most complex, regulates not only digestion but also your brain, central nervous system, and neuromuscular system down to your toes. The Stomach meridian oversees the vagus nerve (CN10), Hypoglossal nerve (CN12), Submandibular Ganglion, and most of the plexus (network of nerves) of the vagus nerve of the GI tract, pulmonary, and testicular/ovarian plexus.

Today's AI further illuminates these interconnections. Note the same teeth are associated with the Stomach and Spleen meridians; see the Tooth-Organ Meridian Chart. These organs and meridians are associated with upper molars #2, 3 and #14, 15, and lower bicuspids #20, 21 and #28, 29. See Figure 20.

Figure 20: Stomach Meridian, Connection to Dental

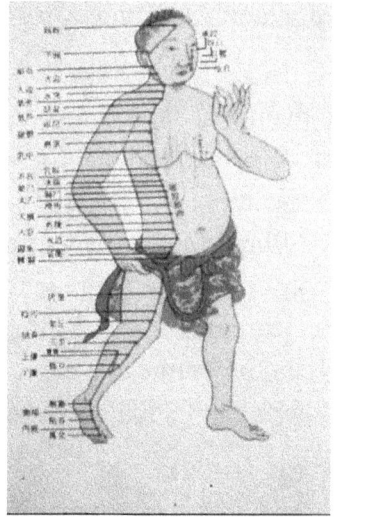
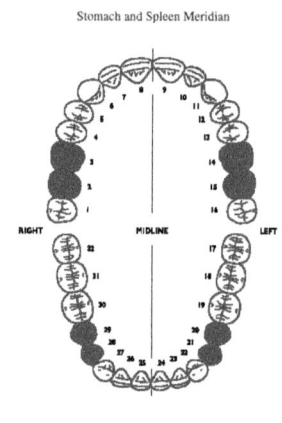

The Stomach and Spleen/Pancreas Meridian functions in the assimilation of Chi (energy) from food through digestion and absorption. Unresolved emotional conflicts or living with someone harboring unresolved feelings can make you more vulnerable in organ systems, according to acupuncture meridian principles. The unresolved emotion linked to the Stomach meridian is associated with "anxiety, dislike, stress, or obsession."

This meridian has been associated with common GI problems such as acidic stomach and reflux, ulcers, occasional esophageal and stomach cancer, and associated anxiety. Infections by *H. pylori* and their connections to ulcers were finally discovered by Dr. Barry Marshall in 1982 when I was a medical resident, debunking the theory that stress was the primary cause of ulcers. It was an infection causing stress, not the reverse.

Medical Acupuncture on Spleen/Pancreas Meridian: Case Studies of Military Officers

In classical acupuncture, the Spleen/Pancreas is considered the principal organ of digestion. It transforms food into nourishment and transports digested foods and fluids from the stomach, distributing them throughout the body. If you cannot supply and feed the whole army of bodily components, the whole military system will collapse with a domino effect.

First Case Study: Military Colonel

A 52-year-old military colonel from Washington, DC, presented with a complex array of symptoms and medical diagnoses. His role involved monitoring drug movements in South America to combat illegal drug trafficking. He fell ill during a field visit to Bolivia, Columbia, and Peru. Despite not having a roadside bomb injury or PTSD, his health was significantly affected.

After being air-evacuated from Bolivia to Walter Reed Army Hospital and later transferred to the Navy Medical Center, he reported a 50 percent improvement. However, he still had a list of lingering symptoms and was working part-time. Figure 21 gives his dozen symptoms and diagnoses when he came to see me.

Figure 21: Symptoms and Diagnoses: Military Officer

Chronic Diarrhea
Chronic Sinusitis/
allergic rhinitis
Empty Sellar Syndrome
Esophageal Reflux
Fever of Unknown Origin
Headache

Insomnia
Irritable Bowel Syndrome
Lumbago/low back pain
Severe Fatigue
Sleep Apnea
Vestibular
Neuritis/Dizziness

Many Imbalanced Meridians Indicate a Risk for Cancer

An Acupuncture Meridian Assessment revealed that 17 out of his 40 meridians were out of balance (Figure 22). The primary issues were with his spleen/pancreas, small intestine, gallbladder, and large intestine meridians. If left uncorrected, these conditions could potentially lead him to a precancerous stage, with the risk of developing tumors in his most immune-deficient organ. A high number of imbalanced meridians, including the spleen/pancreas meridian, often indicate a risk of developing precancerous tumors.

Figure 22: Initial AMA Testing for Military Officer: 17 Meridians Out of Balance

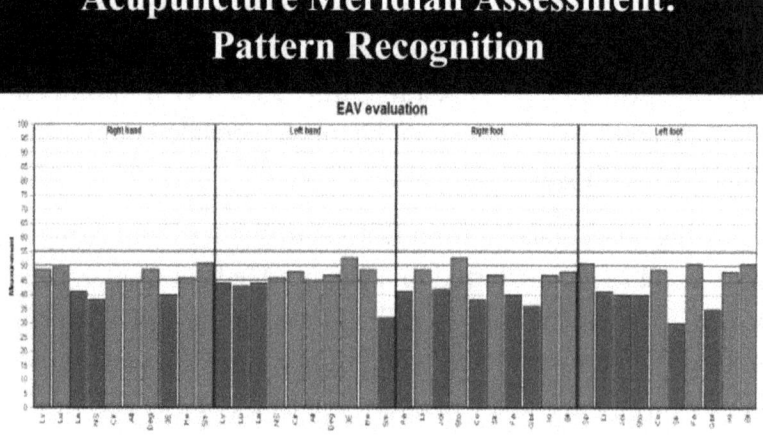

After two rounds of ivermectin and tinidazole, the officer experienced a significant increase in his energy level and overall wellness. For the first time in four years, he felt normal. However, his symptoms started to return, necessitating a different combination of parasite medications. He also had to address dental issues, heavy metal toxicity (mercury, lead, and nickel), and multiple allergies. A dental operation led to severe complications, further complicating his health status. The interconnections between teeth, dental health, and other body systems are detailed in the Tooth-Organ Meridian Chart in Figures 8 and 9 earlier in this book. A color version is on my website, under Resources.

Second Case Study: Retired Brigade General

A retired one-star Brigade General, who had been diagnosed with fever of unknown original (FUO) for several years, sought my help. Despite extensive evaluations at Walter Reed Hospital and the US Centers for Disease Control and Prevention (CDC), his condition remained unresolved. His symptoms included a persistent fever of 102-103 degrees Fahrenheit, bone chills, elevated muscle enzymes, back cramps, lethargy, poor sleep, nocturnal urination, and muscle cramps.

An Acupuncture Meridian Assessment (AMA) indicated that his primary issues were related to the Large Intestine, Gallbladder, Liver, and Spleen/Pancreas meridians. After a ten-day treatment with high doses of ivermectin and pyrantel pamoate, his condition improved significantly. When I saw him a year later in Washington DC, he reported feeling well and his FUO had been resolved. His fever was attributed to parasites.

A combination of ivermectin, pyrantel pamoate, tinidazole, and praziquantel often balances the Spleen/Pancreas meridian, targeting the digestion and immune systems.

Spleen/Pancreas Meridian and Related Teeth

The Spleen/Pancreas Meridian is paired with the Stomach Meridian. The spleen filters blood, stores blood cells, and helps fight infections. It distributes nutrients, maintains muscle tone, and helps regulate blood flow.

The Spleen/Pancreas, the principal organ of digestion, transports nutrients, produces and regulates blood, and transforms food into nourishment. While the Stomach moves things downward, the Spleen filters blood and moves Chi energy upward.

> **While the Stomach moves things downward, the Spleen filters blood and moves Chi energy upward.**

The pancreas has both an endocrine and a digestive exocrine function. It produces insulin and other hormones to regulate blood glucose levels, and it secretes digestive juices and enzymes to help break down food in the small intestine.

Classical acupuncture did not differentiate the spleen and pancreas as a separate independent organ system but refers to the spleen meridian. The spleen is located on the left side of the upper abdomen, and the head of the pancreas begins on the right side, extending to the left side.

> **The spleen is located on the left side of the upper abdomen, and the head of the pancreas begins on the right side, extending to the left side.**

Today's AI further illuminates these interconnections. Note the same teeth are associated with the Spleen and Stomach meridians; see the Tooth-Organ Meridian Chart. These organs and meridians are associated with upper molars #2, 3 and #14, 15, and lower bicuspids #20, 21 and #28, 29. See Figure 23.

Figure 23: Spleen/Pancreas Meridian, Connection to Dental

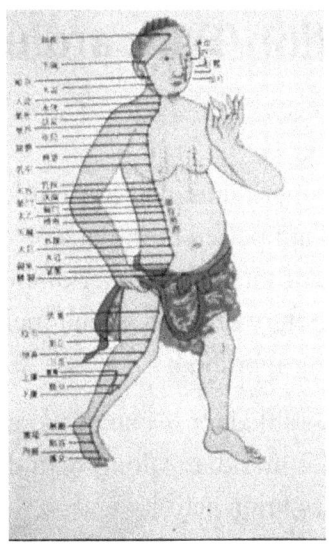
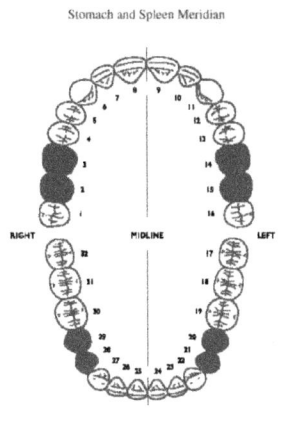

The Spleen/Pancreas meridian is associated with feelings of oversensitivity and a sense of inadequacy, not being good enough. It is not uncommon for pancreatic cancer patients to manifest deficiency in the spleen meridian. This meridian, part of the deep lymph, immune, and digestive systems, seldom shows as the only disturbance in AMA. It is considered the home of thought and influences concentration and learning.

I hope you enjoy my thoughts on UFO and FUO: fever of unknown origin.

Chapter 5 Gallbladder, Liver, Triple Warmer, and Circulation/Pericardium Meridians

The Gallbladder and Liver are paired meridians, and the Triple Warmer and Circulation/Pericardium are paired meridians. Together, they form a complete cycle of interrelated meridian systems. Here are my medical acupuncture articles, which include clinical case descriptions, on these four meridians.

A few introductory comments: The Gallbladder is one of the most fascinating meridians. The Gallbladder meridian, along with the dental meridian, controls and regulates brain activity and neuromodulation via the central, peripheral and enteric nervous system, which also comprise the autonomic nervous system.

Disturbance of the Liver meridian (and gallbladder meridian) is one of the most common findings among chronically ill patients, but it may not translate into liver disease shown immediately in blood tests. It may take many years of overlapping insults from different parasites and toxins to manifest as liver cancer, bile duct (cholangiocarcinoma), or pancreatic cancer.

The Triple Warmer function corresponds to the endocrine system - glands that produce hormones that regulate metabolism, growth and development, tissue function, sexual function, reproduction, sleep, and mood. The Triple Warmer meridian and endocrine system includes adrenal, thyroid, testes, ovaries, and breast-related problems including breast cancer.

The Pericardium or the Master of Heart meridian has a circulatory function without a physical form. The Pericardium/Master of Heart is described as a membrane or sac surrounding the heart and represents the entire circulatory system; its primary function is to protect the Heart from pathogens. Since ancient times, the Pericardium meridian has been poorly defined, since it represents the entire circulatory system, not a specific organ.

The Pericardium and Triple Warmer Meridians are regulators of the sympathetic (fight or flight) and parasympathetic (rest and digest) nervous system, influencing the body's autonomic (automatically regulates bodily functions) and neurovegetative activities, such as sleep, appetite, and concentration, and hormones.

Medical Acupuncture on Gallbladder Meridian:
Therapeutic Illusion on IBS and Autism

Irritable Bowel Syndrome (IBS) symptoms include abdominal pain, bloating, diarrhea, constipation, and changes in the pattern of bowel movement. Your doctor may diagnose IBS based on limited tests and review of your clinical symptoms. The stool test for ova and parasites are almost always negative.

The causes of IBS are not clear. However, there are plenty of theories, including small intestinal bacterial overgrowth, food allergies, gluten sensitivities, GMO food, and genetic factors. IBS is often triggered by an intestinal infection or acute emotional stressful events. There is no cure for IBS according to western medicine. The goal for the treatment is to improve symptoms with dietary changes and use medications to control diarrhea, constipation, and abdominal pain.

About 10-15 percent of the global population is suffering from IBS. There is a tremendous financial interest by pharmaceutical companies to develop the next blockbuster medication. So far, drugs for IBS have had limited impact with too many side effects.

Some drugs, Aldosterone and Tegaserod, were withdrawn in 2007 but there is a stream of new drugs entering the market.

Treating the symptoms of IBS with medication is a "therapeutic illusion." It's like treating a heart patient with cholesterol lowering statin drugs while believing it will prevent the person from having a heart attack. Many IBS patients, despite negative stool tests for parasites, may respond to parasite medications, such as tinidazole, nitazoxanide, and ivermectin, and anti-fungal medications, such as nystatin, fluconazole, or itraconazole.

> **Treating the symptoms of IBS with medication is a "therapeutic illusion" … Many IBS patients, despite negative stool tests for parasites, may respond to parasite and antifungal medications.**

Is it possible that parasites are cloaking themselves to engage in asymmetric unconventional warfare with mankind? Ten years ago, at the Combat Support Hospital in Germany, I saw a retired US Army Special Forces, Warrant Officer, R.D., whom I treated for irritable bowel syndrome. After several previously unsuccessful rounds of combinations of meds from other doctors, she positively responded to parasite medications that I prescribed. She even presented me with a special medallion from the 1st Special Forces Group (Airborne). She spread the word to the network of Special Forces to look for parasite problems for those suffering from IBS.

Within the military, IBS is one of many underappreciated burdens. Many soldiers who serve overseas develop "travelers' diarrhea" which is one of the main causes of illness, lost duty days, and compromised missions. A lot of Special Forces are silently suffering from IBS because they're afraid to speak out about their problems for fear of a medical discharge since there is no cure for it. They may have acquired IBS during their "survival training." It may then have been compounded by overseas operations in many hostile environments and the traumatic stress of combat operations.

Parasite and Fungal Medications Can Help Autism

Another unusual example is Autism. Some years ago, I saw a 39-year-old Registered Nurse from Dallas for weird neurological symptoms with numbness of body, coughing, brain fog, exhaustion, and IBS-like symptoms. My acupuncture meridian assessment indicated 15 out of 40 meridians were out of balance.

One of the main disturbances came from the large intestine, small intestine, allergy, and lymphatic meridian. I started her on parasite medications of ivermectin, pyrantel pamoate, and praziquantel. She noticed a dramatic improvement in her condition with increased energy, no burning sensation, and improved cognition.

Without my knowledge, she decided, out of desperation, to give a part of her parasite medications to her 5-year-old son with severe autism who was diagnosed at age two. He was non-verbal and had focal seizures. The response has been a dramatic improvement in his behavior. He started "talking" after taking his mom's parasite medications.

I had to reprimand the mom for treating her son without a proper medical evaluation. However, I was also impressed by her description of the dramatic improvement of her son's autistic behavior. I finally evaluated the child (after the parasite medication given by his mom) and his gallbladder and nervous system meridian was still out of balance. I put him on different rounds of parasite and fungal medications, nystatin, fluconazole and nitazoxanide, to re-balance the rest of the meridians. He also had very high mercury exposure. This was most likely from his mom who also had a high mercury level.

I then saw them both again. The child's ATEC (Autism Treatment Evaluation Checklist) score dropped from 109 (severe autism) to 4 (considered normal), according to his mom. The ATEC was developed in 1999, not as a diagnostic evaluation but as a way for researchers to evaluate the effectiveness of various treatments for autistic children. ATEC internal consistency reliability was very high (.94 for the Total score) and studies confirm validity of the ATEC Report.

The Gallbladder Meridian Influences Movement, the Autonomic Nervous System, and Cognition

I've written several articles on autism, including, "AutismOne on Healing Autism," and "Autism and Autism Spectrum Disorder." I do not treat Autism. I treat the underlying problems based on acupuncture meridian assessment. Most autistic children have disturbances of intestinal and gallbladder meridians. The Gallbladder meridian is one of the longest and most complex meridians. It partly controls movement, the autonomic nervous system, and cognition.

> **The Gallbladder meridian is one of the longest and most complex meridians. It partly controls movement, the autonomic nervous system, and cognition.**

Disturbance of the gallbladder meridian has been associated with migraine headache, concentration problems, eye/ear problems, neck pain, indigestion, abdominal pain with nausea, and hip, knee, or foot pain. The gallbladder meridian influences our central nervous system from mesencephalon including the center of sleep and waking rhythm, diencephalon sleep center, cranial nerves such as the optic and trigeminal nerves, parasympathetic nervous system including the ciliary optic ganglion, vagus nerve in the medulla oblongata, and the cranial part of the sympathetic nervous system. For more information, see *Voll Electroacupuncture Desk Reference Manual* and related materials from the Occidental Institute Research Foundation (OIRF)[7] and Praxis2Practice.[8]

Gallbladder Meridian and Related Teeth

The Gallbladder and Liver meridians are paired meridians; this means if either is out of harmony, the other can be too. The gallbladder stores and expels bile produced by the liver, which is essential to digestion of fats.

Today's AI further illuminates these interconnections. Note the same teeth are associated with the Gallbladder and Liver meridians, see the Tooth-Organ Meridian Chart. These organs and meridians are associated with upper canine teeth #6 and #11, and lower canine teeth #22 and #27. See Figure 24.

Figure 24: Gallbladder Meridian, Connection to Dental

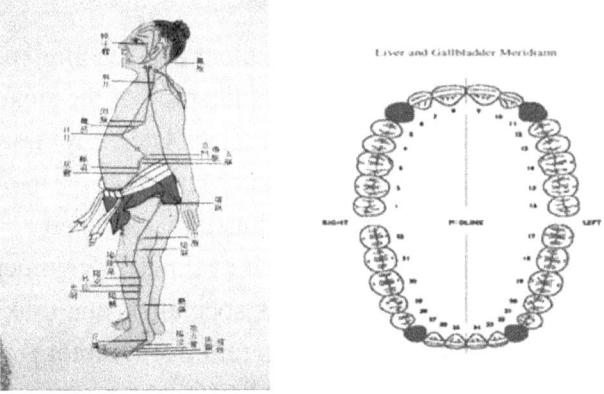

The Gallbladder meridian, along with the dental meridian, controls and regulates brain activity and neuromodulation via the central, peripheral and enteric nervous system, which also comprise the autonomic nervous system.

The Gallbladder Meridian functions with the Liver Meridian to maintain the free flow of Chi and to regulate emotional changes. The gallbladder is associated with feelings of resentment, victimhood, bitterness, and blaming. Fixing the underlying problems and rebalancing or restoring healthy meridians can help resolve these negative feelings.

Medical Acupuncture on Liver Meridian:
Deworming in the Nile Forgotten Art of Preventive Medicine

Schistosomiasis, also known as bilharzia, is a disease caused by parasitic worms, known as Schistosoma liver flukes; see Figure 25 for its complex life cycle, forms, and sites. It is considered one of the most neglected tropical diseases and is not found in the US, according to the CDC.[9] Over 250 million people are infected globally with the second most common parasite after malaria. Several major subtypes of Schistosoma are distributed globally, and the best-known drug therapy is praziquantel 20 mg/kg (up to 60 mg/kg per day) for one day, per CDC guidelines.

I have a problem with the CDC assessment and recommendation based on clinical experience dealing with some of the sickest patients in my practice, which I will address later. My first encounter was about 25 years ago when Mary, a 45-year-old white female came to see me; she was convinced that she had schistosomiasis. She has been seen and evaluated by numerous medical doctors and infectious disease specialists and told her she did not have schistosomiasis. She was told her symptoms were psychological. Her family abandoned her; she lost her children and was living in a women's shelter. I had no experience treating parasites at that time except using some natural herbs.

Common symptoms associated with schistosomiasis include rash, swimmer's itch, fever, headache, muscle pain, diarrhea, constipation, abdominal bloating with pain, shortness of breath, fatigue, enlarged liver and/or spleen, eosinophilia, blood in the stool or in the urine, liver fibrosis, and portal hypertension. Mary had some of the minor list of symptoms.

I did a repeat blood test and stool test for ova and parasites which were all negative. I believed she was telling me the truth despite the lack of scientific evidence with positive proof of schistosomiasis parasites. I tried a therapeutic trial with praziquantel with trepidation based on a medical textbook using the CDC recommended dose. The response was a slight improvement, a disappointment at best. In hindsight, her dose was too low, and she most likely needed a different combination of medications.

Mary was one of my first encounters using prescribed parasite medication based on symptoms and not based on lab test results. Since then, I have tried many different combinations of parasite medication and gained new experience using parasite meds while I was in Bolivia in 2001 for a US Army medical mission. I began using Acupuncture Meridian Assessment (AMA) before the Bolivia mission to detect and connect the dots from a disturbance in meridians to therapeutic trials with parasite medications. Parasite problems are here in every corner of the US; they manifest in different names and diagnoses and become "medically unexplained syndrome" (MUS), as described in my books.

Most chronically sick people do not have one type of parasite but multiple types as a complex bio-ecosystem supporting, communicating, and interacting with toxins, fungi, bacteria, viruses, and prions.

Schistosomiasis has a complex life cycle; the eggs will eventually lodge on the biliary tract in the liver or urinary bladder (see below). Disturbance of the liver meridian (and gallbladder meridian) is one of the most common findings among chronically ill patients, but it may not translate into liver disease shown immediately in blood tests. It may take many years of overlapping insults from different parasites and toxins to manifest as liver cancer, cholangiocarcinoma (bile duct), or pancreatic cancer.

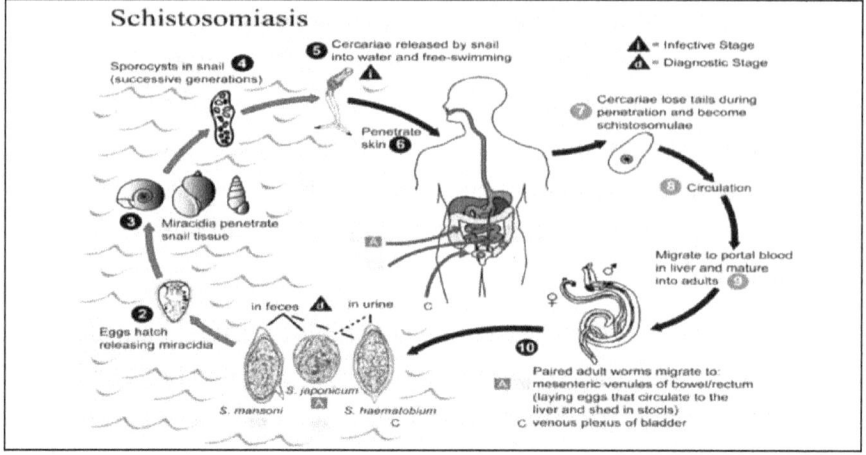

Figure 25: Life Cycle of Schistosomiasis
Source: US Centers for Disease Control and Prevention, DPDx, Schistosoma

When I pick up a disturbance on the liver, pancreas, gallbladder and/or spleen meridian, I am concerned about a possible precancerous condition. Additional problems in the dental, large intestine or small intestine meridians are indications of high risks for developing cancer somewhere in the body before there may be a physical manifestation of a tumor. It can be breast, ovarian, prostate, lung, or brain tumor.

Most chronically sick people do not have one type of parasite but multiple different types as a complex bio-ecosystem supporting, communicating, and interacting with environmental biotoxins, fungi, bacteria, viruses, and prions. I say parasites speak many languages; see the many symptoms they can cause in Figure 26.

A few years ago, I went on a Nile River cruise. Our anthropology tour guide was describing not only ancient Egyptian history and monuments, but frequent Nile River illness: an ancient curse of abdominal bloating, pain, shortness of breath, blood in the stool or urine and gradual demise, not only during ancient times, but also as a current medical problem after the Aswan Dam was built.

I noticed that he had abdominal bloating and became easily winded; he said he was checked for schistosomiasis and tested negative for parasites by his physician. He found out that I was a practicing physician, not retired like most of the tour group, and asked me privately what can be done.

I gave him my small emergency supply of ivermectin and praziquantel, left over from my recent training for physicians on how to use parasite medications with the instruction that if there was some improvement, he would need more medications from his doctors - regardless of tests results, based on his symptoms. I did not evaluate his meridian systems, but his symptoms were consistent with schistosomiasis.

Figure 26: Parasites speak many languages

- Gas/Bloating
- Grinding teeth
- Coughing at night
- Weight loss/gain
- Obesity/underweight
- Lethargy/fatigue
- Sexual dysfunction
- Migraine headache
- Visual problems
- Brain fog
- Food cravings
- Anemia/eosinophilia
- Bruxism
- Allergies
- Suppression of allergies

- Immune deficiency syndrome
- Mental/behavior problems
- Constipation/diarrhea
- Psoriasis/eczema
- Food allergies
- Knee/hip pain
- Abdominal pain
- IBS/colitis
- Night waking/bed wetting
- Night sweats
- Rectal itching
- Muscle/joint pain
- Cyst/tumor

Deworming parasites, most likely Schistosoma liver flukes, and others with ivermectin and praziquantel on the Nile River is a forgotten or neglected art of medicine. After listening to the patient's history, I treated him based on clinical symptoms, not lab reports. Deworming is basic preventive medicine.

Veterinarians know the truth about deworming as a part of preventive medicine and physicians need to be reeducated on the limitations of parasite testing. We need a new way of thinking about chronic problems. We may need to deworm on a global scale with parasite medications. Who knows what else will disappear? Parasite treatment is a forgotten Art of Preventive Medicine.

Liver Meridian and Related Teeth

The Liver and Gallbladder meridians are paired meridians. The liver helps support metabolism, immunity, digestion, detoxification, and vitamin storage. The liver filters all the blood in the body and breaks down harmful substances such as alcohol, drugs and toxins, produces bile that helps digest fats and fat-soluble vitamins, regulates blood glucose levels, metabolizes proteins and lipids, stores vitamins and minerals, and helps in resisting infections via immune factors.

Today's AI further illuminates these interconnections. Note the same teeth are associated with the Liver and Gallbladder meridians; see the Tooth-Organ Meridian Chart. These organs and meridians are associated with upper canine teeth #6 and #11, and lower canine teeth #22 and #27. See Figure 27.

Figure 27: Liver Meridian, Connection to Dental

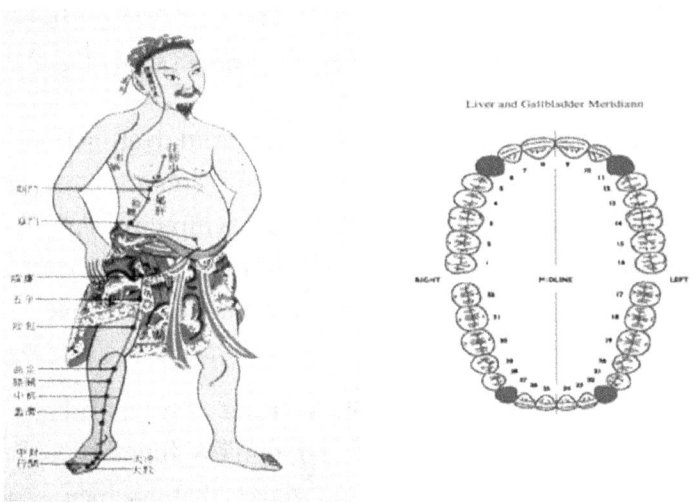

The Liver Meridian controls muscles, tendons, eyes, and genitals, and regulates blood volume and emotional changes. It plays an important role in detoxification.

What do these interconnections mean? Imbalances in any part of the meridian are often associated with problems elsewhere in that system, as seen in the Tooth-Organ Meridian Chart, which shows teeth, sense organs, joints, spinal segments, vertebrae, organs, endocrine organs and tissues, and more.

In TCM, organs and meridians are also associated with feelings. The liver is associated with feelings of anger, frustration, toxic, and stubborn or unyielding behavior. Fixing the underlying problems and rebalancing or restoring healthy meridians can help resolve these negative feelings.

Medical Acupuncture on Triple Warmer Meridian: Adrenal, Thyroid, Lyme, Breast Cancer, Chronic Fatigue Syndrome, CFS/ME, and Dental

Fatigue, often a reflection of adrenal and thyroid dysfunction, is one of the most common complaints during doctor visits, yet most blood tests do not reflect the patients' symptoms. Any infections or environmental toxins will eventually stress your endocrine system, and it will disturb the acupuncture Triple Warmer meridian.

The ancient description of the Triple Warmer (TW) meridian may seem strange to Western medicine, but TW function corresponds to the endocrine system - glands that produce hormones that regulate metabolism, growth and development, tissue function, sexual function, reproduction, sleep, and mood. The TW meridian and endocrine system includes adrenal, thyroid, testes, ovaries, and breast-related problems including breast cancer.

The body is divided into the Upper Warmer, Middle Warmer, and Lower Warmer; called Triple Warmer or San Jiao. In general, simple terms, the function of the Triple Warmer is to circulate the Chi through blood and body fluids, burn food with water, and to harmonize the digestion of solid and liquid foods. TW is considered the path of water and food, the beginning and end of Chi. See the *Textbook of Acupuncture* by Felix Mann.

Most chronically ill, complex patients have multiple disturbances on Acupuncture Meridian Assessment (AMA) and almost always, the TW meridian is out of balance and shows a low reading. An out of balance meridian is like a violin string that is out of tune. You can support them with natural herbs, homeopathic remedies, detox, adrenal and thyroid glandular products, and patients are always grateful to feel better. But often, this natural healing is not good enough to have a long-term benefit.

Investigating further why they have a disturbance in the TW meridian reveals problems such as hidden dental infection, allergy/immune system problems, parasites, toxins and chemical exposures, emotional stress and increasingly, EMF as triggering factors. Depending on the patient's genetic susceptibility and compounding factors, the medical profession may label their symptoms and syndrome as fibromyalgia, Chronic Fatigue Syndrome/Myalgic Encephalomyelitis (CFS/ME), MS, Lyme, cancer, or psychiatric diagnoses.

The Triple Warmer meridian regulates the Hypothalamus which controls thyroid and adrenal functions, Facial nerve (CN7), Glossopharyngeal nerve (CN), and part of the sympathetic nervous system. The Triple Warmer and Pericardium (Master of Heart) meridians are paired meridians, and the Gallbladder and Liver meridians form a continuously flowing, paired meridian circuit. See *Voll Electroacupuncture Desk Reference Manual* from the Occidental Institute Research Foundation (OIRF) website.[10]

Most chronically ill, complex patients have multiple disturbances on acupuncture meridian assessment (AMA) and almost always, the TW meridian is out of balance and shows a low reading.

Case Study: 60-year-old Physician with Lyme

A 60-year-old female physician developed breast cancer, s/p double mastectomy, chemotherapy, post-chemo brain fog, decreased cognition and concentration, and retired on medical disability. She had a multitude of physical pains – in the neck, shoulder, and upper back - and ailments including lymphedema of the right arm, severe fatigue, headache, light sensitivity, shortness of breath, and loss of ability for advanced math. Her physician gave her psychiatric medications to cover her multiple vague symptoms.

An IGeneX Lyme test was done to rule out unsuspected Lyme for her unexplainable physical symptoms; see Figure 28. The test was negative by CDC and New York State (NYS) criteria and positive by IGeneX criteria for its IgM and IgG Lyme Immunoblot test. Note the difference in interpretation for IGeneX and CDC/NYS criteria. A Lyme specialist considered she was positive for Lyme, and prescribed antibiotics.

Figure 28: IGeneX Lab Results for Lyme Blot IgM, IgG

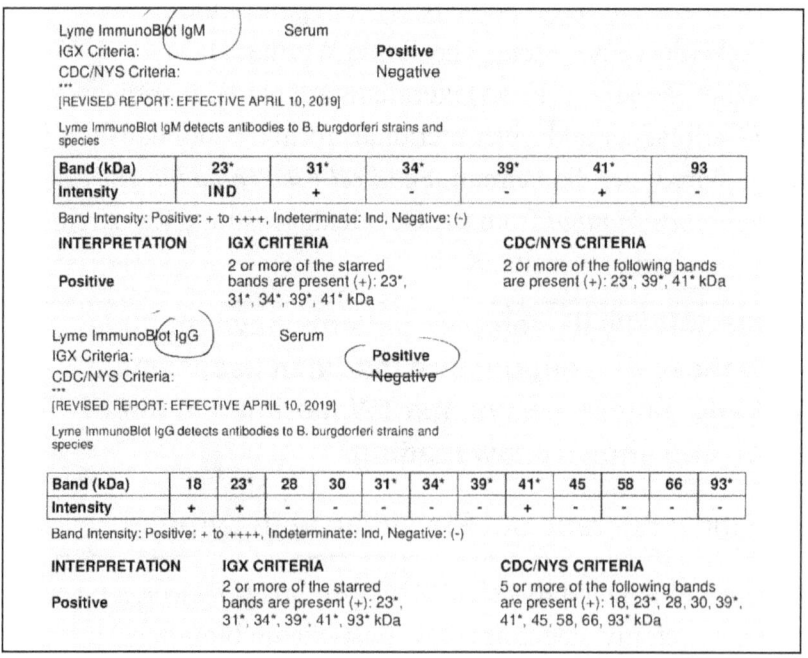

On my AMA evaluation, dental and allergy-immunology points were her dominant problems. Parasites, fungal infections, and mycotoxins were compromising her immune system and were treated with parasite medications pyrantel pamoate and praziquantel, triple antifungal medications, and a detox protocol.

Dental work was done by a biological dentist extracting tooth #30. She also received doxycycline and tinidazole for her dental infections based on AMA evaluation, which is very similar to Lyme treatment. I have seen many "correlations and coinfections" with Lyme and pseudo-Lyme-like dental infections in the last 20 years. Many Lyme patients do not respond to standard antibiotic therapy if they have active dental and parasite infections; you can be the judge when you see her test results. Note: it is important to be out of a moldy environment before dental surgery so it does not enter the site.

She had persistent symptoms and recurring dental infection at tooth #29 despite antibiotics and antifungal meds based on AMA evaluations. It is not uncommon to have multiple endless dental infections. I made a special request to extract tooth #29, right lower second pre-molar bicuspid, which is also associated with mammary glands, lymph vessels, and breast cancer.

See the Tooth-Organ Meridian Chart in Figures 8 and 9 earlier in this book, and on my website. Her dental panorama x-ray was negative and biological dentists refused to extract her #29 tooth. Her condition was deteriorating, and we found one biological dentist to extract the tooth with a special request, "Don't ask why - just pull the damn tooth." A dental DNA test was requested for both dental microbes and for Lyme to rule out overlapping infections, see Figures 29a and 29b.

Figure 29a: DNA Connections Lab Results: Oral Test

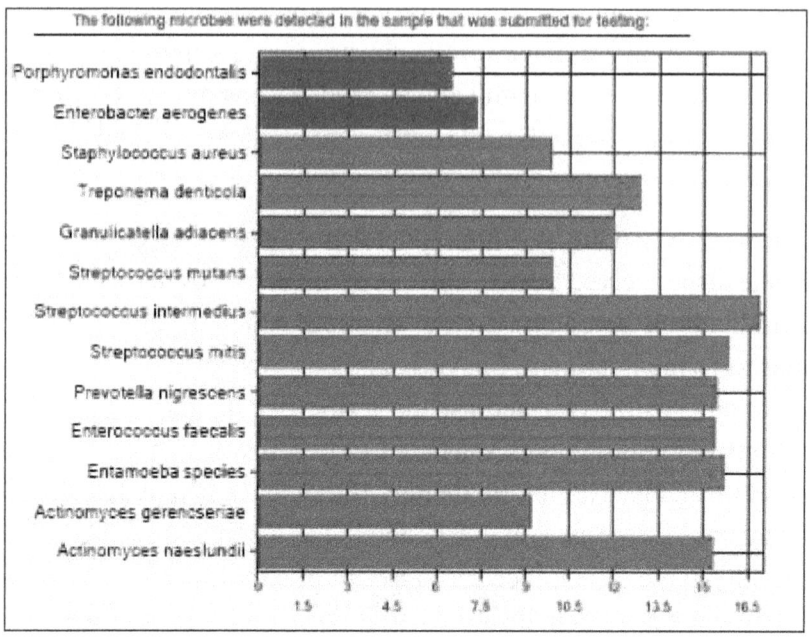

Figure 29b: DNA Connexions Lab Results: Lyme Test

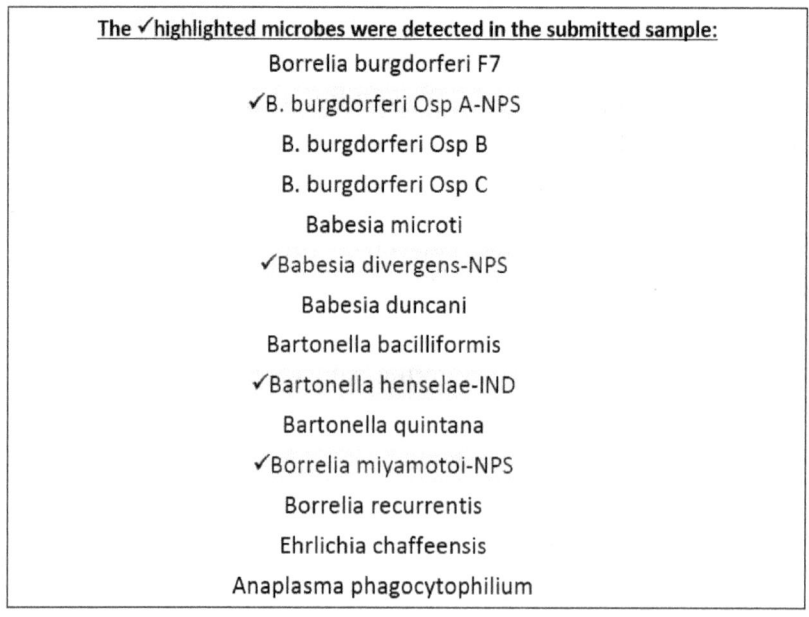

I started her on doxycycline, tinidazole, clindamycin and nystatin to cover infections based on my AMA evaluation before the dental operation. The dental DNA test was positive for the presence of Treponema, Streptococcus, Prevotella, Entamoeba, Enterococcus, Borrelia burgdorferi, Babesia divergens, Bartonella henselae, Borrelia miyamotoi, and more.

You can find the latest DNA test information and costs at dnaconnexions.com; there are savings available on combination test kits. I was already treating the patient for dental infections with the above medications without the DNA test based on AMA evaluation. Important questions include:

1. *How reliable are DNA tests vs. AMA evaluation?* Is it worth spending $1,000 for the DNA tests? Is it possible to treat before getting DNA test results, or too late to treat after the tests are back 10 days later?
2. *What are the limitations of DNA tests and AMA evaluation?* So many unknown factors to consider…
3. *Do these positive DNA tests truly indicate active infectious pathogens*, or an incidental part of microbiome DNA fragments, or molecular mimicry for a false positive DNA test? Or, perhaps, is it possible from the biological evolution point of view, that microbiome DNA incorporated into our genome during evolutionary adaptation? I am beginning to see more positive Borrelia, Bartonella, and Babesia from the dental Lyme DNA test, and more parasites from the dental microbe DNA test, like her case.
4. *Are we treating Lyme disease, or dental infections, or both?* A combination of antibiotics, antiparasitics, and antifungals has helped many of my patients after they have dental surgery for extraction of the problematic

tooth (or cleaning of the cavitation site). Without such additional treatment, infections often recur. Are dental infections the overlooked factor in chronic Lyme, persistent Lyme, Long Lyme, and Post-Lyme?

The patient is also receiving IV UV/Ozone, alternating with high dose IV vitamin C, and I am trying to gradually wean her off psychiatric medications. I am a big believer in natural healing and spontaneous healing, but her recovery will be slow. She may have several additional layers of hidden problems.

Natural healing alone simply is not strong enough to turn her around. Aggressive dental surgery, parasite and fungal medications, antibiotics, and IV UV/Ozone may not be considered "natural healing." Most patients ultimately don't care about the distinctions between natural healing and conventional medicine (prescription drugs and surgery). They just desperately want to get well. As an integrative Internal Medicine physician, I understand the importance of both.

It is time to rethink the importance of the Biological Terrain and our Immune System, which is addressed in my first book, *Accidental Cure*. Perhaps we cannot micromanage our immune system and only target specific microbes. There is always a community of microbes and coinfections, and we need to focus on this larger picture: overlooked and synergistic dental infections, parasites, and fungal infections. These are addressed in second last book, *AcciDental Blow Up in Medicine*.

What can physicians do in the face of chronic fatigue, CFS/ME, and chronic Lyme, also now being called "Long Lyme" in analogy with the persistent unexplained symptoms being called "Long COVID?" Why not integrate the 5,000-year-old "new" disruptive technology called Acupuncture

Meridian Assessment (AMA) into medical practice, and better recognize, identify, and treat the constellation of underlying problems contributing to chronic conditions? It is time to give recognition, credit, and real help to these patients for their struggles and perseverance.

Triple Warmer Meridian and Related Teeth

The Triple Warmer meridian is paired with the Circulation/Pericardium meridian. Unlike other meridians, the triple warmer is not energetically tied to a specific organ in the body. Instead, it helps regulate all the organs and energy systems.

Its function corresponds to the endocrine system - glands that produce hormones that regulate metabolism, growth and development, tissue function, sexual function, reproduction, sleep, and mood. The TW meridian and endocrine system include adrenal, thyroid, testes, ovaries, and breast-related problems including breast cancer.

It regulates the sympathetic (fight or flight) and parasympathetic (rest and digest) nervous system, influencing the body's autonomic (regulates bodily functions), and its neurovegetative activities, such as sleep, appetite, and concentration, and hormones.

Today's AI further illuminates these interconnections. Note the same teeth are associated with the Triple Warmer and Circulation/Pericardium meridians; see the Tooth-Organ Meridian Chart in Figures 8 and 9. These organs and meridians are associated with upper wisdom teeth #1 and #16, and lower wisdom teeth #17 and #32, respectively, as shown in Figure 30.

Figure 30: Triple Warmer Meridian, Connection to Dental

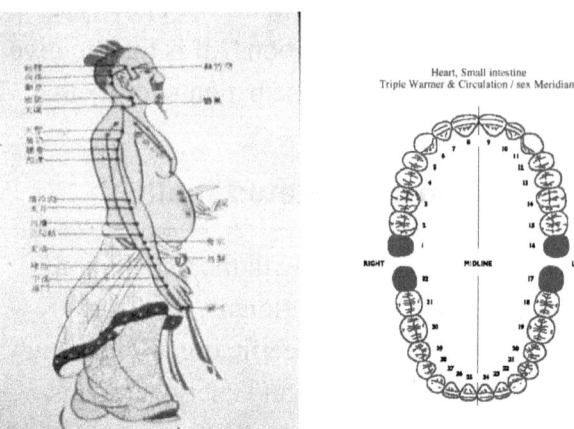

The Triple Warmer Meridian governs hormones, respiration, digestion, and elimination. Imbalances in any part of the meridian are often associated with problems elsewhere in that system, as seen in the Tooth-Organ Meridian Chart, which shows teeth, sense organs, joints, spinal segments, vertebrae, organs, endocrine organs and tissues, and more.

In TCM, organs and meridians are also associated with feelings. The Triple Warmer is associated with feelings of humiliation, indecisiveness, feeling left out, and denial. Fixing the underlying problems and rebalancing or restoring healthy meridians can help resolve these negative feelings.

Medical Acupuncture on Circulation/Pericardium Meridian: Questioning the Scientific Merits of Old and New Medicine

During the last two years of the COVID-19 pandemic, there has been a major shift in public consciousness and questioning of scientific authority in medicine. What is actual – true – science, and who is really in charge? Somewhere between basic medical science and clinical medicine, there are many pitfalls riddled with politics, Big Money, fake science, pseudoscience, less understood natural science, and dubious Energy Medicine and Homeopathy. It gets confusing and complicated. Let me focus on old medicine: medical acupuncture on the Circulation meridian – the Pericardium.

Cardiovascular disease with chest pain, heart attack, congestive heart failure, hypertension, irregular heart rhythm, pericarditis, poor circulation and/or strokes are the leading cause of death in the United States. High cholesterol, diabetes, and chronic inflammation have been the main culprits according to current medical scientific authority, with treatments marketed aggressively by Big Pharma. Treating symptoms with angioplasty, bypass operation, reducing inflammation, and lowering cholesterol levels are the standard of medical care. Big money is at stake. What are the true underlying problems?

This article describes Medical Acupuncture on the circulation meridian, which is often called the Pericardium or the Master of Heart meridian. It has a circulatory function without a physical form. The Pericardium/Master of Heart is described as a membrane or sac surrounding the Heart and its primary function is to protect the Heart from attack by exterior pathogenic factors.

Since ancient times, the Pericardium meridian has been poorly defined; it represents the entire circulatory system, not a specific organ. There are miles of vascular endothelial cells which serve as a protective barrier in blood-vessel walls. It regulates metabolically active vascular endothelial cells, including blood clotting and coagulation. According to classical EAV teachings, allergy-immunology and dental meridian disturbances directly and indirectly affect the circulatory system.

The Pericardium meridian originates in the lateral chest and merges and communicates with the Triple Warmer (Hormonal Regulators) meridian. The Triple Warmer also performs multiple functions without a structure or organs; it is also known as the adrenal-thyroid-pituitary-hypothalamus neurohormonal axis. The Pericardium and Triple Warmer Meridians are regulators of the sympathetic (fight or flight) and parasympathetic (rest and digest) nervous system, influencing the body's autonomic system, which automatically regulates bodily functions and neurovegetative activities, such as sleep, appetite, and concentration, and hormones.

Six years ago, I saw a 58-year-old man from Arizona with palpitations, on-and-off Atrial Fibrillation, hypertension, chest pain, vague GI problems, and fatigue. Acupuncture meridian assessment (AMA) indicated his dominant problems were from parasites, allergies, and dental problems. Most of his symptoms responded to parasite medications, but I still picked up signals that he had persistent dental infections.

A biological dentist felt his dental X-rays were normal and did not extract the three root-canaled teeth as I had recommended. Instead, he had ozone injections. George emailed me and said that he was feeling well and doing great. One year later, I got a call from his wife saying that he had died of a heart attack.

I always wonder if I could have saved him if he had extracted those three perfectly normal looking root-canaled teeth. See the article on my website, "Death Certificate for the Unknown Cause."

> **One year later, I got a phone call from his wife that he had died of a heart attack. I always wonder if I could have saved him if he had extracted those three perfectly normal looking root-canaled teeth.**

I am taking care of a 56-year-old man from Texas with an 8-year history of malignant hypertension, who is not responding to medications. His blood pressure spiked up to 250/150 despite multiple medications. He said he had passed about 140 roundworms last year and still felt crawling movement despite parasite medications, and he is convinced parasites are the cause of his hypertension.

His large intestine, allergy, and dental meridians were his dominant problems. I started him on ivermectin, pyrantel pamoate, praziquantel, and tinidazole for a 30-day trial and his blood pressure dropped from the starting point of 220/140 to 144/99 according to his email. After his trial of parasite meds, his blood pressure rose to 180/115. I resumed his parasite medications and told him he had one root-canaled tooth and an infected lower right jaw cavitation at #32 area that needed to be addressed. I don't want to lose another patient to an overlooked dental infection, or to an aversion to treat it via oral surgery.

Surprisingly, these two cases of cardiovascular problems did not show on their acupuncture points at the classical Pericardium/Master of the Heart meridian. But these problems were revealed in the dental, allergy, and GI-related meridians. Dental and Allergy-Immunology points were first described by Dr. Voll, a German (EAV) physician and acupuncturist 70 years ago, not by classical acupuncture teaching. Dental and Allergy-Immunology meridians regulate and control a whole complex within the biocybernetic matrix. These two recently discovered meridian systems are beyond the current understanding of both ancient classical acupuncture teachings and new western medical science.

Clinical descriptions of poor circulation and an out-of-balance Master of Heart may present as chronic fatigue, vertigo, hypertension, hyperventilation, chest pain, palpitation, and autonomic nervous system dysfunction, etc. According to the teachings of classical acupuncture, *The Yellow Emperor's Classic of Internal Medicine*,[11] the Heart stores the Spirit (Shen), and the Master of Heart carries out the function of Shen. Unresolved emotional trauma may manifest as a broken heart, heart attack, or heart failure without any evidence of cardiovascular disease or cholesterol problems.

Now is a good time to question the merits of science and its limitations, new as well as old. Explore the many unknowns, the uncertainty and mystery of Chi, and the healing powers that we don't fully understand. The Pericardium/Master of Heart and Triple Warmer are paired meridians, and together with the Gallbladder and Liver meridians, are part of the full circuitry of meridians within us. Question the scientific merits of old and new medicine! Let a new, emerging "integrated, science-based medicine" solve the mysteries of Long COVID and cardiovascular problems, one tooth at a time.

Circulation/Pericardium Meridian and Related Teeth

The Circulation/Pericardium meridian is paired with the Triple Warmer meridian. The pericardium is a thin, double-walled sac surrounding the heart and its large vessels; it regulates blood circulation. It helps cushion the heart, holds it in place, keeps it from expanding too much, and protects it from infections.

Today's AI further illuminates these interconnections. Note the same teeth are associated with the Circulation/Pericardium and Triple Warmer meridians; see the Tooth-Organ Meridian Chart. These organs and meridians are associated with upper wisdom teeth #1 and #16, and lower wisdom teeth #17 and #32. See Figure 31.

Figure 31: Circulation/Pericardium Meridian, Connection to Dental

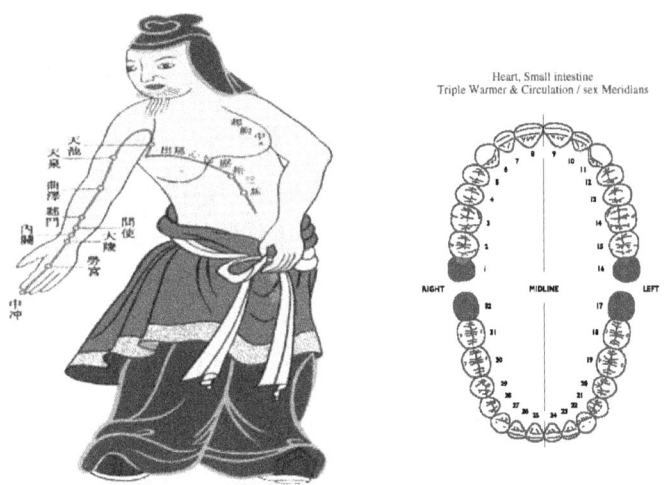

The Pericardium Meridian governs circulation and hormones and protects and regulates the heart. In Traditional Chinese Medicine it is often the best approach to the treatment of heart problems.

In TCM, organs and meridians are also associated with feelings. The Pericardium is associated with feelings of acute grief, shock, broken trust, and remorse. Fixing the underlying problems and rebalancing or restoring healthy meridians can help resolve these negative feelings.

Chapter 6 Heart, Small Intestine, Kidney, and Bladder Meridians

Can a squirrel turn into a dragon? Can a minor tooth injury turn into kidney failure or a heart attack? As you read this chapter, you will see seemingly unconnected events in childhood like falling off a bicycle, or emotional trauma, can shape your body later in life, and manifest as heart problems, kidney failure, cancer, or autoimmune disease. How does your small intestine relate to allergy problems and leaky gut, which can create autoimmune response and eventually immune suppression?

An ounce of prevention is worth a pound of cure. If you don't correct a small problem, you get to correct a big problem. This theme is common throughout cultures, and throughout the systems in your body and your home: $900 for nine squirrels. Here is one of my favorite articles, I hope you enjoy it.

Medical Acupuncture on Heart Meridian:
Portals of Entry for Squirrels and Dragon

I saw a 63-year-old man, Stephan, with his wife, for nocturnal urination problems and elevated PSA of 23. Multiple prostate biopsies were negative for cancer. His wife also told me that he had a sudden heart attack ten years ago while playing sports. He was resuscitated on the field, by emergency response, with electrical shock therapy, and had two stents placed in his heart.

He did not want to come to see me, but his wife dragged him to be evaluated. She felt there was something wrong with him that had not been recognized by medical professionals. She does not want another episode of sudden life-threatening events to happen to her husband. He does not remember the event of his heart attack, resuscitation with electrical shock, and seems to be in denial of what happened to him.

His acupuncture meridian assessment showed imbalances at the lymph/dental/heart meridian and bladder meridian involving the prostate. Is it possible that the heart attack and his urinary problem with elevated PSA are related? It seems squirrely to think there's a connection and to ask how the heart and prostate might be related. However, is it possible a connection exists?

Talking about squirrely questions, I do have a problem with squirrels in our home. We live in a 100-year-old brick house with tall trees and squirrels. These squirrels have been a major nuisance, especially what I call teenager squirrels. These teenager squirrels get into the attic and create major havoc, destroying piles of storage boxes and phone lines.

I wanted to poison or shoot them, but my wife and grandkid protested. They thought it was too cruel. We hired a professional to trap and release them. We caught nine squirrels, and we paid $900 for trapping and release. There is a hole somewhere in our attic and our attic became their playground, especially during wintertime. The solution was only temporary. They came back again.

These teenage squirrels are playful with a certain attitude: smart and sneaky. How do I know? I've lived in the house for over 30 years, and I got to know them well by observing how they play and move around. I couldn't figure out where the hole was in our attic. I needed a professional roofer or repairman to find the portals of entry for these squirrels.

Talking about the portal of entry, in the human body, microorganisms and parasites may penetrate the human body through skin, eyes, nasal cavities and sinuses, pharynx, bronchi, lungs, oral cavity and the teeth, digestive tract, urinary system, and genitalia. Dental, parasites, and fungi have been my major focus in understanding why patients are not responding to standard medical care and are not getting well.

The most common portal of entry is the oral cavity, that is, any dental-related area. The distance between the upper dental to the brain or lower dental to the thyroid is about 10 cm, depending on the location of the dental infection.

Dental problems such as mercury amalgams, root canals, implants, cavitations, and periodontal infections have been dealt with by dentists. Most medical professionals are not looking at dental issues as hidden medical problems.

> **Talking about the portal of entry, in the human body, microorganisms and parasites may penetrate the human body through…The most common portal of entry is the oral cavity, that is, any dental-related area.**

A Swedish neurologist, Patrick Störtebecker, MD, PhD, addressed the principles of the shortest pathway and the portal of entry of infection. In his 1982 book, *"Dental Caries as a cause of Nervous Disorders,"* he described gold crowns as Golden Mausoleums. [12] He also emphatically pointed out that the Cranial-Dental Vertebral Vein and Pelvic Vertebral Veins do not have valves, are a "valve-less vein system," and are susceptible to back flow of venous blood contaminated with infected microorganisms and toxins to the brain/brain stem and lower spinal cord.

Störtebecker described and noted the portals of entry for infections in Figure 32 below: along the trigeminal maxillary, mandibular, and ophthalmic branches associated with the upper and lower dental and eyes.

Figure 32: Störtebecker Diagram

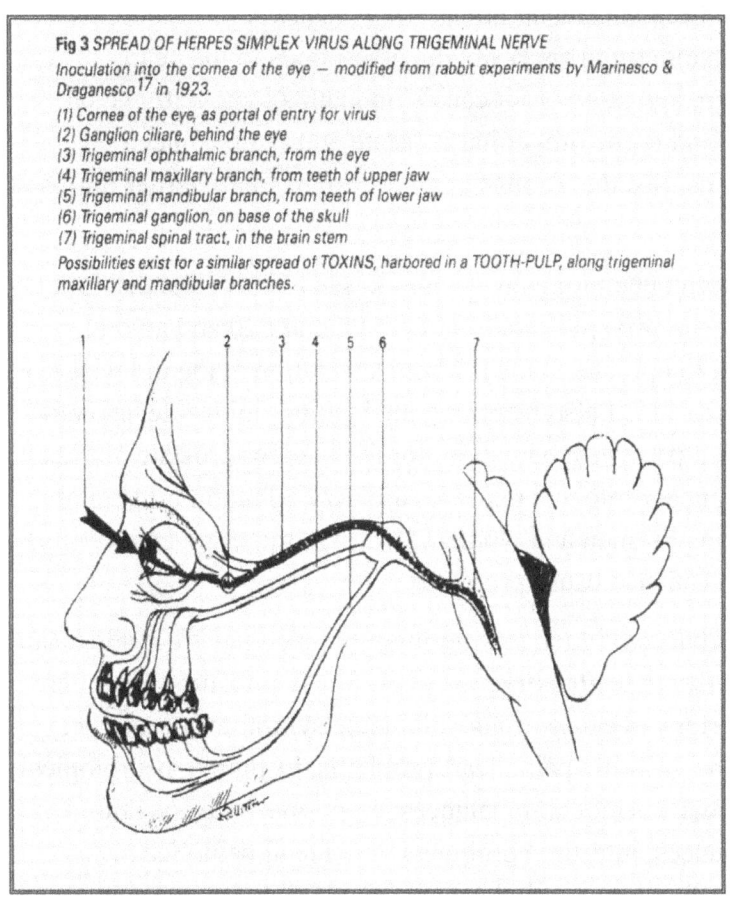

Source: Patrick Störtebecker, Dental Caries as a Cause of Nervous Disorders (1982) Figure 2, p. 39.

Störtebecker's ideas have never been widely accepted by the medical or dental professions, and his book is now out of print.

I bought a copy for one cent. It is one of the best books I've read on dental-medical-neurological connections.

Dental infections and heavy metals have propensities to settle in and cause inflammation in the heart, gastrointestinal and genitourinary tracts, joints, kidney, and the endocrine/nervous system. Stephan had an infection in his jawbone at tooth #17 (old wisdom tooth area) which corresponds to the heart meridian, and at two root canals on teeth #8 and #20, which correspond to the urogenital-prostate and lymph/spleen meridians. See the Tooth-Organ Meridian Chart earlier in this book.

My recommendation was for him to see a biological dentist to remove the two root canals at teeth #8 and #20 and an oral surgeon to operate on his jawbone cavitation at the old wisdom tooth area #17. I also recommended taking tinidazole, an anti-protozoal parasite medication, for the bladder/prostate meridian disturbance. Protozoal parasites are very common urogenital infections for men and women. IUDs (Intrauterine Device) for women can also cause problems.

A disturbance of the heart meridian often comes from silent (no pain) wisdom teeth extraction sites. These infections are often the overlooked cause of unexplainable symptoms of fatigue, headache, arthritic pain, heart problems, insomnia, neurological symptoms, hormonal imbalances, emotional and psychological disturbances, intestinal problems, and facial pain. See my article; "Wisdom Teeth, Undetected Tooth Infections and Incurable Medical Symptoms," on my website.

The Heart and Small Intestine Meridians are paired meridians. Paired circuitry meridians also include the Kidney and Bladder meridians. If you cannot figure out the portal of entry of squirrels in your house, the damage will magnify. It could grow from a squirrel into a dragon.

I am going to call the roof repair man to fix the portal of entry of squirrels into the attic. If you have incurable medical symptoms, I recommend that you see an MD and Biological Dentist "team" who understand the Golden Mausoleums of dental-medical connections.

Heart Meridian and Related Teeth

The Heart meridian is paired with the Small Intestine meridian. The heart pumps blood throughout the body, delivers oxygen and nutrients, carries away waste products to the kidneys, and regulates heart rate and blood pressure.

Today's AI further illuminates these interconnections. Note the same teeth are associated with the Heart and Small Intestine meridians; see the Tooth-Organ Meridian Chart. These organs and meridians are associated with upper wisdom teeth #1 and #16, and lower wisdom teeth #17 and #32. See Figure 33.

Figure 33: Heart Meridian, Connection to Dental

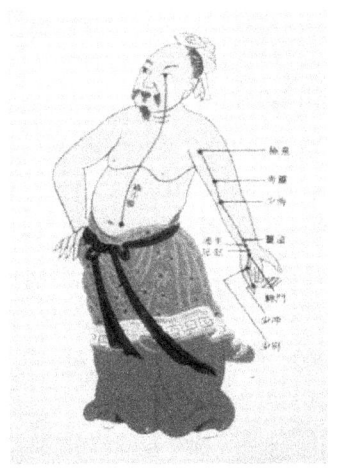
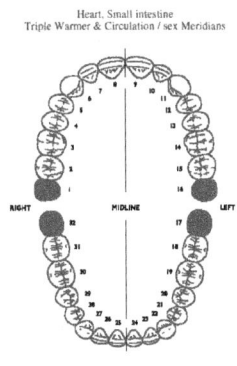

The Heart Meridian governs the heart, circulation, facial complexion, and mental/emotional function. Imbalances in any part of the meridian are often associated with problems elsewhere in that system, as seen in the Tooth-Organ Meridian Chart, which shows teeth, sense organs, joints, spinal segments, vertebrae, organs, endocrine organs and tissues, and more.

In TCM, organs and meridians are also associated with feelings. The Heart is associated with feelings of unlived joy, self-protection, feeling used, and rigidity. Fixing the underlying problems and rebalancing or restoring healthy meridians can help resolve these negative feelings.

If you cannot figure out the portal of entry of squirrels in your house, the damage will magnify. It could grow from a squirrel into a dragon. The same applies to any problem revealed by Acupuncture Meridian Assessment.

Medical Acupuncture on Small Intestine Meridian: From Allergy and Autoimmune to Immune Deficiency

When I detect disturbance on the Small Intestine (SI) Meridian and/or Large Intestine Meridian in my acupuncture meridian assessment (AMA), I will often pick up signals for parasite problems of all kinds, fungus, allergies, and leaky gut. If these problems are not corrected, more autoimmune symptoms will manifest, with eventual immune suppression, immune deficiency, and setting the stage for the development of cancer, via the Gut-Immune connection. A blocked SI meridian may also cause pain along the medial part of the elbow, upper arm, scapula, neck, and ear, and may also cause tinnitus.

Last year, I saw a 64-year-old woman from Oregon who had been feeling poorly for a long time. She had been diagnosed with four well-known autoimmune diseases: 1) Dermatomyositis, 2) Rheumatoid arthritis, 3) Hashimoto's thyroiditis and 4) Interstitial fibrosis of the lung. She was on multiple medications to treat her autoimmune-related symptoms.

What are the odds of developing four separate autoimmune diseases and what is the common denominator for the underlying problems? If you have been following my writing on Acupuncture Meridian Assessment (AMA), it may not surprise you.

> **What are the odds of developing four separate autoimmune diseases and what is the common denominator for the underlying problems?**

Interestingly, her AMA evaluation was not as bad as I thought. Four out of 40 meridians were out of balance: dental, lung, large intestine, and allergy-immunology points. See Figure 34.

She had one infected root canal, parasites, fungi and mycotoxins, mercury heavy metal exposure, and emotional trauma with PTSD, creating a unique condition for the development of autoimmune conditions with four separate diagnoses.

Her food and airborne allergy tests came back negative as if she did not have any allergies; I realized that she was on immunosuppressive medications to treat her symptoms.

Figure 34: Initial AMA Testing for Oregon Woman: Four Meridians Out of Balance

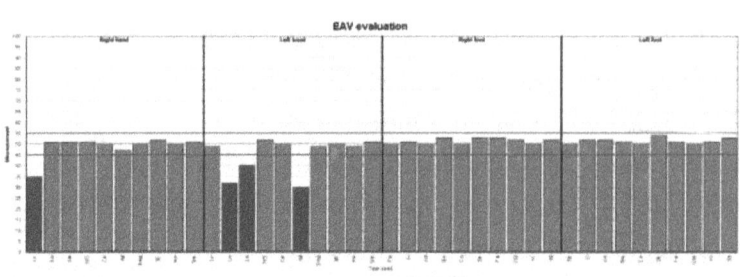

She will have to go through extensive antiparasitic and antifungal medications, dental work, chelation therapy, detox, and nutritional and emotional support therapy for years to reverse her four autoimmune diseases.

If these problems are not corrected, more autoimmune symptoms will manifest, with eventual immune suppression, immune deficiency, and setting the stage for the development of cancer.

From my perspective, naming the clinical diagnosis is not as important as correcting the underlying problems. For most medical practices, medical diagnosis drives the treatment plan, usually drug therapy, followed by insurance reimbursement: the diagnosis-drug therapy-insurance merry-go-round; the triad of the holy grail of the modern health care system.

Recently, I saw a 76-year-old woman from a small town in Missouri with chief complaints of severe fatigue, headache, epigastric pain, bloating, indigestion, and leaky heart valve of unknown cause. She also had four out of 40 meridians out of balance: small intestine, allergy-immunology, and adrenal points on both hands. See Figure 35.

Figure 35: Initial AMA Testing for Missouri Woman: Four Meridians Out of Balance

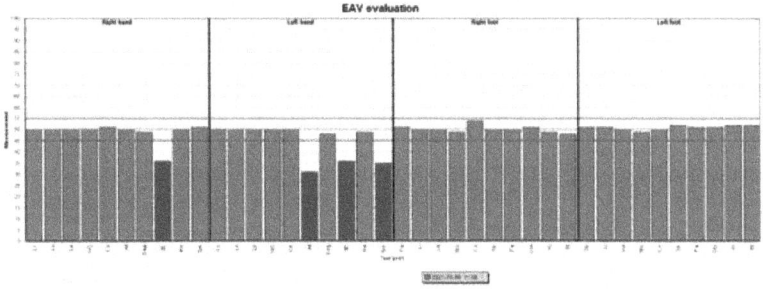

This patient has a history of very high heavy metals of mercury and lead, and leaky gut. I started her on parasite/fungal meds to balance her small intestine meridian, and we will address her heavy metal exposure with chelation therapy. It may take 6-12 months to turn this patient around.

The small intestine processes filtration and absorption of partially digested nutrients from the stomach, and passes waste to the large intestine, kidney, and bladder. It plays a much bigger role than simply a part of the digestive tract. Disorders of the small intestine manifest as rumbling, diarrhea, and disturbed urine excretion. On an emotional level, the metaphor of filtering and sorting is expressed through a difficulty filtering information and sorting facts and conditions to make decisions. Unresolved feelings can manifest as loneliness, difficulty connecting, abandonment, and sense of loss.

How are organs and meridian systems interrelated? The Small Intestine and Heart meridians are paired meridians and paired in a full circuit with the Kidney and Bladder meridians. Often hidden dental infections are tied and interconnected together with the Small Intestine and Heart meridians. The small intestine is an entry to create allergy problems, then develop autoimmune disease, and eventually, immune deficiency and risk for development of cancer, wherever you live.

Small Intestine Meridian and Related Teeth

The Small Intestine is paired with the Heart meridian. It is responsible for breaking down and digesting food, absorbing nutrients, and moving food through the gastrointestinal (GI) tract.

Today's AI further illuminates these interconnections. Note the same teeth are associated with the Small Intestine and Heart meridians; see the Tooth-Organ Meridian Chart. These organs and meridians are associated with upper wisdom teeth #1 and #16, and lower wisdom teeth #17 and #32. See Figure 36.

Figure 36: Small Intestine Meridian, Dental Connection

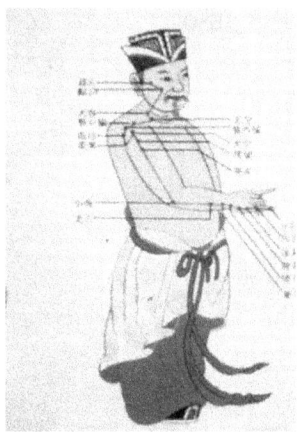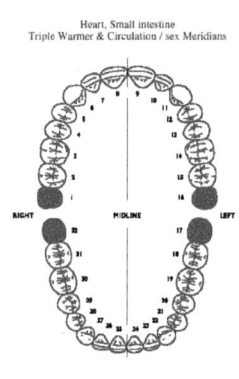

The Small Intestine influences digestion, water metabolism, and bowel function. Imbalances in any part of the meridian are often associated with problems elsewhere in that system, as seen in the Tooth-Organ Meridian Chart, which shows teeth, sense organs, joints, spinal segments, vertebrae, organs, endocrine organs and tissues, and more.

In TCM, organs and meridians are also associated with feelings. The Small Intestine is associated with feelings of loneliness, abandonment, inability to receive, and loss. Fixing the underlying problems and rebalancing or restoring healthy meridians can help resolve these negative feelings.

Often hidden dental infections are interconnected with the Small Intestine and Heart meridians.

Medical Acupuncture on Kidney Meridian:
Acute and Chronic Kidney Disease Saved by Dentists?

Chronic Kidney Disease (CKD) is a common medical condition among aging adults. 15 percent of US adults – 37 million people – are estimated to have CKD, and most do not know they have it. CKD and related problems are exponentially rising. Kidney dialysis centers have been popping up along with cancer and heart centers, two of the deadliest modern diseases.

The most common causes of kidney failure are poorly controlled diabetes and high blood pressure. It can suddenly get worse after taking certain medications like antibiotics or OTC pain meds like ibuprofen, or after medical or dental procedures.

The best ways for older adults to prevent CKD are by controlling high risk factors such as high blood pressure and high blood sugar levels, to have a healthy lifestyle with a balanced diet and physical exercise, and to avoid unnecessary elective surgery or medications that can potentially accelerate kidney damage. Simple blood tests for creatinine and urine testing for proteins in the urine may detect early stages of kidney failure, but most people may not feel ill or notice until

CKD is advanced. As CKD progresses, patients may experience fatigue, anemia, loss of appetite, electrolyte imbalance, swelling, irritability, frequent infections, slow recovery, and/or depression.

Occasionally, there is sudden development of kidney failure without any risk factors such as diabetes or high blood pressure problems among young children and adults. In 2012, I saw a five-year-old boy from Iowa who came to see me with an acute episode of nephrotic syndrome with swelling, extreme weakness, puffy, abdominal bloating and spilling heavy amounts of protein in the urine. His only significant history had been a fall on his face one month before the development of nephrotic syndrome. He was evaluated by a pediatrician and dentist; dental X-ray was normal and had no significant medical findings from the falling incident. Otherwise, he was physically active and in good health before.

On my initial 40-point acupuncture meridian assessment (AMA, also called EAV), I found his dental, allergy-immunology and kidney meridians were out of balance, see Figure 38. I recommended he extract four front teeth – his two front upper and lower teeth. You need to remove the infection from the tooth and surrounding areas, not just the tooth itself, to restore the meridian. See Figure 37.

Figure 37: Initial AMA Reading: Impact of Tooth Injury on Kidney, Dental and Allergy

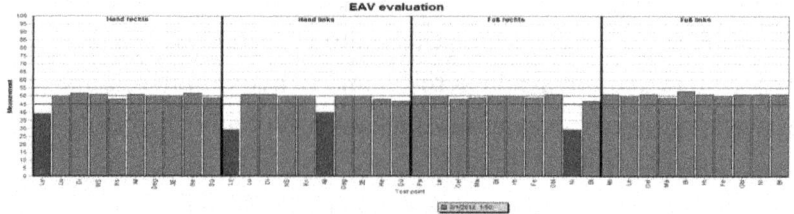

The middle bars refer to normal, balanced meridians; low means chronic "out of balance" meridians. The low bars of "Ly" refers to the lymphatic system of jaw or dental on the left and right side, "Al" refers to the allergy-immunology point on left side, and "Ni" refers to kidney on the right side.

> **You need to remove the infection from the tooth and surrounding areas, not just the tooth itself, to restore the meridian.**

One month after extraction of these four teeth all the meridians were normal, indicating the meridian system is balanced and his entire nephrotic syndrome was resolved. See below.

Figure 38: AMA Reading after Extraction: Impact of Teeth Extraction on Kidney, Dental, and Allergy

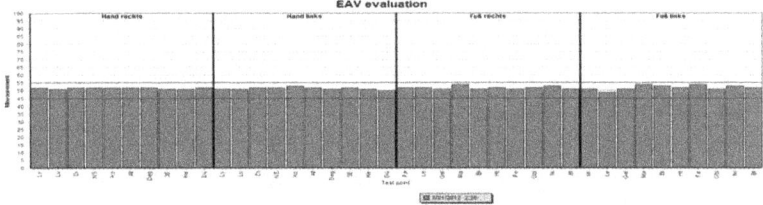

It is not uncommon to see older adults with chronic kidney disease without any risk factors such as diabetes or high blood pressure who are triggered by unsuspected dental trauma from playing sports when they were young, or after dental procedures and gradual development of silent dental infections, especially in the front teeth.

> **It is not uncommon to see older adults with chronic kidney disease without any risk factors such as diabetes or high blood pressure who are triggered by unsuspected dental trauma.**

The front teeth correspond to kidney, urogenital area, bladder, adrenal gland, rectum, pineal gland, back of the knees, front sinus, and other corresponding spines and bones. See the Tooth-Organ Meridian Chart earlier in Figures 8 and 9 in this book and on my website, preventionandhealing.com. Most patients refuse to extract teeth, and prefer root canals or implants, creating impossible no-win situations for medical doctors.

The Kidney meridian is paired with the Bladder meridian, and they have paired circuitry with the Heart and Small Intestine meridians. Acute and chronic kidney diseases can be saved by dentists and sometimes, the other way around. AMA is especially helpful in detecting hidden dental problems and parasite and fungal infections, which I find are often overlooked causes of chronic illness, confounding doctors, dentists, and patients alike.

Kidney Meridian and Related Teeth

The Kidney meridian is paired with the Bladder meridian. The kidneys filter blood, remove waste products and excess water by producing urine, and help balance minerals and hormones. When the kidneys fail, dialysis or a transplant is needed.

Today's AI further illuminates these interconnections. Note the same teeth are associated with the Kidney and Bladder meridians; see the Tooth-Organ Meridian Chart. These organs and meridians are associated with upper front teeth #7, 8, 9 and 10, and lower front teeth #23, 24, 25 and 26. See Figure 39.

Figure 39: Kidney Meridian, Connection to Dental

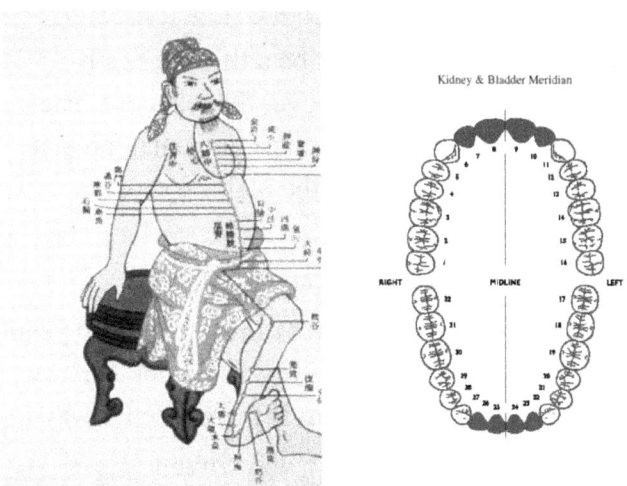

The Kidney Meridian dominates reproduction and water metabolism, it controls hair, bone, hearing, and growth and development. It is not uncommon to see older adults with chronic kidney disease without any risk factors such as diabetes or high blood pressure, that were triggered by unsuspected dental trauma when they were young, or after dental procedures and gradual development of silent dental infections, especially in the front teeth. Acute and chronic kidney diseases can be saved by dentists and sometimes, the other way around.

In TCM, organs and meridians are also associated with feelings. The kidney is associated with feelings of fear, guilt, deep disappointment, and deep exhaustion. Fixing the underlying problems and rebalancing or restoring healthy meridians can help resolve these negative feelings.

Medical Acupuncture on Bladder Meridian:
Two Prostate Cancer Patients

Early detection of prostate cancer can be a life and death situation for many unsuspecting men over 50 years old. The Prostate Specific Antigen (PSA) blood test, a manual prostate exam, and prostate biopsy have been the mainstay for screening tests for the prostate cancer.

During my US Army Reserve military service, I have performed thousands of prostate rectal exams for men 40 years and older during their physical exams. It was a quick cursory exam, and I never enjoyed doing them. Is there a better way to detect prostate-related problems? Is there a role for Acupuncture Meridian Assessment (AMA)?

The Bladder meridian, one of the main acupuncture meridians, is the longest meridian in the body and performs important functions far more complex than urinary water metabolism, as the name implies. Through the Bladder meridian, Chi flows, circulates, interacts and regulates from head to toe, including the eyes, brain, and the entire body.

The Bladder and Kidney meridians are paired meridians, part of the four main circuitries in the body, along with the Small Intestine and Heart meridians. A disturbance of the Bladder meridian has been associated with deep back pain, neck pain, headache, urinary tract disorders from kidney infections, kidney stones, bladder infection, ovary and uterine disease for women, and prostate problems for men.

Prostate enlargement and frequent urination, the older man's nemesis, can progress to prostate cancer - the most common type of cancer for men as they grow old. The prostate, a small walnut-shaped gland in males that produces the seminal fluid that nourishes and transports sperm, begins to enlarge, but may cause no signs or symptoms for many years. Some of the common early signs include trouble urinating, decreased force in the stream of urine, and blood in the urine or semen; and it may progress to bone pain, weight loss, and erectile dysfunction.

Treatment recommendations for prostate cancer have been gradually changing, with less emphasis on aggressive prostate biopsy, total prostatectomy, and more options including localized prostate operation, chemo and hormone therapy, immunotherapy, and targeted therapy based on genetic tests. Some of the progression and complications of prostate cancer and treatment include bone metastasis, incontinence, erectile dysfunction, and change in hormone-related problems in physical appearance and personality.

I have limited experience treating prostate cancer patients. I do not focus on cancer but evaluate cancer patients' acupuncture meridian system, almost like inspecting a fine musical instrument like a violin. I detect, tune, and correct the underlying problems that most oncologists overlook: dental and unrecognized parasite and fungal infections, and checking for environmental toxin exposure.

About 25 years ago, a 60-year-old lawyer came to see me with stage 4 prostate cancer. He had a PSA of 35 (the normal range is up to 4.0), and he had refused prostatectomy and chemo/hormone therapy. He decided to quit his stressful job as a lawyer and retire to a Caribbean Island for the rest of his life. He requested a picture of a healthy prostate so he could meditate with a visual image of healing to restore a normal healthy prostate. Regrettably, I couldn't provide him with one;

a picture was not available at the time. I lost track of him, but most likely he died of old age with prostate cancer, not necessarily from the cancer.

Six years ago, I saw a 73-year-old man from out of town with extensive, multiple joint pain with a diagnosis of Polymyalgia rheumatica; he was initially prescribed steroids. Acupuncture meridian assessment (AMA) showed that his dominant problems were coming from dental infections. A root-canalled tooth was extracted, and two areas of infected dental jaw cavitation were cleaned out by an oral surgeon. He experienced a dramatic improvement in his joint pain. About two years later, his PSA marker for prostate cancer cell activity began rising rapidly on routine blood tests, from 2.0 to 10.0 to 32.6. He came back to see me again for evaluation and treatment.

This time, he also presented with blood clots, leg swelling, a swollen scrotum, and pelvic pain. Based on a new AMA, I started him on parasite and fungal meds and advised more dental work and tooth extractions. He also had high aluminum, cadmium, and lead; and he started EDTA chelation therapy. His PSA rose above 100, which is extremely high, and he saw an oncologist but again refused any therapy. Finally, his PSA reached 995 and then rose to 1,448. He started hormone therapy with his oncologist, began Insulin Potentiation Therapy (IPT) at my practice, and was able to bring his PSA below 100. One time, his PSA dropped to below 10.0, and he was almost feeling normal.

After his dramatic response, both hormone therapy and IPT were stopped to give him a break from weekly travelling. Soon, there was again a rapid rise in PSA and all the markers for advancing cancer: bone metastases and increased bone pain. At the time of this writing, his PSA is around 1,200 and he is experiencing increased general weakness and bone pain. He is still alive - a miracle with that high a PSA level - but time is not on his side. He said he will be ready to die this spring, after taking care to get his house, finances, and affairs in order, for his wife.

You may not think of the prostate-dental connection, but the acupuncture point for the prostate is represented within both the Bladder meridian and Dental meridian, according to Acupuncture Meridian Assessment (AMA). His prostate cancer may have started with dental infections many years ago when he was told he had Polymyalgia rheumatica with multiple joint pain. Breast cancer and dental connection is another common medical and dental (MAD) disconnection, crying out to be told and heard.

> **You may not think of the prostate-dental connection, but the acupuncture point for the prostate is represented within both the Bladder meridian and Dental meridian, according to Acupuncture Meridian Assessment (AMA).**

Bladder Meridian and Related Teeth

The Bladder meridian is paired with the Kidney meridian, and they have paired circuitry with the Heart and Small Intestine meridians. The bladder stores urine and works with the kidneys to remove waste from the blood.

The Bladder meridian, one of the main acupuncture meridians, is the longest meridian in the body and performs important functions far more complex than urinary water metabolism, as the name implies. Through the Bladder meridian, Chi flows, circulates, interacts and regulates from head to toe, including the eyes, brain, and the entire body.

Today's AI further illuminates these interconnections. Note the same teeth are associated with the Bladder and Kidney meridians; see the Tooth-Organ Meridian Chart. These organs and meridians are associated with upper front teeth #7, 8, 9 and 10, and lower front teeth #23, 24, 25 and 26. See Figure 40.

Figure 40: Bladder Meridian, Connection to Dental

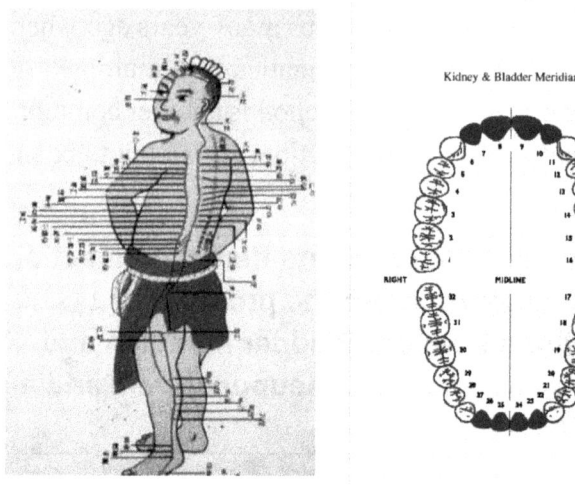

The Bladder Meridian functions with the kidney meridian in water metabolism and excretion.

The Bladder is associated with feelings of shame, not standing up on one's own feet, helplessness, and unfulfilled yearning. Fixing the underlying problems and rebalancing or restoring healthy meridians can help resolve these negative feelings.

Summary

This concludes my introduction and discussion of the 12 classical meridians. In Part 3, I will cover some lesser-known medical acupuncture meridians. In Part 4, the Dental, Allergy-Immunology, and Lymph meridians.

Part 3
Lesser-Known Medical Acupuncture Meridians

Chapter 7 Joint/Cartilage, Skin, and Nerve Degeneration Meridians

Part 2 covered Medical Acupuncture on the 12 main meridians. Ten of these correspond to energetic pathways of major organ systems; while the pericardium sac encircles the heart, and the triple warmer represents the thyroid gland controlling metabolism. These are considered the main meridians of classical acupuncture. I also introduced the dental meridian, as the teeth connect to each of the pathways and systems.

A German medical doctor and acupuncturist, Reinhold Voll, MD, developed a new meridian system about 60 years ago based on the classical acupuncture meridian system. He mapped out well over 500 acupuncture points, known as Dr. Voll's points.

He described new acupuncture points beyond the classical meridian system known to traditional acupuncturists. The most important of Dr. Voll's new classification of the acupuncture system includes the dental/lymph system and allergy/immunology meridians, and other meridians including connective/fibroid tissue, joints, skin/scars, cellular degeneration, fat degeneration, and nerve degeneration meridians. I have not found the cellular and fat degeneration meridians relevant in my practice.

The allergy points are another brilliant discovery by Dr. Voll. I like to call them allergy-immunology points to reflect their true significance. They reflect not only allergies, but the entire immune system. The allergy-immunology points help to unmask not only food and airborne allergies but also hidden toxic metals, environmental toxic chemicals, and fungal mycotoxins. Part 3 will examine these lesser-known acupuncture meridians.

Medical Acupuncture on Joint/Cartilage Meridian: Untangle Rheumatism, Breast Cancer, and Dental Problems

A 38-year-old Australian woman living in the US came to see me with a history of rheumatoid arthritis. She had flare-ups of arthritic joint pain. When I checked 40 points via acupuncture meridian assessment (AMA), her dental meridian was out of balance and her arthralgia pain responded to antibiotics and antiparasitic meds (doxycycline and tinidazole). After a while, I noticed that she came to see me about every six months with another flare-up of joint pain, and each time, responded to antibiotics.

This became a mystery until I asked her about her biannual routine activities. It dawned on her that due to gum problems, she had deep cleaning of her gums every six months, which coincided with flare-up of her joint pain and responding to antibiotics. I advised her to take antibiotics before dental deep cleaning and/or oil pulling for her gum problems. I have not seen her since my last preventive dental care advice.

What did I learn from her case? Routine dental care like deep gum cleaning or drilling might be an unsuspected trigger for infections, inflammation, and biological chain reactions for mysterious medical conditions such as autoimmune response, cancer, and Lyme-like conditions.

Another case is a 47-year-old female with a 10-year history of rheumatoid arthritis, on methotrexate and steroids. Her routine mammogram showed microcalcifications of the right breast, suspicious of breast cancer; she was recommended for biopsy. She also stated that she passed a worm recently that appeared alive and moving in the toilet bowl.

The AMA evaluation showed her gallbladder, large intestine, and dental meridians were out of balance. She declined biopsy and did breast thermography. The report indicated that her right breast thermal heat emissions compared to her left breast was much higher, with TH score of 120 which translate to "abnormal thermal emission and high risk for developing cancer on right breast." The TH scoring system is based on original research conducted by M. Gautherie and Keith published in, *Thermal Assessment of Breast Health*.

Unknown to most medical communities, in December 2001, a major milestone occurred at a workshop held by a group of defense agencies on the use of image processing and thermography to detect abnormal vascular changes – angiogenesis – as an early indicator of breast cancer. See my article, "Medical Infrared Thermography: Heat Recognition from Tanks to Tumors," exploring the use of this technology. For a recent survey article by Mashekova et al, see, "Early detection of breast cancer using infrared technology – a comprehensive review," in *Thermal Science and Engineering Progress* (January 2022).[13]

She went through multiple rounds of parasite and antibiotic medications including ivermectin, mebendazole, praziquantel, doxycycline, tinidazole, clindamycin, and nystatin, and dental work. Her thermography of the right breast gradually improved from high risk, TH-4 to equivocal TH-3, to within normal limit TH-2. See Figure 41 for gradual changes in about five years. One of the benefits of treating her whole body was that her rheumatic joint pain was resolved, as she went from high risk to lower risk for developing breast cancer with diligent dental work, deworming, detox, and nutritional support therapy.

Figure 41: Thermogram of Woman with Dental Infection

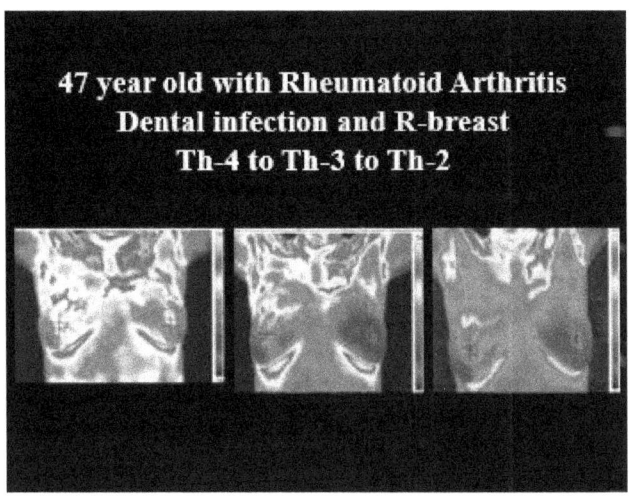

The *Breast Journal* (1998) published a study that showed that mammography's 85 percent sensitivity increased to 95 percent with infrared (IR) thermal imaging and increased to 98 percent with infrared (IR) thermal imaging and physical examination. Y.R. Parisky et al in *American Journal of Roentgenology* (Jan. 2003) published a study in which thermal imaging was performed on 769 subjects with 875 mammographic lesions and compared the results to mammography. Thermography was 97 percent sensitive and showed a 95 percent negative Predictive Value.[14]

The dynamic computerized infrared imaging system significantly increased the accuracy of detecting breast cancer in women who had a suspicious abnormal mammogram requiring biopsy. The conclusion of the study was that infrared imaging offers a safe noninvasive procedure that would be valuable as an adjunct to mammography in determining whether a lesion is benign or malignant.

Medical acupuncture on the articular (Joint cartilaginous meridian was described by Dr. Reinhold Voll in *Electro-Acupuncture according to Dr. Voll* (EAV from Germany. The joint/cartilaginous meridian is located on the second toe, tibial side, mirroring the stomach meridian. Acupuncture meridian channels have their own "complex energy matrix network" and EAV/AMA might untangle the hidden underlying connection among rheumatoid arthritis, breast cancer and dental problems.

Meridians Mimic Medical Syndromes or Vice Versa?

The disturbance of the dental and joint/cartilaginous meridian, not well described by classical acupuncture texts, may mimic Lyme-like, or Ehlers-Danlos Syndrome (EDS, or vice versa, another medical and dental (MAD mystery to be addressed. Almost every dental problem can be associated with joint and connective tissue problems, autoimmune disease, and more.

Medical Acupuncture on Skin Meridian: Better Than Biologics for Eczema, Psoriasis, and More?

Skin care is a big business for cosmetic industries, anti-aging medicine, dermatology, and pharmaceutical giants. New psoriasis and eczema treatments called Biologics are leading many TV commercials. Skin is the largest outer surface sensory organ in the body, metabolically active with the sophisticated immune complex system to protect your body. Changes in skin over time can represent the spectrum from simple normal aging and simple contact rashes to more advanced disease manifesting as melanoma, or a source of chronic migrating parasite infections causing unsightly disfiguring skin lesions.

Have you seen the latest "Biologic" medications for psoriasis and/or eczema that sound like truly a new solution seen in TV commercials? What is a "biologic" medication? These medications alter the immune system in a way that disrupts the disease cycle and improves signs and symptoms of disease within weeks. Eczema is considered a milder version of atopic dermatitis with itchy skin, rash, and often skin irritation from scratching and secondary skin infection. Psoriasis is more severe than eczema with scaly plaques and is often associated with arthralgia (pain), psoriatic arthritis.

Most skin diseases have their origins in unrecognized infections, toxins, or food allergies or sensitivities. Skin rashes that are exacerbated by sugars, fake sugars, gluten, and/or yeasts can develop due to gut imbalances and overgrowth of fungi and yeast. They require healing and restoring a healthy "biological terrain" and microbiome, including the oral cavity, gut, and more. The acupuncture point representing the skin is located on the middle toe and may pick up signals when patients have psoriasis, eczema, or surgical scars. A disturbance of the skin meridian is often associated with concurrent disturbance at the allergy points, circulation, and large intestine (LI) and/or small intestine (SI) meridians. When you balance LI and SI meridians with appropriate parasite medications, skin conditions often improve as a side benefit without using costly biologics.

Most skin diseases have their origins in unrecognized infections, toxins, or food allergies or sensitivities. Before you start a biologic, try…

What is biologic, and are biologic medications safe? Biologic drugs and Biosimilar drugs include a wide variety of products derived from human, animal, or microorganism sources by using biotechnology. They can be manufactured in, extracted from, or semi-synthesized from biological sources. Some examples of biologics include hormones, blood products, cytokines, growth factors, vaccines, gene and cellular therapies, fusion proteins, insulin, interferon, and monoclonal antibody (mAb) products. Patients receive biologics mainly by injection under the skin (subcutaneously) or by intravenous infusion. FDA defines and regulates biologics.

The most well-known biologics for psoriasis include apremilast (Otezla), etanercept (Enbrel), infliximab (Remicade), adalimumab (Humira), secukinumab (Cosentyx) and more. TV commercials are bombarded with new biologics. Some of them are approved for children. I have minimal experience using biologics but there are some concerns for side effects of immunosuppression that can trigger pre-existing conditions or a full-blown medical mystery you did not know you had all along. For example, it could be that a Covid-19 infection or vaccination triggers an unexpected biological chain reaction and autoimmune response for some when on these medications: a high price to pay for a moderate benefit.

Before you start a biologic, you might try parasite cleansing based on Acupuncture Meridian Assessment (AMA), avoiding allergenic foods (e.g. gluten, dairy and GMO products), working with a biological dentist to eliminate incompatible dental materials and hidden dental infections, and also working to detox your entire body, which is important in preparation and follow-up to dental work and treating systemic infections. These steps will gradually strengthen your whole-body immune system, and this multipronged approach may help resolve underlying medical conditions like asthma, chronic fatigue, eczema, fibromyalgia, irritable bowel syndrome, migraine headache, or psoriasis. You may call it an "Accidental Cure."

Be patient! Is healing from within and restoring your immune system better than biologics? You can be the judge - not pharma, FDA, medical journals, or TV commercials. The skin will be the last organ to heal.

Medical Acupuncture on Nerve Degeneration Meridian: ALS, MS, Parkinson's Disease on the Rise!

ALS, Multiple Sclerosis, and Parkinson's disease are often overlooked, poorly understood, serious chronic diseases, after cancer and heart disease. These three neurological diseases are rising at an alarming rate. An aging population, and environmental pollutants and toxins which are often seen as the price of industrialization, are implicated.

Diagnosis of ALS is viewed as a death sentence – with no cure – according to the latest medical science. These three neurologic disorders were rare until post-industrialization and have become more common. Just look around you. It may be someone in your family, a friend, or a member of your community. Lyme disease has also been blamed, but how?

Are we overlooking some of the **"forensic evidence of hidden dental and parasite problems"** that can be easily mistaken as Lyme and coinfections? The nervous system as a meridian system was not well defined in classical Chinese acupuncture. In the 1950s, Dr. Reinhold Voll of Germany described the energetic relationship between meridians and the western concept of the nervous system in his monumental work, *Electro-Acupuncture according to Dr. Voll*.[15] According to Dr. Voll, the Nerve Degeneration (ND) meridian is located on the index finger, mirroring the Large Intestine meridian.

The Nerve Degeneration meridian is influenced by many elements, manifesting through the Trigeminal nerve by the Dental meridian, and through the Vagus nerve by the Gallbladder meridian. These two are the dominant meridians controlling the entire central and peripheral nervous system.

Other meridians that contribute to nerve regulation include the Bladder, Triple Warmer, Governing Vessel, Stomach, Small Intestine, Large Intestine and Kidney meridian. They all interact, regulate, and create a complex neural network beyond the understanding of Western medical science.

I have had a handful of successful responses with ALS patients, and wrote a story about one of them, Ron J, in, "ALS Patient's Unexpected Journey: My Patient as My Teacher." I was invited to give a lecture in Houston at the ALS Summit in 2019.

The slide below indicates he had a Nerve Meridian Disorder, but also his left and right Dental, Allergy-Immunology, Heart, Liver and Gallbladder meridians were out of balance. A middle (45-55) bar means normal; low (under 45) bars mean out of balance. See Figure 42.

Figure 42: 68-year-old with ALS

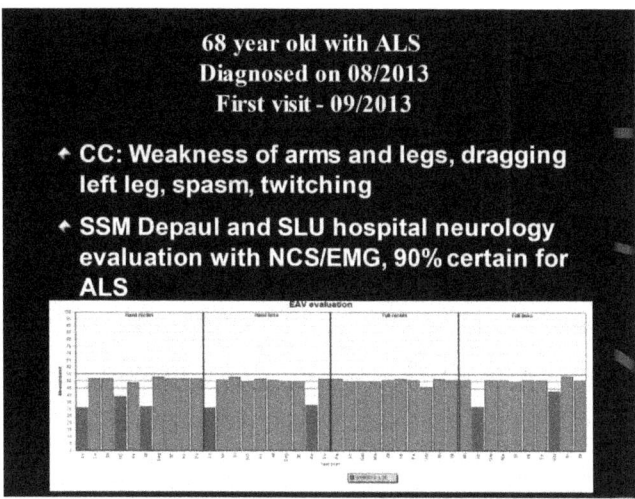

Additional ALS case studies include a dentist, architect, auto mechanic, triathlete, and dental hygienist. Some overcame their ALS, and some died or were lost in follow up. Ron wrote of his experiences in fighting against ALS in his book, *An Unexpected Journey: Searching for a Cause and Finding Hope in the Battle Against ALS*.

His fight against ALS was successful. Initially, his neurologist was 90 percent sure he had ALS and told him he would be in a wheelchair soon. Now almost 10 years later, Ron can ambulate well, and his neurologist said he must have made a mistake, and Ron does not have ALS. This means ALS is a clinical diagnosis, not a death sentence. See the Merwin et al. article, "Organophosphate neurotoxicity to the voluntary motor system on the trail of environment-caused amyotrophic lateral sclerosis: the known, the misknown and the unknown."[16]

I am now taking care of a retired Navy Captain with rapidly progressing ALS; he is in wheelchair. He has 11 out of 40 meridians out of balance, multiple infected teeth under crowns, cavitations in his jawbones, and massive environmental toxins exposure including mercury, perchlorate, organophosphates (herbicides), petrochemicals, and glyphosate; as well as fungal mycotoxins and parasite infections. His recovery will be slow, and he is fighting against time. He understands his enemies and endorses our battle plan to reclaim his health from ALS.

> **The Nerve Degeneration meridian is influenced by many elements, through the Trigeminal nerve by the Dental meridian, and the Vagus nerve by the Gallbladder meridian. These two dominant meridians control the central and peripheral nervous system.**

ALS, MS, and Parkinson's disease are on the rise, and patients do not have time. Time is ticking and they need more than a double-blind placebo controlled random clinical trial (RCT) to find out which medications may help them.

Patients need a real-time focus on understanding, detecting, and addressing major contributing, synergistic factors now. We can detect the missing links - hidden dental and parasite infections and environmental toxins - and connect the dots by applying a modern, disruptive technology called Acupuncture Meridian Assessment (AMA), based on an ancient meridian medical system.

To summarize the main points and observations from my 2019 ALS Summit presentation, we can focus on such areas as:

- Detecting parasites, fungi, and mycotoxins using AMA
- Dental: root canals, anaerobic bacteria and Treponema, Lyme and Lyme-like infections
- Cavitations and biotoxins, dental materials, Bite-TMJ issues, Sleep apnea, galvanic currents

- Trigeminal nerve-brainstem, emissary cranial valveless veins retro flow per Dr. Störtebecker
- Environmental toxins and heavy metals
- Other unknown infections and toxins
- Consider IPT (Insulin Potentiation Therapy) as a part of supportive therapy for ALS
- Focus on Preventive Medicine to give the patient time to heal
- Cluster phenomenon as in military bases or areas of industrial chemical spills

Is the rise of nerve degeneration diseases a product of post-industrial pollutants and toxins and hidden infections, accelerated by modern dentistry?

Dentists and physicians taking care of ALS, MS, and Parkinson's disease patients - and patients themselves with neurological disorders - should read the book by Dr. Patrick Störtebecker, MD, PhD, *Dental Caries as a Cause of Nervous Disorders*.[17] In my personal experience, in most cases, the patient had dental problems despite a normal dental X-ray using the state-of-the-art, Cone Beam CT (CBCT) dental scan. Is the rise of nerve degeneration diseases a product of post-industrial pollutants and toxins and hidden infections, accelerated by modern dentistry?

Most of the main meridians can be balanced with antiparasite, antifungal, and antibacterial medications. What comes next is addressing the dental and allergy-immunology meridians.

Anytime I balance the main meridians, the dental and allergy-immunology meridians will often show persistent and ongoing disturbances. Next, we need to address them.

Part 4
Dental: Portal to Hell or Health?

Chapter 8 Deadly Dental Trap

Unsuspected dental-related medical problems are the most difficult part of recovering from mysterious chronic illness. Hidden dental infections are biological interference fields. They are an important and overlooked factor in progression from acute infections such as Lyme or COVID into chronic post-Lyme or post-COVID and surprisingly progressing into cancer or neurological disease.

Dental recommendations are the number one reason why patients drop out of my practice. Patients want to keep all their teeth and avoid oral surgery at all costs. When you finish this chapter, you will understand why it is important to measure the subtle meridian fields unknown to most dentists. They will not extract the infected teeth without the hard evidence of dental X-ray or Cone Beam CT scan (CBCT), the latest breakthrough in dentistry. CBCT has become the gold standard for detecting a tiny, abscessed tooth or hollow cavitation of jaw infection.

> **CBCT scans can lead to unnecessary dental operations: a double-edge problem of being too sensitive in detecting the hollow space as a presumed infection in the jawbone. It can also miss things which are important.**

American general dentistry is costly, and combining biological dentistry and extensive reconstructive dentistry can be prohibitively costly for many. It is a strong emotional and psychological challenge. Tooth loss is associated with aging, appearance, and inability to chew. There are other options: extraction of infected teeth and partial dentures or bridges. When properly removed and replaced, the meridian is restored.

Live Longer One Less Tooth at a Time: The Secret of Antiaging, Cancer, Lyme and Wellness Depends on Dental...

Eat less – a Calorie Restricted Diet - and you will live longer. This is scientifically proven but not very popular. Extract one bad tooth and it may save your life. This is scientifically unproven and more than despised. Here is a case study: a 40-year-old married man from Florida, came to see me with stage 4 non-small cell lung cancer; he was diagnosed in October 2020, and I saw him in May 2021. The cancer had spread to his brain, liver, bones, and lymphatic system. His metastatic brain had seven large and small tumor lesions with a grim prognosis. His initial symptoms were coughing and fatigue, and he was diagnosed with bronchoscopy, biopsy, CT scan, and PET scan.

He was under the care of a prestigious medical institution in Boston and receiving chemotherapy and immunotherapy. The initial response had been promising, and the tumor was shrinking. He was referred by another alternative medicine practitioner to get a second opinion to rule out any overlooked areas by an academic medical institution, such as parasites and hidden dental infection (my special interests).

On Acupuncture Meridian Assessment (AMA), 12 out of 40 meridians were out of balance. The large intestine, lung, small intestine, and gallbladder meridians were out of balance and dominant problems. He was started on ivermectin, pyrantel pamoate, praziquantel, tinidazole, and nystatin to treat parasites and fungal infections. On panoramic dental X-ray and AMA, he had 3 bad teeth, with a root canal at number 19, while tooth numbers 20 and 29 were not clear-cut but showed evidence of dental infection. See Figure 43.

In his AMA evaluation, a middle (45-55) bar indicates balanced and normal, while a low (under 45) bar indicates chronic degenerative conditions. This technology provides a translation of physiology and biochemistry to frequency (think musical scale) based on meridians, a 5,000-year-old, new disruptive technology.

Figure 43: AMA, Non-Small Cell Lung Cancer Patient

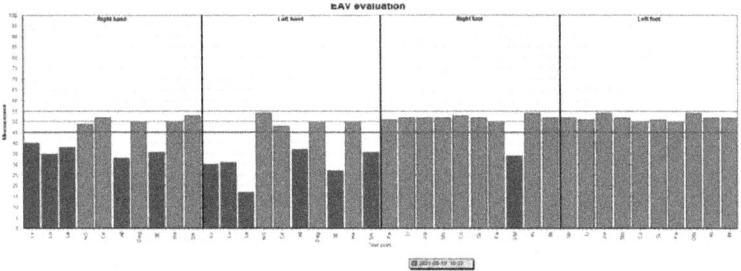

Most of my patients are eager to take parasite medications but are very reluctant to pull a tooth, especially if the dental X-ray does not show clear-cut dental infection. Most patients don't come to see me again when a dentist says the X-ray and dental exam are OK. It is even harder to find a dentist to extract a tooth if the teeth appear fine on dental X-ray and on Cone Beam CT (CBCT) scan.

> **Most of my patients are eager to take parasite medications but are very reluctant to pull a tooth.**

After a long discussion about medical and dental (MAD) disconnections, I told him, if he wants to live longer, get his #19 root-canal tooth out. If he wants to live long enough to see if he will have children and see them grow, also pull tooth #20. If he wants to see his grandchildren grow up, pull all three bad teeth out. He got my message, and he pulled all three teeth.

> **If he wants to see his grandchildren grow up, pull all three bad teeth. He got my message, and he pulled all three teeth.**

His dental operation was uneventful, and he went through multiple cycles of parasite and fungal medications. He was on alectinib, an oral drug that blocks the activity of the anaplastic lymphoma kinase and used to treat non-small cell lung cancer, when I saw him. He did not tell his oncologist that he had extracted three teeth or that he was on parasite and fungal medications. He did not feel comfortable telling his oncologist that he was doing things considered way outside the box.

I had a follow up conversation with his alternative medicine physician recently, and he has been cancer free. The patient also said all the tumors are gone, his cancer marker is down, he is feeling well and doing well. We will never know how much chemo/immunotherapy and dental/fungal/parasite therapy contributed to his remarkable recovery. Cancer is relentless, its cells are metabolically flexible, and cancer stem cells and cancer mitochondria will outwit and survive chemo, radiation therapy and immunotherapy. It can always come back if you do not correct upstream dental and parasite problems.

Professor Thomas Seyfried's book, *Cancer as a Metabolic Disease* (2012) and the latest book by Jane McLelland, *How to Starve Cancer*, provide ample information on how to fight cancer and live longer. Metabolically, cancer behaves like metabolic parasites, according to Tim Guilford, MD. He presented a lecture on glutathione, cancer, and the Warburg Effect at the 8th International Alternative Medical Conference in St. Louis. We are always looking for a new diet or a new cure.

Thomas Seyfried's book extensively covers metabolic management of cancer through a ketogenic diet.[18] Jane McLelland goes beyond ketogenic diet and covers repurposed off-label drug use including doxycycline, mebendazole, niclosamide, ivermectin, and more. I highly recommend reading these two books.[19]

I have been using parasite and fungal medications for well over 20 years with remarkable responses, especially when combined with correcting hidden dental problems in many chronically ill patients - including cancer of all kinds, Lyme and chronic Lyme, neurological disorders, chronic fatigue syndrome/ME and fibromyalgia, IBS, IBD and many unusual, weird symptoms. Dental, fungal, and parasite problems are missing links for medical failure. When you have advanced stage cancer, chronic illness, or neurological disorder, there is no time to drill and repair a tooth, get a crown, root canals, or dental implants.

You may live longer with one less tooth at a time. That is the secret of antiaging, cancer, Lyme, and wellness. Remember that most dentists have no sense of humor, but they can extend your life or shorten it: no laughing matter.

> **Most dentists have no sense of humor, but they can extend your life or shorten it: no laughing matter.**

Autoimmune Disease and Missing Links: A Cure for... Misdiagnosis? Dr. Johann Lechner's Dental Research on RANTES

Do you have one of those autoimmune diseases of "many names" after years of struggling and searching for help with your chronic physical ailments? The rate of Autoimmune Disorders has risen rapidly in the last 40 years and has become one of the most common medical diagnoses with a multitude of physical signs and symptoms. Autoimmunity is a medical enigma and epidemic out of proportion despite advancement in medical science.

One in ten people develop an autoimmune disease (more women than men), and the diagnosis rate is rising. There are now about a hundred classified autoimmune diseases. Among the most well-known are lupus, rheumatoid arthritis, Hashimoto's disease, Grave's thyroiditis, psoriasis, Type 1 diabetes, Crohn's disease, ulcerative colitis, mixed connective tissue disease, chronic inflammatory demyelinating polyneuropathy, and more.

> **The list is growing, and we do not have a clear understanding of the science behind why our immune cells are attacking our own bodies.**

The list is growing, and we do not have a clear understanding of the science behind why our immune cells are attacking our own bodies. Infections, environmental toxins, and genetics are the leading candidates for triggering autoimmune response, but are there other factors that have been overlooked? Did we miss something unknown to us, and in naming the disease based on laboratory test results and physical symptoms, do we overlook the underlying problems? Can we connect the dots, and find the missing links? Let's investigate under our noses, close to our brains, thyroid, and at the opening to the airway and the gut: the oral cavity, for dental-related problems. See Figure 44.

> **Let's investigate under our noses, close to our brains, thyroid, and at the opening to the airway and the gut: the oral cavity, for dental-related problems.**

Figure 44: Inflammation, Infections and Immune Dysregulation

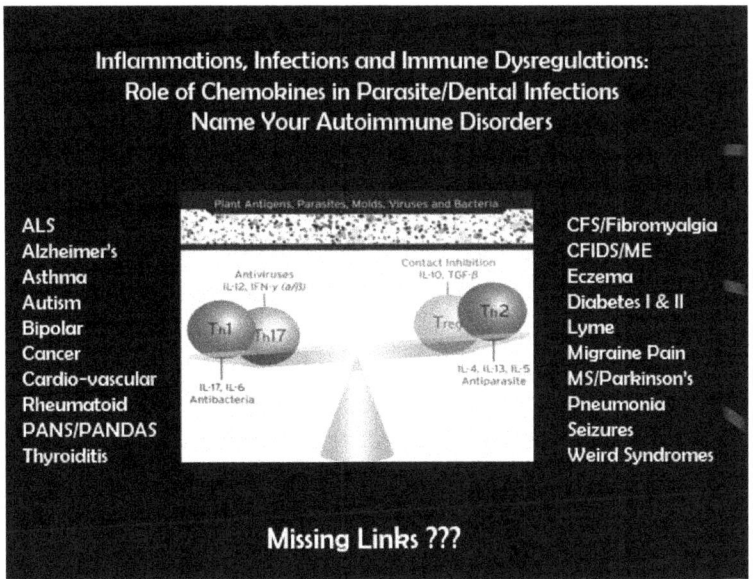

Is it possible that autoimmune disease is a misdiagnosis based on our limitation of medical science? We know one of the hallmarks of this category is inflammation, with some sort of antibodies developed as inflammatory markers to our tissues and organelles, and at the DNA level. As an example, a diagnosis for lupus includes a battery of blood tests, antinuclear antibody (ANA) test, different imaging tests like a chest X-ray and echocardiogram, and skin or kidney tissue biopsy.

Treatment is limited based on your signs and symptoms. It could be ibuprofen, an antimalarial parasite medication like hydroxychloroquine, steroids, immunosuppressant drugs, and new biologics like Rituxan (Rituximab) which can also be used for rheumatoid arthritis and non-Hodgkin's Lymphoma. If you do not correct the true underlying problems, you become a part of the medical system as a permanently labeled lupus patient. Is there a solution to autoimmune disease?

Let me explain. We should not dwell on the diagnosis. Once the diagnosis is made by specialists, the primary focus is to treat symptoms. Sometimes it is better to ignore the diagnosis. Starting with a fresh point of view, I check 40 main meridian points based on acupuncture meridian assessment (AMA) and develop a treatment plan based on addressing the biggest problems first. Lab test results can be used to compare how patients are responding to correcting the underlying problems.

> **Once the diagnosis is made by specialists, the primary focus is to treat symptoms. Sometimes it is better to ignore the diagnosis. Starting with a fresh point of view...**

Over the years, my summary of the main reasons patients are not getting well: neglected dental problems, parasite infections, and environmental toxins including heavy metals and mycotoxins. For example, see a case study of 46-year-old female with lupus, pericarditis, tachycardia, anemia, alopecia and arthralgia in my first book, *Accidental Cure,* and article, "Lupus: Autoimmune Disease and Hidden Pathogens." Elevated ANA, ESR, CRP, and other inflammatory markers all came down as dental work was done on a dental cavitation (jaw infection). Chelation therapy lowered her mercury level, and multiple rounds of parasite medications also helped her to recover from her lupus diagnosis and become asymptomatic, without using immunosuppressive therapy.

> **Over the years, my summary of the main reasons patients are not getting well: neglected dental problems, parasite infections, and environmental toxins including heavy metals and mycotoxins.**

Some people have multiple autoimmune diseases concurrently such as Hashimoto's thyroiditis, rheumatoid arthritis, interstitial pneumonitis, psoriasis, and ulcerative colitis. Unless we can correct the upstream underlying problems, we end up treating symptoms and dealing with the complications of the disease process itself, and the side effects of treatments. See above on how our immune system will tilt based on missing links. In most cases, genetics play a minor role compared to dental problems, parasites, and environmental toxin exposures.

> **Unless we can correct the upstream underlying problems, we end up treating symptoms and dealing with the complications of the disease process itself, and the side effects of treatments.**

Physicians rely on dentists to correct dental problems, and dental issues are the most frequently overlooked missing links. There is a medical-and-dental (MAD) disconnection. The International Academy of Oral Medicine and Toxicology (IAOMT) and International Academy of Biological Dentistry and Medicine (IABDM) have been working to end use of mercury dental amalgams, warning about root canals, and more recently, focusing on the dangers of jaw infection from previously extracted teeth, including wisdom teeth.

Johann Lechner, DDS of Germany is a leading researcher on dental infections, especially jaw infections with osteonecrosis, known as fatty degenerative osteonecrosis of the jaw (FDOJ). He finds immune dysregulation, with overexpression of an inflammatory cytokine called RANTES (short for regulated upon activation, normal T-cell expressed and secreted), see Figure 45 below. High RANTES has been associated with osteonecrosis of the jawbone (cavitation), and with breast cancer, chronic fatigue syndrome, neuropathy, and rheumatic diseases, among many medically unexplained conditions.

Figure 45: Jawbone Osteonecrosis and Inflammatory Cytokine RANTES

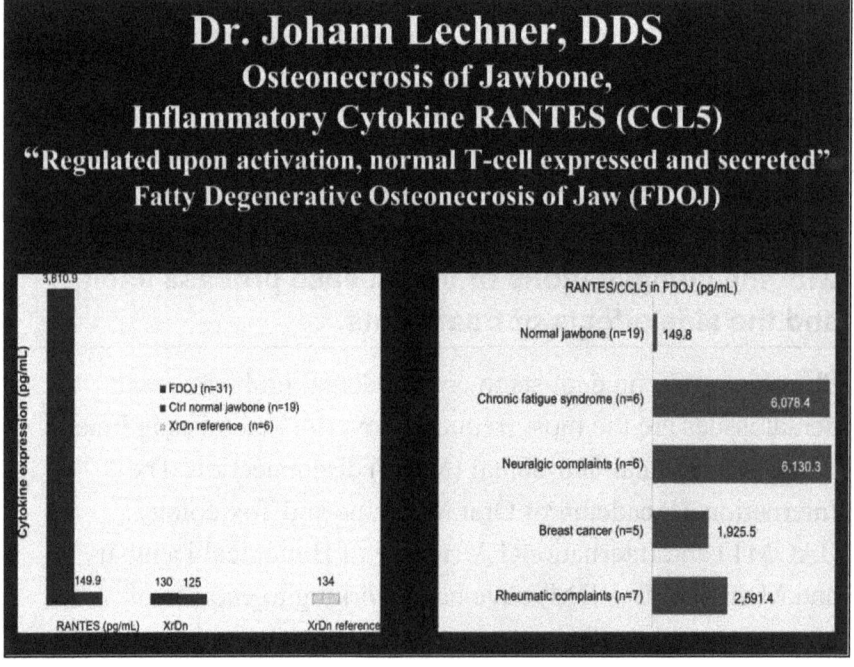

One of the major cruxes of the problem is that routine dental X-rays will not reveal jaw infections until there is significant bone damage. Even Cone Beam CT dental X-ray (CBCT), the gold standard, may miss osteonecrosis of jawbone unless there is 10-15 percent bone destruction or more. The early warning signs for dental and jaw problems can be picked up based on energetic evaluation using acupuncture meridian assessment (AMA).

> **If we understand energy medicine, a cure from autoimmune disease is possible and this is not an accidental cure.**

If we understand energy medicine, a cure from autoimmune disease is possible and this is not an accidental cure. My book, *AcciDental Blow Up in Medicine: Battle Plan for Your Life*, will guide you in treating misunderstood autoimmune diseases. IAOMT and IABDM are the leading biological dental organizations. A strong physician-dentist team can connect the missing links of medical and dental problems and go beyond (misdiagnosis) to treatment. Success or failure in your recovery is often based on dental work done correctly, a missing piece of the puzzle for autoimmune diseases.

Toothless in St. Louis, God Forbid – Toothless in Vienna: Fairy Death Tale from Berlin

On my way from St. George's Klinik near Munich to International Holistic Medical Days in Vienna – for my lectures and training on acupuncture meridian assessment (AMA) – I visited Dr. Helmut Retzek's clinic in Voecklabruck, Austria for a few days, and I saw some patients for fun. Dr. Retzek announced that I would be visiting his clinic and signing up for an evaluation for anyone who was interested. He has a large following through his website, ganzemedizin.at, which has extensive high-quality research materials; most of them are in German but some are in English (Google's browser will translate all of them for you).

One of the patients was a 65-year-old man from Berlin with a history of prostate cancer. I did my usual 40-point meridian assessment and told him he needed to take parasite medications and have extensive revision of his dental work. He apparently read my book, *Accidental Cure*, and was excited and eager to take parasite medications based on my recommendations – but he was not happy that a lot of dental work needed to be redone. His expression and demeanor were not a happy face from Berlin. Disgruntled patients are expected when I tell them they need to redo their dental work.

While he was putting on his shoes, he asked me why I was not dead yet! I know I can annoy my patients with my dental revision recommendations, but not to the point of threatening to kill me, at least, not yet. He said he has been following medical politics in the United States and was aware of the many disappearances of integrative/alternative medical doctors by sudden death from suspicious suicide. His last comment was that maybe "they" leave me alone because I was a retired US Army medical officer, and I am not claiming or am discrete about undermining the medical-pharma establishment. To make a long story short, it is like a Fairy Death Tale from Berlin – not well-known in America. By the way, I didn't think he was emotionally ready to do the dental work.

My dental recommendations go from bad to worse and seem almost cruel to some patients. It is not uncommon for me to recommend a new patient extract an infected tooth rather than have a root canal procedure (or a past root canal redone), bridge work, or a dental implant. It takes a lot of nerve for most people – like you – to lose a tooth, especially when you do not have a horrible toothache, and/or your dentist told you that your root canal is in good shape, and there are no signs of active infection on x-ray.

However, a dental x-ray may not reveal damage until bone destruction has reached the 20-30-40% level and is finally visible on X-ray consistent with x-ray or X-ray throughout. Dental infections often have multiple microorganisms including parasites, fungus, bacteria and viruses. They will migrate to any weak links, especially joints, heart, kidney, breast, sex organs, spinal cord, and brain. They also produce biological toxins. I highly recommend reading the work of Swedish neurologist, Patrick Störtebecker, MD, PhD; in the United States, see the work of Boyd Haley, PhD, Nick Meyers, DDS, and Thomas Levy, DDS.

As described in Chapter 2, a few years ago, a 52-year-old engineer with squamous cell carcinoma of the right thumb died after complications of the tragic bungling of dental-medical-oncology-radiation misadventures. When I saw him, his biggest problem was a dental infection at tooth #10, but his dental x-ray did not show any sign of dental infection. I was not able to convince him or his dentist to extract the tooth for over a year. Meanwhile, his tumor was growing rapidly, and the oncologist recommended amputating the whole thumb and undergoing radiation therapy. Every time I evaluated him, the dental problem was his priority problem, and he and his dentist finally agreed to extract tooth #10 under the condition that he sign a waiver that he would not sue the dentist. As a part of the agreement, a dental DNA test was done to provide forensic evidence of any infection that was not detectable by x-ray.

His DNA test finally came back for multiple infections at the normal-looking tooth showing Entamoeba (protozoal parasites), Prevotella, Serratia, Enterobacter, Staphylococcus, Haemophilus, Actinomyces, and Cytomegalovirus. After the tooth extraction, he had radiation therapy, but it was too late. His cancer spread and he eventually died. I may or may not have been able to help him, but without forensic evidence of a DNA test, we would never have guessed how badly his tooth was infected, well before it would show up visible on x-ray.

Recently, I saw a 36-year-old woman from Hawaii with recurrent cancer of the left breast. She was diagnosed at age 29 and had a mastectomy and chemotherapy. The cancer came back two years ago, it was resected, and it came back a third time and was rapidly growing in size. According to my AMA evaluation, her priority problem was a dental problem, followed by parasite and fungal problems. She had three bad teeth; tooth #20, a left premolar tooth, corresponds to her left breast where she had recurrent cancer. I told her three teeth need to come out eventually, but tooth #20 should come out first, and she should take parasite and fungal medications as part of rebalancing her meridian system.

She will be flying back home with one tooth less from St. Louis, but her immune system will be much stronger to fight the recurrent breast cancer. I told her that on the airplane, she should tell people that she is from Ozark Mountains – a hillbilly from the Arkansas side (a politically incorrect Missouri state joke) - and that it's common to be missing a tooth. She did not appreciate my sense of humor.

Is it better off being one tooth less, or toothless, in St. Louis? In Vienna, the center of fine art and culture in Europe, God forbid, toothless is forbidden! I evaluated many medical doctors from Vienna, and they all had dental-root canal and parasite problems. Even a culturally refined, cosmopolitan city like Vienna is not immune to the two most overlooked medical enigmas that keep the medical-dental-pharma industry rolling. The story of death from my Berlin patient may have some truth to it, so let's keep it quiet as if you have never heard of it...

Dental Parasites, Fungal and Bacterial Infections: Dreaded Periodontal Surgery is like Oral What?!

Have you ever had periodontal surgery for gum disease? It is so unpleasant that Canadian dentist Murray Vimy calls it oral circumcision - a bad Canadian joke, I guess. The initial oral surgery results appear favorable, but the benefits usually do not last very long unless you can correct the underlying problems. Dentists often blame the patient for poor oral hygiene: not flossing enough and not brushing properly.

"The Mouth is the Mirror of all Disease," according to Sir William Osler, one of the original founders of Johns Hopkins. Current Western medical education was shaped by his teaching, but this wisdom somehow got lost in the specialization of medical professions, and the importance of the dental/oral cavity has been ignored.

Dental infections and periodontal gum disease reflect systemic disease from eating a processed Western industrial diet, according to Dr. Weston Price's classic book, *Nutrition and*

Physical Degeneration. The prevalence of physical degenerative diseases such as skeletal malformations including jaw/mandibular atrophy, caries and tooth loss are due to periodontal infection.

Today, medical doctors are busy taking care of patients with heart disease, rheumatism, kidney disease, Lyme, cancer, Alzheimer's disease, dementia, chronic fatigue, fibromyalgia, IBS, and neurological problems like MS, Parkinson's disease, and ALS. As physicians, we treat diseases based on symptoms, labs, and diagnostic tests, and often get lost because proper dental evaluation as a cause of chronic illness is not a part of medical evaluation.

> **As physicians, we treat diseases based on symptoms, labs, and diagnostic tests, and often get lost because proper dental evaluation as a cause of chronic illness is not a part of medical evaluation.**

Canadian dentist Trevor Lyons published an important but underappreciated book, *Introduction to Protozoa and Fungi in Periodontal Infection: A Manual of Microbiological Diagnosis and Nonsurgical Treatment,* in 1989. He covers how and why dental pathogens are the culprit not only for dental infections, but for creating systemic infections and a multitude of chronic medical conditions. Simply put, advancing destructive periodontal disease involves oral protozoal parasites. This is confirmed by S. Fadhil Ali Malaa et al. in a 2022 article stating, "*Trichomonas tenax (T. tenax)* and *Entamoeba gingivalis (E. gingivalis)* are two oral protozoan parasites that are universal and found in patients with poor oral hygiene, as well as chronic and periodontal diseases."[20] I would add fungal Candida to that list.

Parasites, Fungi, and Bacteria in Periodontal Infections

Bacterial infections may play a smaller part than originally thought in periodontal disease, while parasites and fungi play a larger part. Once established in the oral cavity, parasites become the dominant organism in periodontal gum pockets. With no known enemies, they are hidden kingmakers of most modern chronic "incurable" diseases.

> **Once established in the oral cavity, parasites become the dominant organism in periodontal gum pockets.**

Simple gum and gingival inflammation and infections can transform into deep periodontitis, causing loss of teeth or deep jaw infection, and unintended consequences of periodontal surgery, including root canals and dental implants, and eventually demise of your health. Amoxicillin or Augmentin are typically prescribed by dentists, but they do not cover anaerobic infections or spirochete infections well.

I have found a combination of doxycycline (or azithromycin), tinidazole, and clindamycin, along with antifungal nystatin, better covers the broad spectrum of dental infections, and also Lyme disease hiding under the teeth. John Coombs, MD from Ottawa, noted that gingival treatment benefits patients with chronic fatigue, anxiety, depression, panic attack disorder, and rheumatism from *E. gingivalis*.

> **A combination of doxycycline (or azithromycin), tinidazole, and clindamycin, along with antifungal nystatin, better covers the broad spectrum of dental infections, and Lyme disease hiding under teeth.**

For most health professionals, including dentists, the field of parasitology is not a well-known entity, and oral parasites are not on the radar for differential diagnosis of chronic illnesses or medically unexplained symptoms. The beliefs that patients will not become infected with parasites because parasites are a third world problem, and parasite infections only happen when inadequate hygiene practices are observed, are outdated – an unrealistic intellectual exercise. We are living in the setting of global migration, frequent travel, and global warming - creating unique opportunities to spread parasite infections that we as medical and dental professionals are not prepared to deal with. See the many articles I have written on this subject in my books, *Accidental Cure*, and *AcciDental Blow Up in Medicine*.

> **Most parasites can ensure survival by having a resistant form as either cysts or eggs with complex lifecycles, and interaction with our good and not-so-friendly microbiomes.**

Most parasites can ensure survival by having a resistant form as either cysts or eggs with complex lifecycles, and interaction with our good and not-so-friendly microbiomes. They have unique biological adaptations to the environment, follow moon cycles to hatch eggs, and may get assistance from bacteria to hatch eggs. It will take multiple cycles of different combinations of parasite, fungal, and antibiotic medications that can last over a year while correcting one's diet, nutrition, biological terrain, and metabolism.

When you get rid of one dominant parasite, less dominant parasites will arise. The patient will have to go through treatment of many layers of smaller parasites, fungi, single-celled protozoal parasites like *Entamoeba*, intracellular parasites, bacteria, and viruses. Parasites are masters of deception, using camouflage, hiding, confusion with antigenic variations or coinfections; they engage in counter-defense by disabling the host's immune response.

> **It will take multiple cycles of different combinations of parasite, fungal and antibiotic medications that can last over a year while correcting one's diet, nutrition, biological terrain, and metabolism.**

E. gingivalis and *Actinomyces* species are known to cause inflammation and necrosis in the female genital tract, havoc via destructive periodontal lesions, and fatigue, headaches, foul smelling breath (halitosis), and frequent flu-like infections. *Entamoeba* ingests red blood and white blood cells, sucking out the cell contents, often resembling a multinucleated giant cell (think of lymphoma), per Lyons. They also go after fatty tissues like brain and breast tissue.

> ***Entamoeba* ingests red blood and white blood cells, sucking out the cell contents, often resembling a multinucleated giant cell (think of lymphoma). They also go after fatty tissues like brain, thyroid, and breast tissue.**

T. tenax is another common oral protozoal parasite and is associated with female vaginal foul-smelling discharge and itching, or painful urination. These parasites often harbor bacteria and viruses, even Legionella bacteria. *Entamoeba histolytica* is a close cousin of *E. gingivalis*, and it is associated with intestinal problems. They produce and store toxins within their bodies and release them to control their environment.

When these parasites die, they release enzymes (elastase) and biotoxins into the tissues, which results in further necrosis, destruction and gum bleeding. This provides a source of food for the succeeding wave of invading daughter cells and perpetuates the cycle of infection. The White Blood Count (WBC) outnumbers *Entamoeba* by a 100:1 ratio and triggers WBC to produce and release elastase, destroying its own soft tissues and triggering autoimmune responses.

E. gingivalis is the epitome of parasites since the parasite commands the host to destroy its own tissues to promote blood flow for the sole purpose of feeding the invading organism. Think of how many cancerous cells' behaviors are like metabolic parasites, and often respond to antiparasitics, antifungals and antibiotics. See my article with Frederick (Tim) Guilford, MD, "Antiparasitic and Antifungal Medications for Targeting Cancer Cells Literature Review and Case Studies."[21] You can read the full article on the Publications section of my website. The abstract is at the end of this article, along with a perspective he shared on his experience with AMA.

Candida will not colonize unless there has been a preexisting protozoal or bacterial infection. Left untreated, the protozoa may ultimately be suppressed by the presence of fungi and mycotoxins. Candida can switch forms, known as "dimorphic": from a long filament called hyphae to yeast, and release fungal toxins. It can transform into spores if the environment becomes unfavorable for it and turn into thick-walled cells that look swollen, called chlamydospores. This is a disseminating form, often a silent infectious stage.

When eliminating oral parasites, Candida is the most frequent organism to overgrow and create superinfection. It is important to treat parasites and fungus concurrently and in alternating sequences, while correcting the biological terrain with diet, nutrition, and detoxification.

> **It is important to treat parasites and fungus concurrently and in alternating sequences, while correcting the biological terrain with diet, nutrition, and detoxification.**

Even the act of chewing can send showers of bacteria and parasites into the bloodstream. Living with oral parasites and fungus may be like living with a ticking time bomb. Defuse this biological dental bomb from creating a chain reaction of explosive inflammatory reactions.

Start by treating intestinal GI tract-related large parasites first with medications like ivermectin, pyrantel pamoate, and praziquantel; next treat dental parasites and fungi with doxycycline, tinidazole, and nystatin. Follow with fluconazole and itraconazole to cover deep fungal infections. Reinfection is very common; change your toothbrush frequently, oil pull daily with sunflower seed oil, and brush with salt and baking soda.

Two Case Studies

First case, a 60-year-old physician with adrenal burnout, breast cancer, Lyme, and dental infections. AMA testing showed disturbances on the Triple Warmer (TW) meridian, which corresponds to the endocrine system. These are the adrenal, thyroid, and reproductive glands that produce hormones that regulate metabolism, growth and development, tissue function, sexual function, reproduction, sleep, and mood. An oral DNA test on her extracted infected tooth was positive, with multiple pathogens including *Entamoeba*. A Lyme panel showed *Borrelia, Babesia, Bartonella,* and other coinfections hiding in the tooth. See Figure 46.

Figure 46: Case 1 - Physician with Dental Infections

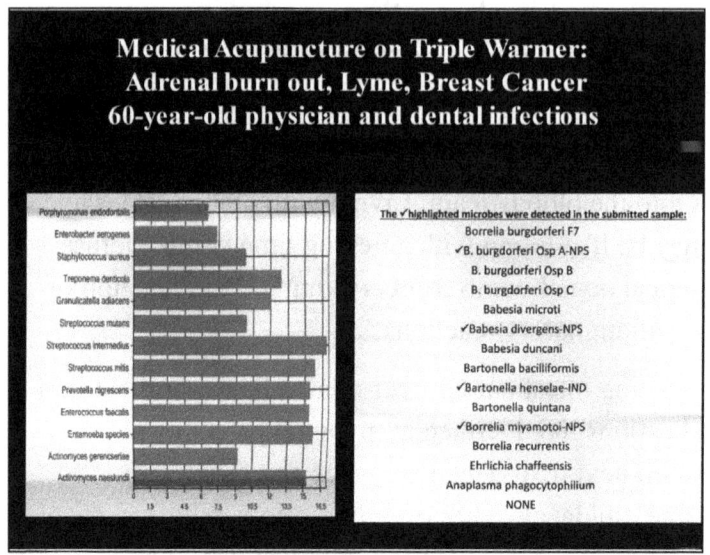

Second case, a 57-year-old with ALS. His oral DNA and Lyme panel reveal *Borrelia* and various infections in a former wisdom tooth cavitation site. See Figure 47.

Figure 47: Case 2 - Man with ALS and Dental Infections

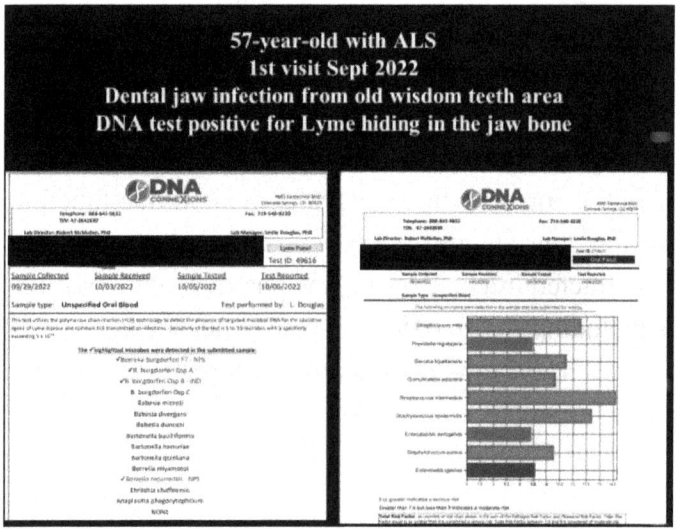

In summary, I have briefly reviewed and hopefully renewed interest in Dr. Trevor Lyons' lifetime work and his landmark book. Good news: hold off on oral circumcision or periodontal surgery just yet. Instead of relying on periodontal surgery and antibiotics to control periodontal disease, combine antibiotics with antiparasitic and antifungal medications, oil pulling and proper brushing, and improve your diet and nutrition. DNA Connexions testing is now available, and it confirms Dr. Lyons' findings about dental-medical connections for chronic fatigue, thyroid and adrenal hormone imbalance, cancer, Lyme, neurological diseases, and much more.

It is time to connect the dots between dental and chronic, mysterious medical problems. Acupuncture meridian assessment (AMA) can help connect the dots by detecting the subtle energy disturbances described in ancient civilizations called acupuncture meridians. Oral circumcision is optional.

Physician Perspective: Tim Guilford, MD

"Ten years ago, I chose to become a client of Dr. Yu, even though I had no specific diagnosis, but was motivated by a family history of cardiovascular disease and cancer. For a short time, I had elevation of PHI as Dr. Yu discusses in his first book, *Accidental Cure*. About 5 years ago, I developed debilitating foot pain and inflammation, similar to gout. After a series of evaluations, he determined the cause of the foot inflammation might be related to a tooth with an old crown harboring infection. As the foot pain was progressing, I decided to remove the tooth even though the tooth appeared normal to my dentist. After tooth removal, the pain no longer occurred and has not recurred in over 2 years.

My visits to St. Louis gave me a chance to interact with many of Dr. Yu's clients in various stages of therapy. After a few visits, we decided to write a scientific paper on treating cancer like a metabolic parasite and sharing Dr. Yu's results in our joint article, "Antiparasitic and Antifungal Medications for Targeting Cancer Cells Literature Review and Case Studies."[22]

A dramatic example of cases I've seen at Dr. Yu's clinic is a man with biopsy and photographic proof of cancer of the upper jaw, a lesion with which I was familiar as a Head and Neck Surgeon.

The individual declined a major surgery recommended by a well-known cancer hospital and elected to follow Dr Yu's advice. A bit more than a year later, the jaw lesion had resolved, and he was happy to follow up with occasional intravenous vitamin C infusions.

About two years ago, I referred to Dr. Yu a 40-year-old woman who had a recurrence of breast cancer. Evaluation at a major cancer hospital prior to beginning work with Dr. Yu revealed the breast cancer had spread to involve the bone of the sternum, a Stage IV Breast Cancer. In addition to being placed on antiparasitic and antifungal medications and undergoing insulin potentiation therapy, she was found to have two wisdom tooth cavitations requiring debridement. A year and a half later, I met her again and she reported follow up evaluations revealed no cancer.

After my interactions with Simon Yu and his clients, I have no doubt about the choice of therapy I would make if confronted with a cancer diagnosis."

The abstract of our article follows, and it is also on Dr. Yu's website under Publications.

Frederick T. Guilford, MD

Antiparasitic and Antifungal Medications for Targeting Cancer Cells Literature Review and Case Studies

Frederick T. Guilford, MD; Simon Yu, MD

Alternative Therapies in Health and Medicine, **2019 Jul; 25(4):26-31.**

ABSTRACT

Context • Chronic inflammation is a new catch phrase for the explanation of all chronic degenerative diseases, from asthma, arthritis, heart disease, auto-immune disease, and irritable bowel disease to cancer. Occult infections from oncovirus, bacterial, and fungal infections as well as from lesser known parasitic infections are driving forces in the cellular evolution and degeneration of cancer cells. An approach using currently available medications that target both fungal and parasitic metabolism appears to interfere with the metabolic synergy that is associated with tumor growth and aggressiveness.

Objective • The review examined whether antiparasitic and antifungal medications that interfere with the metabolism of cancers, can be useful in cancer therapy by treating cancer as an infectious disease and as a metabolic parasite. Design • The research team searched the National Center for Biotechnology Information (NCBI) PubMed database databases, using different keyword combinations, including repurposed drug, antifungal, antiparasitic, cancer, parasite, anti-cancer repurposed.

Setting • Prevention and Healing, St Louis, MO, USA.

Results • The literature search identified a number of studies, including in vitro, in vivo and clinical, which support the use of antifungal and antiparasitic medication in the treatment of cancer. In the clinical area, the authors observed benefit from the use of antifungal and antiparasitic medication in the treatment of a variety of cancer cases.

Conclusions • Due to the complexity of the behavior and biology of cells, scientists' primary focus should be on detection and elimination of sources of inflammation. Antiparasitic medications, and also antiviral, antibiotic, and antifungal medications should be thought of as underrecognized, underappreciated, and forgotten medications that can be part of cancer therapy. The information offered in this review suggests scientists should think of cancer not only as a metabolic disease but also as a metabolic parasite and should consider using antiparasitic medications under a new understanding of the role of inflammation, infection, and mitochondrial dysfunction in development of cancer cells.[23]

Frederick T. Guilford, MD, is the Medical Director at Your Energy Systems, LLC, located in Palo Alto, CA, USA. Simon Yu, MD, is the Medical Director at Prevention and Healing, located in St Louis, MO, USA.

Bite, Breathing, Brainstem (BBB), and More:
Better Bite, Better Life

Orthodontists who specialize in TMJ and bite issues are a rare breed within the dental profession. When I think of orthodontics, I automatically think of preteens and teenagers wearing braces to correct crooked teeth for cosmetic reasons, and for a beautiful smile. There are even fewer orthodontists focusing on bite, breathing, sleep apnea, unexplained pain syndrome, and brainstem connections. Let me introduce some offbeat upbeat odd dentists who can change your health far better than many MDs.

Albert Einstein said, "The world we have created is a product of our thinking; it cannot be changed without changing our thinking. If we want to change the world, we have to change our thinking... no problem can be solved from the same consciousness that created it. We must learn to see the world anew." I got this quote from Paul Greenacre, DDS from Ottawa, Canada from many of his writings on Bite, Breathing, Brainstem, Breastfeeding, and the Biofeedback neurological concept of dental distress.

We have been corresponding on why proper dental bite is vital. I am familiar with these subjects and have written many dental-related articles, see my last book, *AcciDental Blow Up in Medicine*, and the dental category articles in my blog. I am not a dentist and cannot fix dental problems. We need offbeat orthodontists who think differently about bites, breathing and brainstem.

> **We need offbeat orthodontists who think differently about bite, breathing, and brainstem.**

Here is a list of the benefits of correcting misaligned dental bite which correspond with those of A.C. Fonder, DDS, founder of holistic dentistry, and author of, *The Dental Distress Syndrome*:

1. Better breathing so less airway distress, less snoring and less sleep apnea.
2. Improved head posture and spinal alignment after palatal expansion and jaw realignment. Improved scoliosis, kyphosis, and less back pain.
3. Neckaches and tension improved.
4. Learning difficulties improve and less ADHD.
5. Eliminate migraines and chronic morning headaches and other trigeminal nervous system issues like scalp pain or head itchiness.
6. Fewer menstrual difficulties and less erectile dysfunction. Improved fertility.
7. Improved autonomic nervous system functioning resulting in better digestion, less constipation and GI problems. Improved ability to relax, refresh and restore bodies and minds.
8. Faster recovery from PTSD, concussions, whiplash, sports trauma, and car accident injuries.
9. Recovery from fatigue, anxiety, depression, and mental or mood disorders.
10. Warmer hands and feet; may improve thyroid function.
11. Recover from some trigeminal neuralgias and reduce epileptic seizures.
12. Improved balance and equilibrium.

13. Improved ENT related problems and ear pain.

14. Improved athletic and scholastic performance.

15. Improved pregnancy outcomes.

16. Less jaw related TMJ and facial pain.

17. General relaxation and feeling of reduced stress.

Past ENT specialist Henry Uhlemeyer, MD wrote, as reported by Greenacre, that if the mandible (lower jaw) is not physiologically positioned, stress hormones are automatically stimulated, muscles tense, blood pressure rises to overcome resistance, pulse quickens, respiration is shallow and loses efficiency. The body raises blood sugar to fuel response to emergency, release adrenaline, and increase the pain threshold. In his opinion, the mandible is the electrical control coordinator for the whole body: the mandible must be in a physiologically balanced relationship to make the entire body work as one balanced unit.

> **The mandible is the electrical control coordinator for the whole body: the mandible must be in a physiologically balanced relationship to make the entire body work as one balanced unit.**

In addition, the trigeminal cranial nerve from the brainstem is where the nerve circuitry for breastfeeding begins. The motion of breastfeeding activates the touching of the tip of the tongue, which contains the 3rd division of the trigeminal nerve. This is the basis of the neurological connection of mother and infant, with the trigeminal nerve helping activate the dominant cranial nerve in the brainstem.

When the trigeminal nerve is under stress, it releases substance P, a noxious neurotransmitter factor affecting cell membrane function, metabolic disruption and involved in chronic pain. The trigeminal nerve travels all the way down the cervical spine, as far as C4, and is right next to the vagus nerve in the brainstem. The tongue is innervated by the trigeminal, vagus, and cranial nerves 7, 9, and 12.

But wait, there's more! I have witnessed Gary Wiele, DDS from St. Louis, and Donald R. Moeller, MD, DDS from Georgia, correct the bite of Parkinson's-like patients with severe hand tremors almost disappearing. Dr. Moeller wrote, "Intraoral devices with specific modifications are able to rapidly modify the gait, stability and posture of some patients." Moeller coauthored a dental journal article on how similar intraoral devices can reduce nightmares, headaches and sleep disruptions in PTSD patients.[24]

> **"Intraoral devices with specific modifications are able to rapidly modify the gait, stability, and posture of some patients." – Donald R. Moeller, MD, DDS**

I additionally thank Dr. Felix Liao, DDS for his book, *Six-Foot Tiger, Three-Foot Cage: Take Charge of Your Health by Taking Charge of Your Mouth,* which connects the dots between mouth structure and total health.[25] "Six-foot tiger" is the medical, dental, mood, and financial consequences of a "three-foot cage" — a mouth that's too small for the tongue. Oxygen deficiency, poor sleep, and more can result.

This may be more than you want to know about bite, breathing, and brainstem. The position of the bite influences and affects many physiological manifestations and requires specialized orthodontic dentists to evaluate and correct dental distress signals that can significantly improve your health.

Acupuncture Meridian Assessment (AMA) can easily detect bite-related problems, which are often exaggerated by parasite infections causing bruxism - grinding teeth - showing up in the lymphatic system of the jaw. Parasites, dental distress, vagus-trigeminal nerve disturbances, and the brain are inseparably interconnected. This is a new concept of "thinking differently" about medical-dental connections, thanks to Dr. Greenacre, Dr. Moeller, and other offbeat upbeat odd dentists.

Guidelines for Treating Dental Infections

Based on my experience, here are some key guidelines for treating dental, oral, and jaw infections. AMA indicates which teeth or jaw areas have problems, and which medications help rebalance them.

- Bacterial infections may play a smaller part than originally thought in periodontal disease, while parasites and fungi play a larger part.

- Once established in the oral cavity, parasites become the dominant organism in the periodontal pocket. With no known enemies, they are the hidden kingmaker of most modern chronic "incurable" diseases.

- Amoxicillin or Augmentin are typically prescribed by dentists, but they do not cover anaerobic infections or spirochete infections well.

- A combination of doxycycline (or azithromycin), tinidazole and clindamycin (beware of potential side effects), along with antifungal nystatin, covers much better the broad spectrum of dental infections, and Lyme disease hiding under teeth.

- Most parasites can ensure survival by having a resistant form as either cysts or eggs with complex life cycles and interaction with our good and not-so-friendly microbiomes.

- It will take multiple cycles of different combinations of parasite, fungal and antibiotic medications that can last over a year while correcting one's diet, nutrition, biological terrain, and metabolism.

Dental work is costly. My advice to patients is that all dental work should be done in stages, with heavy metals and infection cleared and areas well healed before considering tooth replacement options. This is a lower risk strategy than a comprehensive plan that combines all treatment and restoration and assumes success before it is demonstrated to work for you over time. You can also consider using different dentists for various parts of your work.

Mercury fillings (dental amalgam is 50 percent mercury) should typically be removed first as mercury impairs immune response and has neurological impacts. This should be done by a biological dentist who uses the Safe Mercury Amalgam Removal Technique (SMART) protocol, thesmartchoice.com. It is advisable to have a biocompatibility test to inform your selection of crown materials and bonding agents to replace fillings.

Extractions should be performed by an experienced biological dentist or oral surgeon. As explained in my articles, infection is not always visible on X-ray or CBCT scans. If there is an energetic disturbance it is an indicator of chronic degeneration or acute infection, and it must be addressed to restore a healthy terrain and lower the burden on the immune system. Some dentists call this "restoring the meridian."

Many biological dentists are taught and consider surgery along with ozone and platelet-rich fibrin (PRF), along with vitamin C, sufficient to clear infections during extraction or cavitation surgery but in my experience, that is not always the case.

Use AMA medication testing to determine which combination will address the many oral pathogens and start treatment right before or after surgery. Pathogens can be documented by use of a dental DNA test like DNA Connexions; the results take a few weeks so start treatment with extraction or oral surgery.

Figure 48:
Acupuncture Meridian Assessment Before and After Test Plate with Tinidazole/Ivermectin

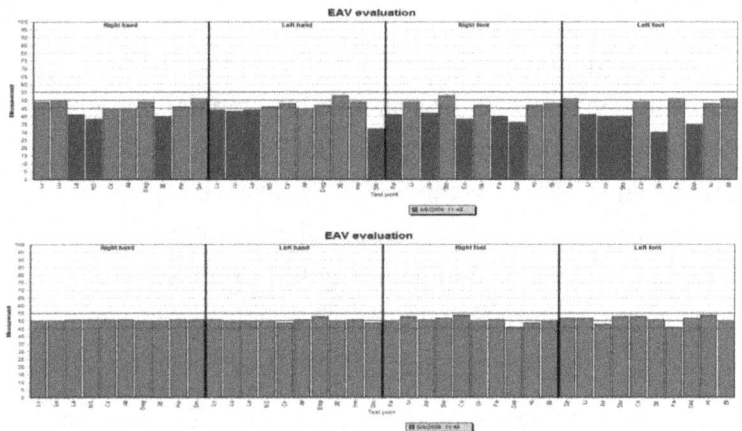

Part 5
Cancer: Infection, Inflammation, and Mitochondrial Dysregulation

Chapter 9 Cancer: Who is Afraid of Cancer?

Don't let fear control you when you are diagnosed with cancer. Big pharma sells fear for profit. Fear is a big selling tool for patients to go through chemotherapy, radiation therapy, immunotherapy and radical surgery. The cancer industry, like the military-industrial complex, is a big lucrative business and needs a perpetual war on cancer. The War on Cancer is misdirected and misguided. There are a lot more options to choose than you may think.

Cancer rates are increasing, especially among younger people. We don't see or witness all the changes in our environment, soil, food supply, additives, processing, etc. The rise in EMF throughout our homes, schools and workplaces put additional stress on our immune systems. New synthetic biology for delivery of drugs and vaccines further confuse our immune systems and create metabolic, mitochondrial, and immune dysregulation. This chapter will cover options to augment and strengthen your battle plan for cancer.

Metabolic Therapy for Cancer: Theory and Practice - Keys to Longevity

Theory: Metabolic therapy is an important part of overall cancer therapy but not a cure for all cancer. Let me explain. Metabolic therapy for cancer has been championed by Professor Thomas Seyfried from Boston College in his book, *Cancer as a Metabolic Disease* (2012).[26] He validates Dr.

Warburg's theory for the origin of cancer with its monumental finding: most cancer is a singular disease of mitochondrial respiratory abnormality coupled with compensatory fermentation. The Warburg effect involves the continued fermentation of glucose in the presence of oxygen.

There has been momentum in the integrative medical community to promote this concept of metabolic therapy as a viable, safer cancer therapy with a strict ketogenic diet and "press and pulse" concept using supplements and medications to attack vulnerable, abnormal cancer cells' mitochondrial function. I have known Dr. Seyfried for many years; we both gave talks on several occasions at medical conferences. He spoke about "Cancer is a Metabolic Disease" on cancer cell biology and ketogenic diet, and my lectures addressed dental, parasites, and fungal infections connected with most chronic diseases and cancers.

Chronic inflammation has been linked to carcinogenesis by a cascade of cellular signals of cytokines, nitric oxide, transforming growth factor (TGF-beta), etc. This leads to eventual injury to mitochondrial function and mitochondrial respiratory abnormality, responsible for the development of cancer. Many underlying factors are driving inflammation; see the figure below for stresses on metabolic function of mitochondria.

A calorie-restricted ketogenic diet will put more stress on cancer mitochondria and slow the progression of cancer cells' development and metastasis. Dr. Seyfried's book covers this in detail. Below is a diagram adapted from Dr. Young Hee Ko, PhD of Johns Hopkins, who developed 3-Bromopyruvate (3-BP) from her lecture on multiple sources of stressors to mitochondrial abnormality and metabolic dysfunction.[27]

Eventually, cancer cells are metabolically challenged, gasping for glucose and glutamine for energy and cannot effectively use ketones for energy in the early stage of cancer.

Figure 49: Multiple Causes of Mitochondrial Damage

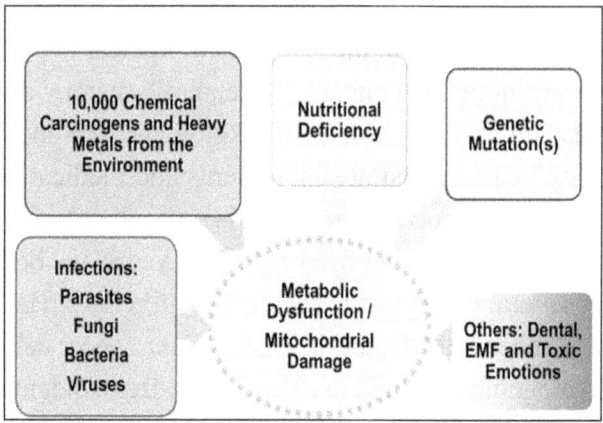

Source: Adapted from Y.H. Ko et al.[28]

> **A calorie-restricted ketogenic diet will put more stress on cancer mitochondria and slow the progression of cancer cells' development and metastasis.**

Practice: Previously, I covered Seyfried/Warburg's work on cancer from the point of view of the human body as a matrix of meridians; we can measure the immeasurable and invisible acupuncture meridians as described in several of my articles. These include: "Cancer is an Infectious Disease as if Cancer is Metabolic Parasites" and, "Metabolic Therapy for Cancer, Theory and Practice: Keys to Longevity – What Can Sabotage a Ketogenic Diet?" describing a calorie-restricted Ketogenic Diet (KD) for cancer therapy. Here are a few important tips:

A) There is no one simple cause and solution to cancer or chronic illness. A combination of factors is in play; each must be addressed in sequence. I use acupuncture meridian assessment (AMA) to help determine the underlying causes in each patient and how to address them. Today's medicine overlooks the role of several vital factors in chronic disease and cancer: parasite infections, fungal infections, dental problems, chemical exposures, and heavy metals. The greatest resistance among patients is reluctance to follow my dental recommendations, for a combination of cost and psychological factors. In addition, dental, parasites, and fungal infections impact the gut and microbiome, and can complicate diet and nutrition strategies.

> **There is no one simple cause and solution to cancer or chronic illness. A combination of factors is in play; each must be addressed in sequence… You will not get well using one therapy alone.**

B) You will not get well using one therapy alone, whether it is standard of care surgery, chemo and radiation, diet, dental procedures, detoxification, prescription drugs, supplements, homeopathy, mind-body, or electrical devices. In some cases, the standard of care can be curative or needed as a last resort. Diet and nutrition alone will not succeed in cancer and chronic illness; they must be addressed in combination with other key factors to restore a healthy biological terrain and immune system.

I have been getting a steady request for consultations from Dr. Seyfried's online referrals, and I simply cannot handle email requests for guidance and consultations without seeing patients. My evaluation consists of a hands-on evaluation including acupuncture meridian assessment (AMA) to map out disturbances in the energy flow through the meridians. My focus has been detecting two main factors that conventional academic medicine has overlooked for many years: parasite-fungal infections and dental problems driving hidden chronic inflammation. Parasites can sabotage metabolic therapy, and a ketogenic diet becomes less effective. Let me explain.

This is my quick overview of a metabolic therapy diet based on Dr. Seyfried's work and my interpretation of his recommendations. I want to thank Dr. Seyfried for reviewing this article; for more information see his blog at tomseyfried.com/blog, and faculty profile at Boston College. There are also helpful materials on the website of Alicia Halakas, PA, who collaborates with Dr. Seyfried.

The following recommendations are part of my Internal Medicine/Integrative Medicine practice:

1) Dr. Seyfried does not claim a ketogenic diet will cure cancer, but it is important to understand that cancer cell biology and cancer cells depend largely on glucose and glutamine metabolism for survival, growth, and proliferation. Exploiting the weakness of cancer cell mitochondria by restricting caloric intake with a ketogenic diet, lowering blood glucose, and raising ketones, gives brain cancer patients with glioblastoma multiforme better survival outcomes and extends survival rates, not necessarily a cure. Most patients have significant asymptomatic dental infections and parasite infections in my clinical observation that must be addressed ASAP.

> **Most patients have significant asymptomatic dental infections and parasite infections in my clinical observation that must be addressed ASAP.**

2) To start a calorie-restricted ketogenic diet, you need to buy a glucometer and ketone meter and start measuring glucose and ketone. Measure your blood sugar and ketone levels in the

morning, before and after meals. After a while, you will get the feeling of interconnection between what you eat and your blood glucose and ketone levels. Ketone strips are rather expensive, and these can easily add up in cost.

3) Start your diet slowly. You can eat two meals per day and eventually one meal per day plus small keto snacks. You may consult a dietician/nutritionist who can guide you individually. My clinic does not have an in-house dietitian, and my staff are not trained to give recommendations. I have written several articles on nutritional therapy for cancer and general dietary guidelines; see for example, "Diet, Nutrition, Weight Loss and Longevity." If you want to jumpstart a keto diet, start with a water fast for 5 days. Sugar accelerates cancer growth! It is not easy to do a 5-day fast if you are not used to fasting. I tried it, so I know!

4) Start by setting your intake to 50 percent fat, 30 percent protein, and 20 percent carbohydrates. Then, start adjustment of fat and carbohydrates first, then protein. You can adjust and increase consumption of fat up to 70 percent while lowering protein to 20 percent and carbohydrate to 10 percent based on your blood glucose and ketone levels. Unless you are highly motivated, you need a dietician or nutritionist to help you with calorie counting. The goal is to starve glucose-glutamine-dependent cancer cells and support the whole body on a calorie-restricted keto diet.

5) Hair tissue mineral analysis is highly recommended in my practice. Hair tissue mineral composition and the ratios of macro-minerals (calcium, magnesium, sodium, and potassium) provide a measure of your unique metabolic state for the last several months. Metabolic typing as a fast oxidizer or slow oxidizer predicts what kind of diet you need, can indicate

mineral deficiencies, possible heavy metal exposures, etc. Most cancer patients have significant heavy metal toxicity and need a DMPS/EDTA chelating agent to provoke and unmask hidden heavy metal exposure, which is much more sensitive than hair tissue mineral analysis.

6) Food allergy testing (IgG delayed response) is also highly recommended. You will be surprised: you might be allergic to mushrooms, asparagus, or broccoli. The most common allergens are wheat, corn, soy, peanuts, and dairy. You may not realize it and try to eat more when you are not feeling well, and then feel worse, and you cannot guess because it is a delayed IgG response.

7) Know your glucose/ketone ratio if you are serious about metabolic diet therapy. Try to bring your sugar level below 80-90 and continue to lower the level to 60-70 and raise the blood ketone level to 3 or higher. (You need to convert blood sugar level to mmol/liter: mg/dL = 18 x mmol/L). For example: blood sugar of 100mg/dL divided by 18 will give you 5.55 mmol/L. If your ketone level is at 3, your glucose/ketone index is 5.55 divided by 3 = 1.83. The goal is to bring the glucose/ketone index below 2.0 and ideally 1.0, if possible, especially for brain tumors like glioblastoma. You may add commercial ketone supplements to achieve a better ratio. This is not easy to follow without any dietician or nutritional assistance. Different types of cancer require an individualized, modified ketogenic diet.

8) Don't be too hard on yourself if you cannot bring your blood sugar level below 80 or ketone level above 3. Intermittent fasting is another option. You still have a chance to recover from cancer by addressing other factors. Many of my patients will not commit, give up, or lose too much weight. Some are

too focused on the ketogenic diet and denial on dental problems, parasite infections, and environmental toxins. Ketogenic metabolic therapy has become well-known to the public, often with unrealistic expectations. The impact of parasite infections and dental problems with cancer is relatively unknown to the public and academic medicine.

9) Medications that can potentially target aerobic glycolysis include 2-deoxyglucose (2-DG), 3-bromopyruvate (3-BP), dichloroacetate, and resveratrol. The "press and pulse" concept is seeking to lower glucose levels with a calorie-restricted keto diet followed by a glucose-like compound or glutamine-like compound. I have problems getting these and they are not part of my regimen. The glutamine pathway inhibition recommended by Dr. Seyfried using the glutamine analog drug, 6-diazo-5-oxo-L-norleucine (DON) is only available to researchers. I tried but couldn't obtain it. The side effects can be serious; it is not recommended for general practitioners.

10) You may use more natural glutamine inhibitors containing Ursolic Acid, Caffeic Acid, Hesperidin, and EGCG marketed in Europe; search the internet for natural glutamine inhibitors. Ursolic Acid is found in Rosmarinus, Caffeic Acid is found in Propolis, Hesperidin is found in Bitter Orange, and EGCG is found in green tea. The Keto Diet reduces tumor cell proliferation, glycolysis, inflammation, and angiogenesis in tumor cells and their microenvironment. Other potential medications targeting cancer cells include metformin and antibiotics such as doxycycline and azithromycin; antiparasitic medications, e.g., ivermectin, albendazole, mebendazole, praziquantel, niclosamide; and antifungal medications, e.g. itraconazole and fluconazole.

Think Differently. All chronic diseases, cancer and neurological diseases may benefit from a modified ketogenic diet. Inflammation will improve, weight loss is expected, resulting in better management of diabetic patients and obese patients. It is not easy to follow a strict diet for prolonged periods, but it will be a good start to stabilize your metabolic state, and support mitochondria function. Consider a food allergy rotation diet and hair tissue mineral analysis for metabolic typing and vitamin and mineral replacements. To have a successful ketogenic diet, you need family support and commitment to change. I send you my encouragement to stay on course: don't be discouraged and find a good dietitian/nutritionist to guide you.

Is there a skeptics' view of metabolic therapy for cancer? Most oncologists do not embrace for various reasons and will discourage you from trying. Peter Pedersen, MD of Johns Hopkins, another giant in the field of tumor mitochondria and the bioenergetics of cancer, points out that Warburg never stated that a generalized structural defect in electron transport was responsible for the origin of cancer, but rather "insufficient abnormal respiration" was responsible. But, how? The subtle differences may have profound implications for the management of cancer patients in the future. Stay tuned for more scientific debates.

My quick summary on Metabolic Therapy for Cancer: Eat Less and You May Live Longer. Monitor your glucose and ketone levels. Keep glucose levels below 80 and ketone levels above 3 to 4, and glucose/ketone ratio 2.0 or below, if possible, especially for brain tumor patients. Parasites trigger inflammation and may control your mind. They can make you crave sweets and sabotage metabolic therapy for cancer.

You may want to start with parasite-fungal meds first and then you may have an easier time lowering your glucose level. If you are interested in my approach, review my website, make an appointment, and see me in person. It is essential for my clinical evaluation and recommendations. I do not do teleconferences or telemedicine and cannot respond to individual emails or general questions.

The Holy Grail of Antiaging is in your hands:
Biohacking Wnt signaling pathway to beat cancer

What is the Wnt signaling pathway and why would you want to unlock its secrets?

What on Earth is Wingless-Int-1 (Wnt)?

In cellular biology, the **Wnt signaling pathways** are a group of signal transduction pathways which begin with proteins that pass signals into a cell through cell surface receptors. The name Want, pronounced "wint", is a portmanteau created from the names Wingless and Int-1…Wnt signaling was first identified for its role in carcinogenesis, then for its function in embryonic development.

Source: Wikipedia

The Wnt/beta-catenin ("Wnt" for short) signaling pathway can be applied to antiaging, cancer, and many chronic degenerative diseases. The Wnt signaling pathway is a complex, complicated network of proteins and peptides known for its role in regulation of proliferation, differentiation, migration, regeneration, polarity, and gene expression from embryonic stems to development in adult tissues.

Wnt was discovered in 1982 by cancer researchers. In 2012, K. Hoffmeyer et al published an article in *Science*, "Wnt B-Catenin signaling regulates telomerase in stem cells and cancer cells.[29]" Big pharma is racing and betting on who will first develop the molecules that will control the Wnt signaling pathway. Billions of dollars are at stake for developing and marketing blockbuster drugs, potentially bigger than statins and Ozempic combined.

For the last 25 years, I have been writing about parasite medications successfully treating many different medical conditions beyond parasite infections, describing the phenomenon as an "Accidental Cure." It might be asthma, MS, autoimmune diseases of all kinds, Lyme, CFS/ME, cancer, etc. Is it possible that parasite medications are doing more than just killing parasites? Most well-known parasite medications like ivermectin and niclosamide have been proven to regulate the Wnt signaling pathway. Is this an unintended, ultimate, somewhat accidental biohacking, or just plain dumb luck?

Biohacking is citizen "do-it-yourself" biology: making small, incremental changes in diet, exercise, lifestyle, supplements, etc. to catalyze small improvements in health and well-being. Changes in blood chemistry, blood pressure, body weight, energy level, heart rhythms, blood, cholesterol, sleep patterns, and more provide calibration of measurable impacts to improve health. There are different types or forms of biohacking, including nutrigenomics, DIY biology, and more. Early leaders such as Dave Asprey have fueled a growing movement for health self-improvement.

People have also been hacking the medical system and taking parasite meds on their own for vexing, unexplainable medical conditions when their physicians could not help them.

Fenbendazole has been very popular with cancer patients after Joe Tippens' testimonial for his terminal lung cancer.[30] A young MIT engineer figured out how to use parasite meds to heal herself from unexplained illness. I wrote about her in my article, "Parasite Treatment Hacked by an MIT Engineer: Think Small, Dream Big for Pandemic." You can visit her website, Debug Your Health, at debugyourhealth.com.

Understanding the complexity of biochemistry, metabolic pathways, and immune system regulations is intimidating, making it almost impossible to micromanage each pathway without the consequence of unpredictable chain reactions and side effects. It needs some assistance from AI.

At Medical Week 2024 in Baden-Baden, Germany, I gave a lecture, "Parasites, Fungal, Dental Infections and Cancer: Unconventional Diagnostics and Therapies." My thesis is there is a simpler way to regulate the Wnt signaling pathway by incorporating unconventional diagnostics to navigate and bypass complex biochemical-metabolic pathways using acupuncture meridian assessment (AMA). It is like inspecting the body's bioelectrical frequencies like a violin and tuning them to a harmonious musical scale, using the meridian system based on ancient intelligence.

Figure 50 below depicts the Wnt signaling pathway controlling cell differentiation vs. proliferation. Figure 51 lists parasite medications that also target cancer cells. Niclosamide, on the top right side of the graph is a common parasite medication, downregulating the Wnt signaling pathway. Niclosamide, mebendazole, praziquantel, and ivermectin (white color) work well in synergy for GI-related cancer.

Figure 50: Wnt Signaling Pathway

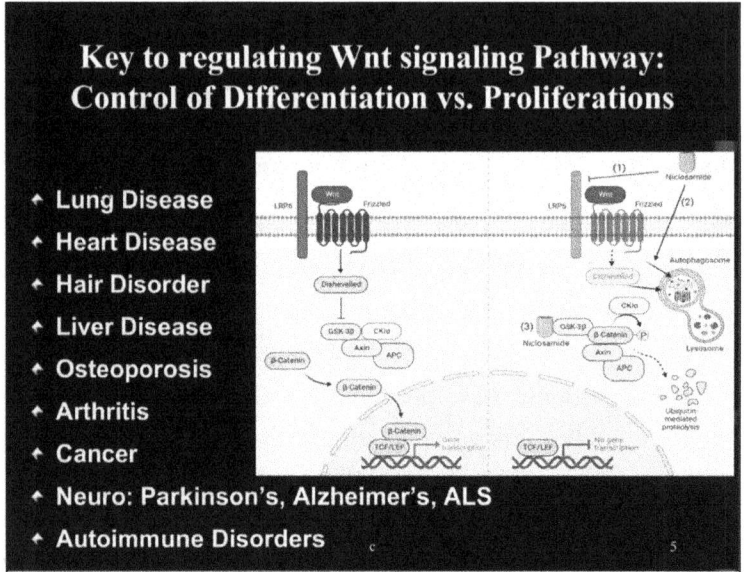

Figure 51: Medications Targeting Cancer Cells

Parasite-Fungal Medications Targeting Cancer Cells

Ivermectin	12mg	tid to qid 2-3-4 wks
Mebendazole	100mg	
Praziquantel	600mg	
(Niclosamide)	500mg	
Azithromycin	500mg	
Tinidazole	500mg	
Nystatin	500,000ug	
Followed by		
Doxycycline	100mg	tid to qid 2-3-4 wks
Fluconazole	100mg	
Itraconazole	100mg	
(3-Bromopyruvate)		

Dental related infections are covered by azithromycin, and by tinidazole or metronidazole and nystatin (orange color). Doxycycline for intracellular parasites (orange color) and fungal infections are covered by fluconazole and itraconazole (bottom white color). Dr. Tim Guilford and I published an article on this topic, "Antiparasitic and Antifungal Medications for Targeting Cancer Cells: Literature Review and Case Studies," in *Alternative Therapies in Health and Medicine*. (Jul 14, 2019).

My Medical Week lecture was videotaped soon after in my clinic and is available on YouTube.[31] Biohacking using Acupuncture Intelligence (AI 2.0) involves more than just taking parasite medications as listed in Figure 51:

- These are what I use 80 percent of the time with slightly different combinations of natural remedies, homeopathic and prescription medications.
- Diet and nutritional support are also important. Typically for cancer patients, I recommend a diet with 50 percent good fats, 30 percent protein and 20 percent carbohydrates, with the selection of foods based on a food allergy test and blood type diet.
- Hair tissue mineral analysis provides information on your metabolic type and on nutritional support needed based on mineral levels and ratios.
- Detoxification is important, I recommend a gallbladder/liver flush once per month for 6-12 months.
- Dental infections and environmental toxins are separate but overlapping issues that must be addressed concurrently.

The Wnt signaling pathway is an ancient, evolutionary-based pathway for survival. Aberrations in the Wnt signaling pathway are associated with birth defects, and a multitude of chronic diseases and cancer. The meridian system and acupuncture have been known for thousands of years, practiced throughout Asia, and are now widely practiced globally. However, most acupuncturists who do pulse-diagnosis do not actually measure the meridians as a system. Dr. Reinhold Voll, MD, of Germany developed Electro-acupuncture according to Dr. Voll (EAV, which I have simplified and adapted as Acupuncture Meridian Assessment (AMA.

It is time to embrace ancient, authentic intelligence (AI 2.0 to outsmart artificial Intelligence (AI and enhance biohacking. Apply parasite and antifungal meds based on AMA to simplify, correcting upstream problems and revealing commonly overlooked dental problems and environmental toxins that burden the immune system. Regulate and control the Wnt signaling pathway to bypass and streamline complex biochemical interactions, metabolic pathways and immune regulations by using antiparasitics, antifungals, and antibiotics. Biohacking with the guidance of AMA or other forms of energetic testing is like uncovering the Holy Grail of antiaging, chronic disease, and beating cancer in your hands, working with your physician and biological dentist as a guide.

Patient Story: Prostate Cancer Treatment

I started having problems with my prostate. My pain increased so I went to my urologist. He said I needed a biopsy and after this procedure I found out I had stage 4 advanced cancer. I started external radiation treatments, and during this time my blood work showed my PSA level rising to a high level. I did another biopsy which showed that the cancer had spread to my bladder. They couldn't do more operations or seeding, which is placing radiation pellets in your prostate, because it had spread. Cut and burn were my treatment choices. When you do this procedure, they warn you not to have any pets or children sitting in your lap due to the risk of radiation poisoning.

Just after radiation treatments my cancer doctor told me that the best option was to have my prostate and bladder removed. I told them I'm an old man and that the operation would be very hard on me, and I wanted to think about it. My doctors were very concerned that I didn't understand this is what I needed.

I went online to research and read the book, *World Without Cancer*, by Edward Griffin, and started to learn more about cancer. I found Joe Tippens' account about parasites causing cancer symptoms. I started taking fenbendazole, ivermectin, and chlorine dioxide. Within a month, my PSA level started dropping to a low level. I told my doctors what I was doing. Two of them didn't want to know any more about it; one seemed interested, and I gave him a copy of the book.

Now the weird stuff: while urinating during the radiation treatment, I found a lot of objects being released. I captured most of those and showed them to my urologist, and he said, "Oh Joe, that's just scabs from the biopsy." I bought a microscope to look at these scabs; they were not typical scabs but very strange looking objects, and some had what I consider worms on them. One day I felt something large coming out. I was very scared of what was happening. I captured it, it was pointed at both ends, larger in the center, segmented, and a dull white color. It was 3 mm long and 1 mm larger in the center. To my eyes it looked at a worm.

I told my doctors about this, and they didn't seem to be interested. None of the doctors I saw had a microscope, so I brought mine with me with samples for them to look at. They didn't want to. One doctor said, "Joe, I don't know what you're doing, just keep doing it." My cancer doctor told me that it looks like I am in remission. Over a year and a half later I still feel fine, with no pain.

On a side note, I ordered fenbendazole and ivermectin from India. When it got to New York City, Customs confiscated it and sent me a letter saying they were returning it to the sender in India. I wrote back and told them it is sold over the counter in USA for pets. They sent another letter saying they were still sending it back. I wrote them again and said I needed to know under what section and article the FDA has that authority.

Later my neighbor came to me and said, "Joe, it looks like this box belongs to you." It was my order from India, but my name had been blocked with a pen. There was barely enough of the address visible for the post office to deliver it but to a nearby wrong address. When I ordered it from India, I tried to use my credit card, but it was denied, though I have plenty of credit. I used Bitcoin and that went right through. I want people to know that there are other options besides cut and burn, and they should do their own research and understand that there could be other ways of handling this problem.

Leukemia and Lymphoma: Simple Solution A Possibility?

In August 2022, I saw a 56-year-old man from Chicago with diagnosis of chronic myelogenous leukemia (CML) in 2019. He said he had every test under the sun, including a bone marrow biopsy and genetic testing. He received chemotherapy and developed cardiac atrial fibrillation, had a minimal response to chemo, and switched to Spryrcel (dasatinib). His original white blood cell count (WBC) was 82,000 (normal range: 3,400 to 10,800); his blood counts were stabilized, not rising but not normalized yet. Is there a simple solution for an overlooked area that can lead to blindsided misdiagnosis and mistreatment of leukemia and lymphoma cases?

Leukemia and lymphoma are malignant blood-forming cancers, proliferating in the bone marrow and lymphoid tissues, respectively, and spill over to peripheral blood and infiltrate lymph nodes and other tissues. Leukemias are classified into two main types, myeloid or lymphoid; and acute or chronic. Treatment and prognosis are different depending on age, stage, and type of leukemia. The cause of leukemia is not known in most patients, although genetic and environmental factors are driving the proliferation of lymphoid or myelogenous (bone marrow) blood cells according to mainstream academic medicine.

The physical exam for the 56-year-old man from Chicago with CML was normal. He did not appear in any distress. His dental X-ray showed three root canals, and AMA assessment showed 14 out of 40 meridians were out of balance. See Figure 52.

Figure 52: Initial AMA Evaluation

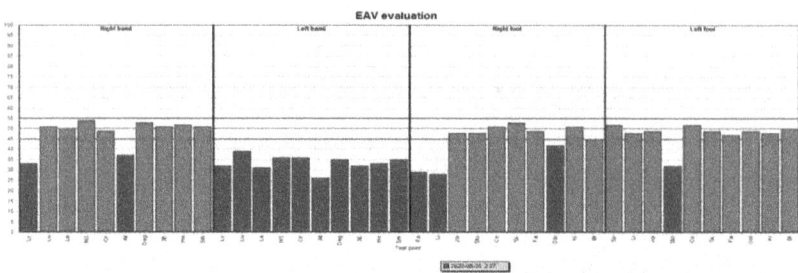

The figure shows 10 readings each from his right and left hands and feet, a total of 40 points. The middle (45-55) bars are within normal range. Low bars (under 45) are chronic, out of balance. Each meridian has been known and described in detail for thousands of years and this is not new information.

I started him on ivermectin, mebendazole, praziquantel, niclosamide, doxycycline, tinidazole, and nystatin plus homeopathic and nutritional support therapies based on EAV-Acupuncture Meridian Assessment (AMA). Five months later, all his root canals and dental amalgams were out. He finished multiple rounds of parasite and fungal meds, and his white blood cell counts were normal at 3,800. It is too early to tell if he is cured. Perhaps his new med, Spryrcel (dasatinib) became more effective after taking care of dental and parasite problems. Coincidence, or a simple solution for potentially life-threatening medical problems with leukemia?

I call this EAV-AMA evaluation, a 5,000-year-old (new) disruptive technology. For more information, see my article, "Acupuncture Meridian Assessment – "New" Medicine Based on Ancient Principles."

Previously, I wrote about two cases of chronic lymphocytic leukemia; both patients were physicians. One responded after extraction of infected teeth, parasite/fungal medications, and chelation therapy for heavy metals. Also, his diabetes mellitus resolved, and severe psoriasis/eczema disappeared. The other physician did not respond and continued to progress. Later he found out he had a massive environmental toxic exposure from growing up on Long Island near a toxic dump. He was not aware of the early life environmental toxin exposure, and he did not respond to my therapy. See my article, "Environmental Toxic Chemicals and Mysterious Illness: A Tale of Two Leukemia Patients."

I recently saw a 65-year-old man with lymphoma with very enlarged lymph nodes around his neck from Florida. He refused the recommended chemotherapy. My recommendation was to extract root canals, remove five dental mercury amalgams, do chelation therapy with DMSA and DMPS chelating agents for mercury toxicity, and take parasite medications.

His lymphoma disappeared shortly after all his dental work was done. He tried explaining it to his oncologist, who was not interested in knowing what he did. Too much of a paradigm shift to accept another alternative therapy. I was not treating the cancer but trying to rebalance his 40 meridians and let the body heal itself. See Figure 53, all 40 meridians are in normal range.

His lymphoma disappeared shortly after all his dental work was done. He tried explaining to his oncologist, who was not interested in knowing what he did.

Figure 53: Post-Treatment AMA Evaluation

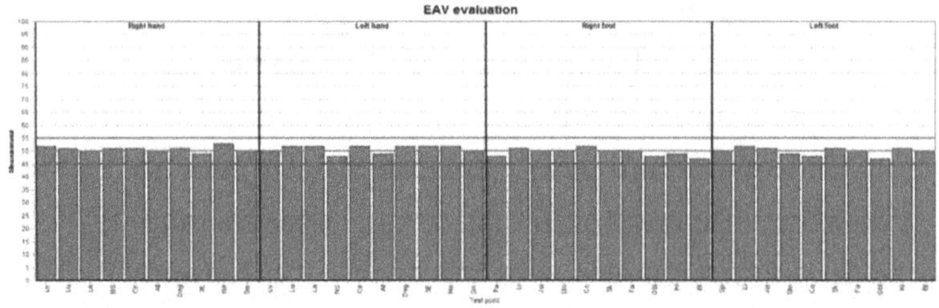

These are not isolated rare cases, but frequent repeatable anecdotes when you can rebalance all 40 meridians. If we can measure, translate, and read the energy field of the individual "unique pattern" based on ancient teaching of the acupuncture meridian system, we can cure the incurable by measuring the unknown. Healing comes from within by going beyond Western Newtonian science and embracing the concept of balancing the subtle Energy Medicine.

In leukemia and lymphoma, it is time to look for simple solutions - addressing overlooked parasites, environmental toxins, and dental problems which are not a part of our medical education - to integrate into our current medical knowledge database. Medical diagnosis can be misleading. A simple solution may come from exploring the ancient wisdom of acupuncture meridian assessment.

> **Medical diagnosis can be misleading. A simple solution may come from exploring the ancient wisdom of acupuncture meridian assessment.**

Patient Story: Mantle Cell Lymphoma

In early 2019 I noticed that I had three swollen lymph glands in my neck. I disregarded them until June, when I decided I should see a doctor. My general practitioner referred me to a surgeon who took them out for biopsy in July. The biopsy revealed I had mantle cell lymphoma. An MRI revealed I had Stage 3 lymphoma.

I was scheduled in September to have a port installed in my upper right chest. Before that surgery I studied the pros and cons of chemotherapy. On the very day the installation of the port was scheduled, I awoke early and read some more on the Internet. I decided against chemotherapy and made the appropriate calls to cancel the surgery. I elected to go a different route, to discover what else could be done without the dangerous side effects of chemotherapy.

In early 2020, I found a local herbalist with a PhD in nutrition. She had unfortunately developed cancer at a young age and had worked up a program to treat herself. She runs her own business and lives a very active lifestyle. Under her instruction I changed my diet to as many organic foods as were available, purchased a water filtration system, and added supplements, vitamins, minerals and herbs to my intake. I gave up sweets, gluten, and lactose. I bought a far infrared sauna for my home use. I made a point of continuing my exercise regimen every day to keep the lymph fluids moving. At the time of my diagnosis, I weighed about 145 pounds at five foot nine inches tall. At this time, I weighed about 120 pounds.

Even so, I remained active and vital. However, there was no sign of overcoming the lymphoma. I began a search for another practitioner, hoping to find a medical doctor who could help me. My wife supports me very strongly, and she had a friend who was seeing and recommended Dr. Simon Yu. In addition, my wife discovered Dr. Dietrich Klinghardt on the Internet. Dr. Klinghardt confirmed in one of his podcasts that Dr. Yu was a colleague. We contacted Dr. Yu's office and scheduled an appointment in April 2021.

Dr. Yu has treated me for the underlying causes of the lymphoma. I have received treatments and medicines to cleanse my body of parasites, heavy metals, and toxic molds. However, Dr. Yu insisted that dental problems had to be rectified before I had any hope of overcoming my illness. The remaining two swollen lymph glands in my neck were unchanged.

I had a dead tooth removed by a biological dentist in Dothan, Alabama in the summer of 2021. In October of 2021 I saw Dr. Wiley Green, a biological dentist in Frankfurt, Indiana. I had three silver/mercury amalgams taken out of teeth on the left side of my mouth and replaced by a nontoxic substance. In November 2021, on the Monday before Thanksgiving, I had the two on the right side of my mouth removed.

Within ten days of the second set of procedures, the swollen lymph glands in my neck were back to normal size. Urine and hair samples have since been analyzed and reveal I am still shedding significant amounts of mercury. Dr. Yu prescribes medicines that facilitate the detox process.

I am absolutely convinced that the removal of the toxic silver/mercury fillings are the key to my recovery. My body is now free of a constant source of a dangerous toxin but can instead focus on fighting lymphoma. I live a full, active life, and look forward to many more years, God willing.

Glioblastoma Multiforme (GBM) Case Studies: Biological Dentistry in Oncology Care

Patients who consult me are typically aware that my specialty is not confined to a specific field within medicine; rather, it encompasses General Internal Medicine and Integrative Medicine. Despite this, I consistently see cancer patients seeking second opinions, who are interested in Acupuncture Meridian Assessment (AMA) to determine potential parasite issues or dental-related problems. I always emphasize that I am not an oncologist—I do not specifically treat cancer, but rather, I treat the whole patient. Two areas often overlooked in medicine are hidden dental infections and parasite infestations.

On occasion, patients inquire about my success rate for specific medical conditions. For instance, I recently consulted with a physician's wife diagnosed with stage 4 colorectal cancer, with metastases to the liver and lung. I explained that I do not specialize in cancer treatment, that I am a solo, private practitioner—not a cancer institution—and that my approach is to address underlying issues rather than directly targeting cancer cells. I also informed her that I do not have statistical data to provide my success rate.

Unsatisfied, she pressed for a success rate. After some thought, I told her that patients willing to extract their infected teeth generally had a better response, a higher survival rate regardless of the choice of therapies she chooses, than those who do not adhere to my dental recommendations, which often involve the extraction of all problematic teeth. From my perspective, the more extractions of bad teeth, the better. However, such recommendations can deter patients who are not prepared for such measures. Her crowned tooth looked normal on dental X-ray, but it was affecting her large intestine and lung, as indicated by AMA and the Tooth-Organ Meridian Chart. As expected, she did not return for follow-up.

The case ended there—no action was taken, no harm was done, but was it the best outcome for her?

The cause of glioblastoma is largely unknown. The prognosis is generally poor, with survival following diagnosis averaging about one year, regardless of whether standard medical care—which often includes craniotomy with brain tumor resection, radiation therapy, and chemotherapy—is administered.

The term glioblastoma multiforme was introduced in 1926, based on the belief that the tumor originates from glial cells. It has a highly variable appearance due to the presence of necrosis, hemorrhage, and cysts.

Over the past two years, I have seen several cases of advanced-stage Glioblastoma Multiforme (GBM). Three of these patients, from Michigan, Washington, and Canada, agreed to extract their teeth. They are still surviving against all odds.

Figure 54 summarizes these cases, which I presented at a cancer talk at IGMEDT in Vienna in 2024. The common denominators included dental problems, parasites, and fungal infections.

Each patient extracted their problematic teeth, took cycles of antiparasitic and antifungal medications, and had insulin potentiation therapy (IPT), along with IV UV/Ozone, IV vitamin C, and chelation, if indicated.

Figure 54: Three Glioblastoma Multiforme Patients

> **Glioblastoma Multiforme**
> **Parasites, Dental Parasites - 3 cases**
>
> - 65-year-old oncologist, s/p craniotomy, chemo and radiation from Washington state
> - 46-year-old Canadian, s/p craniotomy, chemo and radiation
> - 61-year-old from Michigan, s/p craniotomy, s/p *E. coli* infection in the brain, 2nd brain operation, no chemo/radiation
>
> Common Denominators: dental, parasites, IPT, fungal, etc.

Figure 55 below shows the three patients' Acupuncture Meridian Assessments (AMA), translating their medical conditions into unique meridian-based frequency scales.

Figure 55: Initial AMA Readings for Three Glioblastoma Multiforme Patients

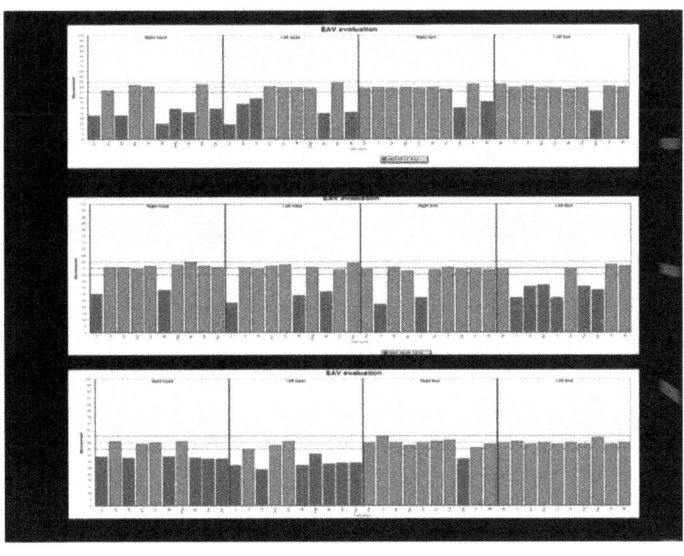

While the shared diagnosis is Glioblastoma Multiforme, each patient exhibits a unique meridian frequency pattern, indicating which meridians were impacted. Medication testing was conducted to see which medications were indicated for each patient. AMA was repeated at each visit to monitor progress and adjust additional treatment.

Below, see each patient's dental panoramic X-rays, marked with stars where teeth were to be extracted, in Figure 56. Although their X-rays appeared normal, my AMA energetic testing indicated infections in all of these cases: 1) two upper root canals and two lower bicuspids, 2) one baby tooth, and 3) one upper and one lower molar.

Figure 56: Panoramic X-rays for Three Glioblastoma Multiforme Patients

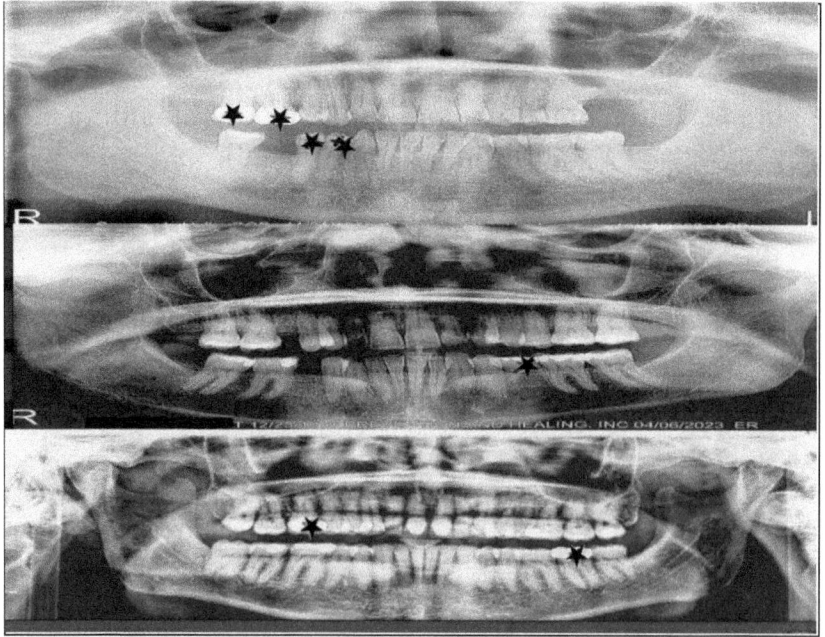

All three beat the odds for their disease, at least for a while.

Case Study: A 46-Year-Old Canadian Patient with Glioblastoma Multiforme (GBM)

This case involves the same 46-year-old Canadian patient who was first diagnosed with glioblastoma in 2022, in more detail than in the previous case study. Following a resection of the frontal lobe, chemotherapy, and radiation, the tumor initially shrank. However, it returned in 2023. When I first saw her in April 2023, she had difficulty speaking and displayed a flat affect with no facial expressions, though she was able to understand and respond with nods. At that time, 13 out of 40 meridians were out of balance.

A significant step in her treatment was the extraction of an infected baby tooth. One year later, she exhibited normal spontaneous expressions, and her speech was articulated. There were no midline shifts in her brain, and all 40 meridians were balanced. She provided me with an old MRI from 2023 (Figure 57) and a new one from May 2024 for comparison (Figure 58).

Figure 57: MRI of Recurrent Tumor, Pre-Visit, April 2023

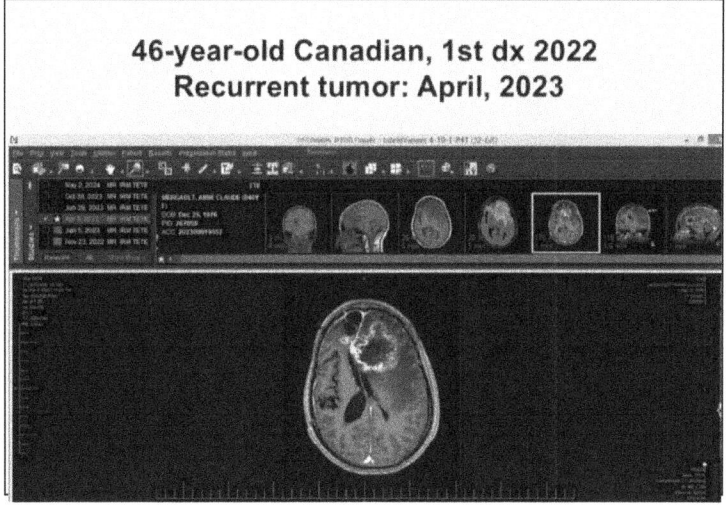

Her treatment regimen included an alternating cycle of ivermectin, pyrantel pamoate, praziquantel, tinidazole, doxycycline, and wormwood for 10 days, followed by oregano oil, nystatin, itraconazole, and fluconazole for 10 days. She was also exposed to high levels of fungal mycotoxins, Ochratoxin A and Mycophenolic Acid.

This cycle was repeated for one year, and she continues to take antiparasitic, antibiotic, and antifungal medications. She underwent insulin potentiation therapy (IPT) twice, IV UV/Ozone, and IV vitamin C, as well as DMPS chelation therapy for high levels of mercury, lead, and gadolinium. Her diet consisted of 50 percent fat, 30 percent protein, and 20 percent carbohydrates, and she followed a food rotation diet based on an allergy test and a blood type O diet.

Figure 58: MRI of Recurrent Tumor, Post-Treatment, May 2024

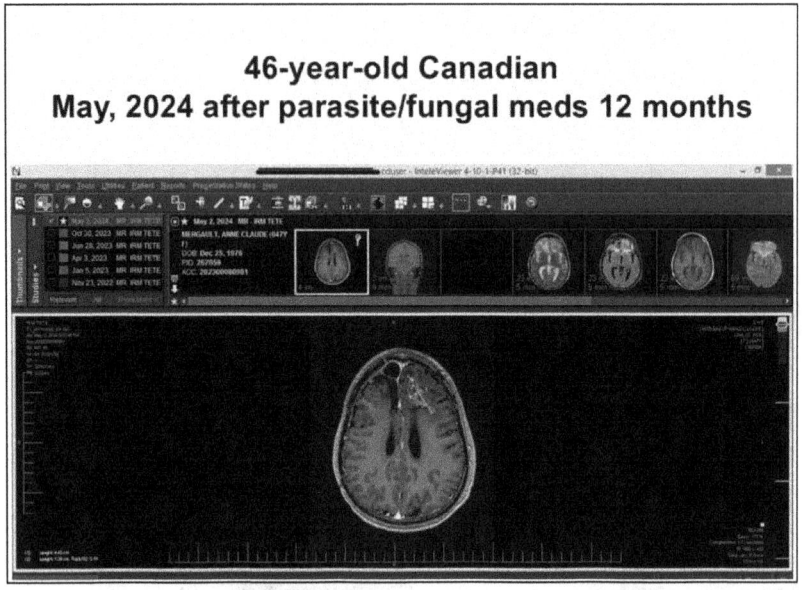

Figure 59: Pre- and Post-Treatment AMA for Canadian Patient

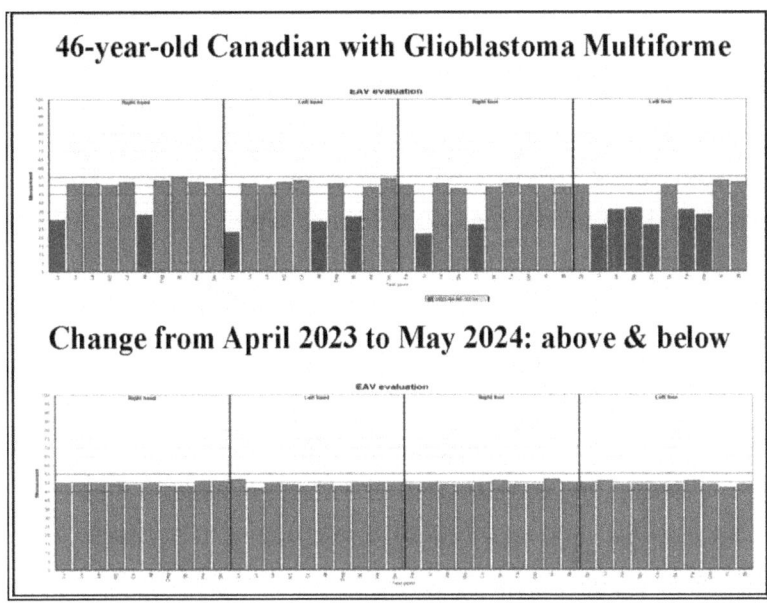

Figure 59 depicts the progress she made. From my perspective, the most crucial step was the extraction of her infected baby tooth, which appeared to be normal on a dental X-ray. This dental infection had been a constant source of infection and inflammation near the brain for many years. Without a biological dentist willing to extract the tooth, her chances of overcoming this deadly brain tumor would have been slim.

Now more than ever, we need biological dentists for all chronically ill patients: those with cancer, Lyme, autoimmune problems, and neurodegenerative diseases. Choosing a biological dentist is like choosing between a red pill or a blue pill—you don't know what you're getting into. I recommend contacting IAOMT or IABDM for a referral to a local biological dentist. Choose your dentist wisely. Biological dentistry is an integral part of oncological care.

Patient Story: We are thankful her mass is resolved

At the suggestion of her doctors, my wife and I made four trips to see Dr. Yu. We believe Dr. Yu was instrumental in her healing. Here is the full story: In April 2022, my wife, who never smoked, had a 2.9 cm x 3.9 cm mass in her left lung. The mass was described by the radiology MD as highly metabolically active, with a glucose uptake value of 27.6, and likely a malignant carcinoma (cancer). The scan showed several lymph nodes "lighting up." The mass was determined to be inoperable by a thoracic surgeon.

My wife underwent no conventional treatment, no biopsy, surgery, chemotherapy, or radiation. She chose instead to work with an internal MD and an integrative oncologist in our area, using natural therapies such as high-dose IV vitamin C, among many other therapies for detoxification and strengthening the immune system.

Dr. Simon Yu identified some small mercury fillings my wife did not realize she had. Dr. Yu treated my wife for both parasites and fungus. Through her experience, we learned that lung masses are often misdiagnosed as lung cancer; and parasites, fungus, and cancer are often present in the same mass. This can create an overwhelming burden on the immune system, making it harder for the body to deal with cancer.

With Dr. Yu's protocol, approved and welcomed by her local doctors, her parasitical and fungal infections were resolved. We believe her body's immune system was then able to attack and destroy the inoperable mass in her left lung, using no chemotherapy or radiation. Her local doctors were also treating her at the same time as she was undergoing Dr. Yu's protocol.

In July of 2023, my wife had a follow-up PET Scan. The radiology MD now described the previous mass as having been completely resolved. Because she had received no chemotherapy or radiation, the radiology MD commented that the mass was most likely non-malignant. We are not sure if we agree with this, however we are very thankful her mass was resolved.

On our first visit with Dr. Yu in St. Louis, quite by chance or otherwise, I met an 80-year-old gentleman who had eight years prior been diagnosed, via a biopsy, with stage-4 inoperable lung cancer. He was given 18 months to live. He was treated by Dr. Yu and is still alive and well, 10 years later. He also had several mercury-filled molars extracted as part of his treatment protocol.

I cannot get into as much detail as I would like to in this review. However, in May of 2022 my wife and I were praying and searching for answers, direction, and truth. We believe God led us to Dr. Simon Yu, along with her local doctors, as we had decided not to get any conventional cancer treatment whatsoever, including a recommended biopsy to "see what the mass was to prescribe the best treatment available." My wife and I highly recommend Dr. Simon Yu and his Prevention and Healing practice. I believe his books will give you some hope and encouragement.

Part 6
Pathogens Hijacking the Genome and Other Unexpected Encounters

Chapter 10 Russian Genetic Roulette, Epigenetic Reprogramming, and Other Topics

Environmental changes are happening rapidly with and without human action and intervention. Genetic engineering and synthetic biology are new phenomena. The consequences are unknown. What are the impacts of genetically modified organisms (GMO) on our food crops and on our health? We are about to find out as subjects of these experiments.

When a single gene is inserted, up to five percent of gene expression is modified. One out of twenty genes in the organism had increased or decreased or shut off their protein creation altogether based on a single gene insertion. When soy burgers and soy milk were consumed, three of seven volunteers developed herbicide-resistant bacteria in their guts. The gene had transferred from food to the bacteria in a single meal, according to *Seeds of Deception and Corrupt Science* by Jeffrey Smith.

It is now well recognized that people with certain common genetic mutations do not metabolize certain nutrients as well as others, and do not detoxify and excrete heavy metals or toxic chemicals as well as others. Children and adults with such mutations are more genetically susceptible or vulnerable to a wide range of diseases, from autoimmune conditions and autism to heavy metals poisoning and neurological diseases.

Ehlers-Danlos Syndrome (EDS) and More:
Pathogens Biohacking and Reprogramming the Epigenome?

Is it possible Ehlers-Danlos Syndrome (EDS) is the final manifestation of reprogrammed host DNA or epigenome by bacterial pathogens? Hippocrates described "excessive mobility" in 400 B.C. Hypermobile joints are old news; naming it Ehlers-Danlos syndrome (EDS) is new.

Ehlers-Danlos syndrome (EDS) was first described over 100 years ago and is now recognized more often with 13 subgroups of classification. EDS is considered a genetic-related hereditary connective-tissue disorder. Common symptoms include hypermobile loose joints, joint pain, stretchy velvety skin, and it is associated with cardiovascular problems including aortic dissection, joint subluxation and dislocation, scoliosis, chronic pain, and a growing list of symptoms.

Recently I saw a young woman with vague chest pain and hypermobile joints. She was told she had cardiovascular related Ehlers-Danlos syndrome (EDS) by an EDS specialist from the east coast. My evaluation indicated she has hidden dental infections in old wisdom teeth extraction sites based on acupuncture meridian assessment (AMA) that was affecting her chest pain. Her dental X-rays were normal.

I sent her to an oral surgeon to clean out the old infected dental and jaw socket areas and her chest pain was resolved. I also sent her to see a rheumatologist for a second opinion; the rheumatologist told her she did not have EDS. This case makes you think about over diagnosing Ehlers-Danlos syndrome, possibly mimicking EDS-like symptoms from other factors.

Dental Infections Mimic Many Medical Diagnoses

Hidden dental infections are one of the most common denominators for mimicking hundreds of medical diagnoses. Common problems include chronic fatigue, arthritis, fibromyalgia and chronic pain, cardiovascular problems including chest pain and stroke, kidney problems, autoimmune disorders, neurologic disorders, and many unknown symptoms including EDS from my personal clinical observations. Several patients I have seen for other medical problems also had EDS as a part of their medical history, and they also had hidden dental and parasite infections.

> **Hidden dental infections are one of the most common denominators mimicking hundreds of medical diagnoses.**

Currently, EDS is considered a genetic disorder that occurs due to variations of more than 19 genes that are present and defects in the structure or processing of the protein collagen. Diagnosis is often based on symptoms and genetic testing or skin biopsy. There is no cure since EDS is considered a genetic disorder. Treatment is supportive therapy including physical therapy and braces to support the joints and muscles.

As I saw the young woman with EDS-like symptoms resolve after dental work, I began to explore the connections between hidden dental infections and EDS with limited information.

EDS may make you more susceptible to periodontal infection, but not the other way around. Periodontal involvement may lead to the diagnosis of underlying systemic EDS condition, but there is no literature supporting that dental-periodontal infection might be the culprit of EDS. Periodontal EDS is a rare disorder characterized by soft, hyperextensible skin, abnormal scarring, easy bruising, and generalized periodontitis with early loss of teeth.

Is it possible that some unrecognized infections may trigger genetic expressions, and we assume that the EDS is solely a genetic inherited disorder?

> **As I saw the young woman with EDS-like symptoms resolve after dental work, I began to explore the connections between dental infections and EDS.**

Pathogens Hijack the Epigenome

I came across a 2014 article by Silmon and Kim in *The American Journal of Pathology* titled, Pathogens Hijack the Epigenome: A New Twist on Host-Pathogen Interactions.[32] They state, "Pathogens have evolved strategies to promote their survival by dramatically modifying the transcriptional profile and protein content of the host cell they infect. Modifications of the host transcriptome and proteome are mediated by pathogen-encoded effector molecules that modulate host cells through a variety of different mechanisms... Host gene regulatory mechanisms may be targeted through cytoplasmic signaling, directly by pathogen effector proteins, and possibly by pathogen RNA."

A 2018 case report by Mozayeni et al. in *Medicine* indicated systemic Bartonella infection associated joint hypermobility mimicking EDS, type III and to consider systemic bartonellosis as a differential diagnosis for EDS.[33] Modulation of host signaling pathways, targeting host nuclear proteins, post-translational modification, and molecular mimicry of nuclear proteins by pathogens and immortalization and oncogenesis, etc. are a part of biohacking of epigenomes that we are beginning to accept with some limited understanding.

Here is a case of a chronic fatigue and fibromyalgia patient (not Ehlers-Danlos syndrome) with a multitude of symptoms. She was referred to cavitation surgery. The DNA Connexions test results of her dental biopsy indicated many hidden dental infections, see Figure 60. In my experience, dental problems are often a driving force for inflammation, in effect biohacking epigenomes into many different medical diagnoses.

Figure 60: DNA Connexions Result of Dental Biopsy

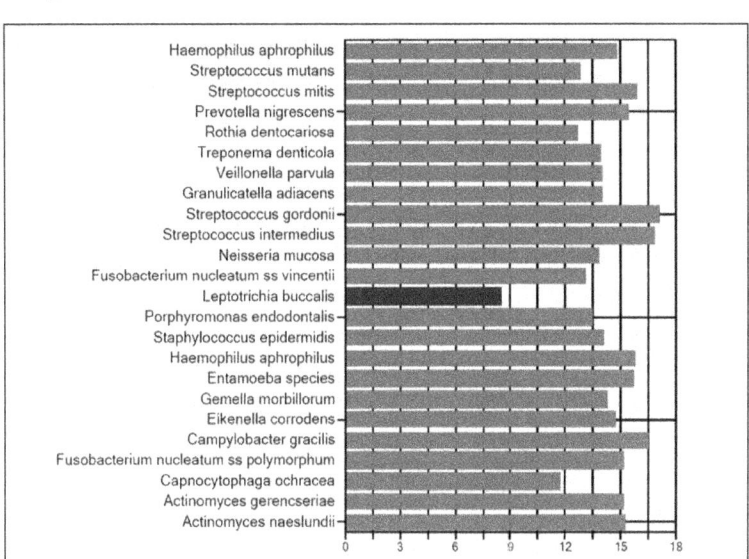

Hypermobile joints have been around for many years, but the diagnosis of EDS has been only recently recognized with subclassifications based on individual symptoms. Many medical specialists are managing their patients' unique symptoms with support therapies. There is no cure for EDS.

Some chronic disease patients with EDS symptoms have been treated for other underlying risk factors - such as dental infections or Bartonella, parasites or fungal infections – and have improved their EDS symptoms; maybe there is a true genetic EDS and a secondary non-genetic EDS. Treat the underlying infections and it may modify the expression of epigenomes and stop their bio-hijacking. For me, a treatment plan is based on acupuncture meridian assessment (AMA) and balancing the meridians, not based on medical diagnosis. For EDS, Lyme, or chronically ill patients, hidden dental infections and parasites are the most often neglected medical conundrum.

Patient Story: Pain Free after Ankylosing Spondylitis

I cannot thank you enough for all you have done for me. I have never felt better and never imagined that I would be able to live a pain free and medication free life.

In August 2007 I was diagnosed with Ankylosing Spondylitis which is a form of arthritis. I had constant pain in my hands, feet and back. I also had sharp pains in my chest that would take my breath away multiple times a day.

This diagnosis came as a shock to not only me but my family. I grew up as a very active kid and played soccer through my freshman year of college. The pain that I dealt with on a daily basis had taken me away from my active lifestyle and left me wanting to do nothing but lie in bed.

On top of the pain I felt from the arthritis, I was also starting to have side effects from the medication I was taking through my rheumatologist. I had constant stomach pain and nausea that turned out to be ulcers from all the steroids and medication that I was taking to deal with the arthritis pain.

I was starting to wonder if all this medication was worth the side effects. This is when I decided that a lifetime of pain and constant medication was not going to make my life any better. I wanted my healthy and active life back.

In May 2010 I was introduced to Dr. Yu. After various testing, diet changes, supplements and parasite cleansing, Dr. Yu found something that didn't seem right with both my lower jaws. I was then referred to Dr. Moreland for more testing and it was confirmed that something was not right.

After my first oral surgery there was already some improvement and Dr. Yu continued treating me with antibiotics, supplements, vitamins, and procedures to extract toxins. August 2011 was my 3rd and final oral surgery with Dr. Moreland to clean out the lingering bacteria in my jaw where my wisdom teeth had been removed in 2001.

I felt better after each surgery and was able to slowly reduce my medication from my rheumatologist after each surgery. As of September 2012, I have been medication free, pain free and have been considered in remission by my rheumatologist. While I evidently have the genetic marker for Ankylosing Spondylitis, it seems to me that the infection in my jaw simply overwhelmed my immune system.

If it had not been for Dr. Yu and Dr. Moreland, I would have continued to get worse as the medication from my rheumatologist was just masking the symptoms, as best they could, and the underlying cause would have never been addressed. I now have my life back and could not be happier!

Accidental Cure for Macular Degeneration:
Vision Loss Affects 37 Million Americans

Going blind with impaired vision is one of the most common fears of losing independence as we grow older. Vision loss affects 37 million Americans over 50 years, and one in four who are over 80. Low vision is defined as central vision acuity of 20/70 with the best correction. Legal blindness is defined as central visual acuity of 20/200 or worse with correction. Visual field size is also an important criterion of vision loss.

Vison loss in the older adults is associated with increased risk of falling, inability to drive, loss of independence, depression, and an increase in all-cause mortality. The most common causes of vision loss and blindness in older patients are (1) age-related macular degeneration, (2) glaucoma, (3) diabetes mellitus retinopathy, and (4) age-related cataracts.

The US Preventive Service Task Force (USPSTF) concludes that current evidence is insufficient to assess the balance of benefits and harms of screening for impaired visual acuity in adults older than 65 years, that is, there are no conclusive benefits of universal eye screening in older adults. That means you are on your own to protect your vision and eyesight. Comprehensive eye examinations every one to two years for all adults are recommended by the American Academy of Ophthalmology. (*American Family Physician*; August 2016).

Vitamin supplements (lutein, zeaxanthin, and omega-3 fatty acids) may lower the risk of the progression of age-related macular degeneration but do not prevent the development of macular degeneration. Vitamin supplements are a highly controversial topic among nutritionists, alternative medical doctors, and allopathic physicians.

Occasionally, I see patients for a particular complaint like IBS for which I treat the underlying problems with parasite medications. Sometimes, I get unexpected responses like the resolution of lifelong asthma, anemia, chronic fatigue, fibromyalgia, psoriasis, etc. I described this phenomenon in my book, *Accidental Cure*.

I'll share one discovery of an accidental cure for macular degeneration. I saw a 65-year-old physician, Doctor J. from North Carolina, for the chief complaint of Parkinson's disease with a tremor of his right hand for over one year. He also has neuropathy, intermittent atrial fibrillation, and a recent diagnosis of macular degeneration.

He has been practicing integrative medicine for over 30 years. In fact, we share a patient. She was suffering from "Delusional Parasitosis" with so many unusual somatic complaints. He referred her to me for a medical evaluation to rule out potential parasite problems. He did not dismiss her like most physicians in North Carolina. After great difficulty treating her with multiple parasite medications and extensive dental work, finally, she was stabilized. He decided to come see me for an evaluation for himself.

Acupuncture meridian assessment indicated 10 out of 40 meridians were out of balance. His main problems were dental infection on lymphatic system, parasite problems from large intestine meridian, and fungal problems from allergy-immunology points. He was treated for parasites with ivermectin and pyrantel pamoate. On the second visit he was treated for flukes with praziquantel based on disturbance of the gallbladder meridian. On the third visit he was treated for fungal problems manifested in allergy-immunology point with itraconazole. Part of the dental work was also done by an oral surgeon during that time.

He could not see me for follow-up for several months due to a family situation, but we discussed his status over the phone. He told me there was no improvement on his tremors. He had great expectations that his tremors would improve after parasite medications and dental work. I was also disappointed. However, by serendipity, he saw his ophthalmologist recently for a follow up and the eye doctor seemed befuddled when he was examining Doctor J.'s eyes. He could not see any sign of macular degeneration.

Doctor J. asked me a question like any curious physician, is it possible to cure macular degeneration with parasite medications? I told him I don't know. However, many patients often say their eyesight improved after taking parasite medications. River blindness in Africa is treated with the parasite medication ivermectin.

During his diagnosis of macular degeneration and his follow up appointment, the only therapy he took was taking parasite medications as a part of rebalancing his large intestine and gallbladder meridians for his Parkinson's disease. The Gallbladder/Liver/Stomach/Bladder meridians regulate eye-related function according to acupuncture meridian principles. He still has tremors from Parkinson's disease, but macular degeneration is not there anymore.

Is it possible to cure macular degeneration with parasite medications? At least for this patient, it was possible. Neurological disorders like Parkinson's disease may take many years to slow down the progression of the disease and stabilize the condition. He had a relatively early stage of macular degeneration. He responded to specific parasite medications at the right dose, right sequence, and right combinations based on meridian assessment. If he was older and in a more advanced stage of macular degeneration, I do not expect he would have responded to the medications because the damage would have been too far gone beyond repair.

By treating the underlying problems rather than focusing on treating the symptoms, disease, or diagnosis, reversal of the macular degeneration was possible at an early stage in this situation. Let's call that an accidental cure for macular degeneration. Medical professionals interested in learning how to measure the subtle energy fields with acupuncture meridians to detect parasites and hidden dental problems can check my website for special training seminars on these subjects.

Excerpt: Lyme and Post-Lyme Syndrome:
Forensic Case Study from New York

Who else committed the Crime of Post-Lyme? If Lyme spirochetes and co-infections are treated with aggressive IV antibiotics and patients still have symptoms, can we solve the mystery of Post-Lyme Syndrome by applying the analogy of forensic science? Let us investigate what happened after aggressively eliminating Borrelia spirochete infection.

Forensic science is the application of science to criminal and civil laws, mainly during criminal investigation, as governed by the legal standards of admissible evidence. Assuming the Borrelia is dead, mutated, transformed, or hiding as a cyst form; Lyme specialists look for coinfections like Babesia, Bartonella, Ehrlichia, Anaplasmosis, Mycoplasma, and Rocky

Mountain Spotted Fever (RMSF) as a culprit for persistent post-antibiotic Lyme symptoms.

Let me introduce 60-year-old Sharon, a college professor from upstate New York, a classic post-Lyme syndrome patient as a forensic case study. The patient had a tick bite in 2013 and was treated with doxycycline. In 2014, she was officially told she had seronegative Lyme disease. In 2016, she experienced vision loss with white clouding of her vision, but her eye exam was normal. Since then, she has experienced right eye pain, pins-and-needles-like pain, needs an eye patch to read, and has seen 13 physicians.

She had a spinal tap in January 2017 and was positive for Borrelia. She was officially diagnosed with CNS neurologic Lyme disease. An infectious disease specialist started her on a 28-day course of IV ceftriaxone, with no improvement. She was told her Lyme disease was treated, and she now had post-Lyme syndrome. She experienced persistent tingling arms and legs, incontinence, low back pain, fibromyalgia pain all over, severe fatigue, appetite loss, weight loss, and severe insomnia.

She went to a Lyme clinic in Arizona and received a 10-week course of IV antibiotics and six weeks of insulin potentiation therapy (IPT) but developed pancreatitis during treatment. Next, she had oral surgery in Colorado for four cavitations and replaced two amalgams. She "crashed" according to her words. She also had a coffee enema, during which she passed "two different kinds of parasites" – the admissible evidence – and came to see me for parasite problems.

Acupuncture meridian assessment (AMA) showed that 8 out of 40 meridians were out of balance. Her gallbladder, allergy/immunology and small intestine meridians were the dominant problems. She started on parasite meds: ivermectin, pyrantel pamoate, and praziquantel; followed by anti-fungal meds: fluconazole and itraconazole; and other support therapies.

On her next visit, she reported feeling much better, and all her 40 meridians were balanced. She will be on multiple rounds of alternating parasite/antifungal meds. This is a long process of eliminating several layers of infections – Borrelia burgdorferi and coinfections – with IV antibiotics, dental cavitation (jawbone infections with oral surgery, and finally, parasites and fungal infections with potent prescribed medications.

It may be premature for me to say she is healing from Post-Lyme Syndrome yet. Time will tell. From the forensic science of who committed the crime, her missing links between Lyme disease and Post-Lyme Syndrome were her dental infections (four jawbone cavitations) and parasites/fungal infections.

Palladium, not Polonium! Am I Dead?

What can we learn from my palladium poisoning misadventure? The year 2018 was a shock for me when I found out in my yearly routine checkup that I have been poisoned with palladium. It did not show up on previous heavy metals tests. I have never seen that extremely high level of palladium. Among the thousands of patients I have seen during the last 25 years, only a few patients had palladium toxicity. They all had cancers and all died, and my palladium level was much higher than their levels.

Keep in mind that there are fast and slow acting poisons. You may have heard of polonium as a deadly poison used to assassinate an ex-Russian spy, Alexander Litvinenko, in

London in 2006. Polonium-210 was spiked in his tea at a business meeting. A rare, short acting deadly radioactive metal discovered by Marie Curie, polonium can be delivered through inhalation, swallowing or broken skin.

Toxicologists estimate that one gram of polonium-210 could be enough to kill 50 million people and harm another 50 million people from radiation sickness. Treatment includes supportive care for radiation related symptoms of nausea, vomiting, anorexia, hair loss, low white blood cell counts, diarrhea, and bone marrow suppression. Chelation therapy agents such as DMPS, DMSA, and penicillamine have been used to bind to polonium and eliminate it from the body. I wrote on this subject in my first book, *Accidental Cure*, and in short articles, "Chelation Therapy," and "Chelation Therapy for Heavy Metal Toxicities Even When Least Suspected."

The Russian government denied wrongdoing but then, most governments deny wrongdoing anyway. I would not mess around with Russians!

The most common heavy metal toxicities I have seen in my practice are mercury, lead, tin, tungsten, aluminum, nickel, and cadmium. Hair mineral analysis is a good screening test for toxic metals. Provoking chelating agents like DMPS, DMSA, or EDTA are the most accurate ways of detecting deeply embedded toxic metals in tissues.

Heavy metal poisoning is a lot more common than you may think. Unfortunately, it is not a part of standard medical school training. But have you heard of palladium poisoning? Palladium is used as an industrial metal as a catalyst and in dentistry but is not a common medical problem. Twenty-five years ago, I had two separate accidents with a broken mercury thermometer and acute mercury poisoning. Luckily, I was just trained in how to measure heavy metals and using chelating agents; I was able to treat myself. Since then, I have been checking for heavy metals (20 different metals) on all my patients with chronic, medically unexplainable problems, and I get a yearly update on the heavy metal test for me. See Figures 60 and 61 for the common symptoms associated with mercury and lead.

Figure 61: Symptoms Associated with Mercury

Mercury

- Depression
- Dizziness
- Fatigue
- Hyperactivity
- Immune system dysfunction
- Insomnia
- Irregular heartbeat
- Irritability
- Lack of concentration
- Memory loss
- Metallic taste
- Migraine headaches
- Mood swings
- Muscle tremor
- Nervousness
- Numbness/tingling
- Rashes, skin
- Salivation, excessive
- Thyroid dysfunction
- Urinary problems
- Vision loss
- Weakness, muscle

Figure 62: Symptoms Associated with Lead

Lead

- Anemia
- Anger
- Anxiety
- Alzheimer's
- Arthritis
- Cancer
- Concentration low
- Confusion
- Convulsions
- Depression
- Dizziness
- Dyslexia
- Epilepsy
- Fatigue
- Headaches
- Hyperactivity
- Hypertension
- Impotency
- Indigestion
- Infertility
- Insomnia
- Irritability
- Learning disability
- Muscle pain
- Psychotic behavior
- Tooth decay
- Tremors

My initial reaction to my extremely high palladium toxicity was, "Am I Dead?" Am I going to get cancer and die like many of my patients in the next few years? Is somebody trying to poison me? Russia? Big Pharma? After all, whenever one of the alternative integrative medicine physicians dies under suspicious circumstances, I get a phone call from my patients checking on me. My mind goes through wild spinning, and I take a deep breath, check my pulse, and do a reality check.

When the level is far outside of normal range, you need to verify by re-checking the level. I checked three times, and the level was climbing even higher. I checked again: both my pulse and the reality check. I am not dead yet. I started calling some of my physician friends. One antiaging physician asked me to check my hormones. My hormone levels were perfect, and he could not help me. He was envious of my hormone levels. I figured I may die from palladium poisoning with perfect hormone levels. What a comforting thought! The other physician asked for a genetic test for detox pathways. The genetic test was normal for all detox pathways including MTHFR genes.

What is the next step? Palladium is highly toxic to the kidneys, liver, and nervous system, and I began to have muscle cramps and spasms and stopped exercising. I have seen too many patients die from over-exercising. Palladium is also toxic to many enzyme functions including carbonic anhydrase, a zinc dependent enzyme. Palladium can block carbonic anhydrase in the cells and build up carbon dioxide at the cellular level, like a "slow cellular strangulation" of mitochondrial metabolism. Carbonic anhydrase converts carbon dioxide to carbonic acid and is highly sensitive to many toxic metals.

All my cancer patients who died from palladium toxicity also had dental problems, parasites, fungal, bacterial infections, and other heavy metals exposures. The next step was checking my cancer profile. My phosphohexose isomerase (PHI) level, which can indicate a shift in glucose metabolism by cancer, was very elevated: it suggested my cellular respiration was switching to an anaerobic cancer-promoting metabolism. I started DMPS chelation therapy.

My palladium level is gradually coming down and my PHI level is coming down to the normal range, indicating cancer metabolism can be reversed; otherwise, cancer may manifest 3-5 years down the road. My palladium level is far from safe yet but at least it is coming down slowly with chelation therapy.

I tell my fellow physicians training in acupuncture meridian assessment (AMA) that if I die within next few years, I want to make sure they know that I died from palladium, not polonium poisoning. Hopefully, my tombstone will say, "Palladium, not Polonium: Prevention and Healing is Golden," many, many years later. I hope we all can learn from my unexpected palladium poisoning misadventure. I will become an expert on palladium toxicity by default. How did I get palladium???

> Update: Following 5 years of chelation therapy, my palladium level came down from 500 to 6 µg/g creatinine; anything above .3 is considered too high. It may be a lifetime commitment to free myself from palladium toxicity. I am out of the danger level, but not yet at an optimal safe level.

Toxoplasmosis Parasite Deceiving Medicine:
Reversing Unsuspected Mental Illness?

Is it possible to reverse engineer unsuspected mental illness? Several years ago, I saw a 59-year-old nurse from North Carolina with chief complaint of parasites coming out of her oral cavity through her teeth and gums. Nobody believed that she had parasites. Her family wanted her hospitalized in a psychiatric unit for evaluation and treatment of mental illness, suspecting acute mania or schizophrenia. She told me, "I'm not crazy. I just have a parasite problem." My patient also had chronic fatigue, fibromyalgia, brain fog, IBS, GERD, chronic diarrhea, Hashimoto's thyroiditis, history of hepatitis C from a needle stick, and was unable to work as a nurse. She had insomnia, fungal enteritis and mold exposure. In addition, she had many severe rotting dental cavities.

Parasites can be an underlying cause of hundreds of mysterious medical and mental illnesses. For example, toxoplasmosis, caused by the parasitic protozoan Toxoplasma gondii – a unicellular parasite, similar to Babesia or Malaria – commonly infects cats, cattle, poultry, sheep, goats, and more. It can also infect humans, where toxoplasmosis effects may range from asymptomatic to severe disease. Transmission can come from handling cat litter, eating undercooked meat, and congenitally from mother to fetus. With a US prevalence of about 11 percent, asymptomatic infection occurs in the general population. In congenital infection and immunosuppressed individuals, more severe forms of the disease may occur, but the blood test for Toxoplasma is not always reliable.

Lymphadenitis (lymph node swelling), fatigue, and malaise are some of the most common clinical symptoms of the disease. I have very limited experience with Toxoplasma, but perhaps I have overlooked many more toxoplasmosis cases, according to German physician Dr. Uwe auf der Strasse. He recently published, *The Toxoplasmosis Handbook: A parasite deceives medicine and makes us sick – Recognize and treat Toxoplasma gondii*. Toxoplasmosis is fairly common in Germany; infection rates rise from 20% to 77% for increasing age cohorts.[34] The book is now available in German and English under a slightly different title; I got this information from my good friend, Dr. Helmut Retzek of Austria.

From Retzek's blog post, Dr. Uwe auf der Strauss – the hero-physician of 2019: "Starting from the case of a woman who has been ill for 50 years and who was temporarily significantly improved with a special antibiotic (clindamycin), he was able to identify the underlying infection being toxoplasmosis, worked up the scientific literature on toxoplasmosis, successfully treated 150 similar patients and thus gave us a very detailed picture of one disease that is almost always misinterpreted as Lyme disease, rheumatism or chronic fatigue syndrome or fibromyalgia in patients that have not been successfully treated so far."

"The parasite occurs in several forms: The tachyzoite is the official vegetative form, but the body forms antibodies in about 70% of the cases, which pass with long-term infection. In the human body the tachyzoite transforms into the spore form bradyzoite, which multiplies much more slowly and experiences a change in the cell membrane so that the human immune system no longer recognizes this "spore". We currently have no antibody diagnostics against the bradyzoites and so the disease can no longer be detected in the case of prolonged infection. Bradyzoites live above all in muscle cells and in the brain."

Toxoplasmosis Symptoms, Questionnaire and Scoring The symptoms described by auf der Strasse are very clear, as summarized by Retzek. The percentage after a symptom refers to the share of toxoplasmosis patients presenting that symptom.

"**A**" symptoms:
- Great tiredness and exhaustion after minimal effort, high need for sleep 100%
- Strong muscle pain after minimal exertion, takes days to release and relax 100%
- Concentration disorders 93%
- Sweating, especially at night 78%
- Shortness of breath with little exertion, fast high pulse with exertion, feeling of pressure on the heart or chest, especially with exertion; infection of heart muscle or diaphragm; patient typically had previous examinations by a cardiologist and/or pulmonologist 67%
- Listlessness 63%

- IgG against Toxoplasma 60%

"**B**" symptoms:
- A. Irritability 59%
- B. Visual disturbance, blurred vision, unclear vision 44%
- C. Dizziness 37%
- D. Depression 41%
- E. Fears 33%

"**C**" symptoms:
- Morning stiffness 30%
- Water retention (especially of the hands and feet) 33%
- Sleep disorders 38%
- Coordination disorder, runs into objects, gait insecurity
- Abdominal pressure
- Headache
- Joint pain
- Lymph node swelling

Because the blood test is not reliable against all stages and forms of the disease, Dr. auf der Strasse uses a Toxoplasmosis questionnaire as an aid to diagnose and trial medications. If no more than three of the A symptoms are present and the other symptoms are normal, then there is probably no toxoplasmosis. If there are at least three A symptoms, and three from B or C, there is probably toxoplasmosis. Tiredness was the leading symptom that was present in all reported cases. Dr. Strasse uses clindamycin initially as a trial and then adds Pyrimethamine plus sulfadiazine and other combinations. Pyrimethamine is also used for Malaria, Pneumocystis carinii, and Babesia.

I treated my nurse from North Carolina with multiple parasite medications including ivermectin, pyrantel pamoate, praziquantel, tinidazole, doxycycline, and antifungal meds based on acupuncture meridian assessment (AMA). In collaboration with Dr. John Wilson, her Integrative medicine physician, we added pyrimethamine, sulfadiazine, and folinic acid based on a blood test with a very high IgG antibody titer of 102 (above 8.8 is considered positive for toxoplasmosis).

While it may sound farfetched, I have learned from my patients that parasites can affect and control your mind, as well as muscles, organs, nerves and more. See my articles, "Parasites and Mental Illness: Delusions of Parasitosis," and "Parasites and Mind Control," on my website.

This patient is now doing much better physically and emotionally and is going through the process of reconciling with her estranged family after multiple rounds of different combinations of parasite meds. Her biggest challenge was dental work. She said she spent over $20,000 on dental revision work, still had parasites coming out of her oral cavity, and was unable to see me due to financial hardship for more than two years. Last month, I saw her again. She still had residual parasite-related symptoms. I told her she needed more parasite medications, and to extract seven infected teeth for the potential of a full recovery. Dental-related parasite problems are an often-overlooked part of dental-related medical problems.

In summary, when patients are suffering from unusual complex chronic conditions, both parasites and dental problems must be considered as they have been deceiving medical professions for many years. Do not treat based on the latest expensive lab test or follow new fads for your symptoms or diagnosis. Do not treat for a single parasite, i.e. Toxoplasma gondii alone. Most patients have multiple parasites, coinfections and dental problems that must be addressed in the right sequence, in addition to environmental toxins and allergy-immunology dysregulation. This is a multi-year project for reversing unsuspected medical and mental illnesses or any complicated medical and dental (MAD condition, including chronic fatigue, fibromyalgia, rheumatism, or neurological diseases such as ALS, MS, Parkinson's disease, and more.

Three Million Dollar Kentucky Woman's Case: Adrenal Burnout, Lyme, Seizures and More

Recently, I saw a 40-year-old patient from Kentucky with myriad symptoms too long to list, including Lyme, seizures, severe fatigue, neuropathy, migraine headache, and chronic pain. She told me that she had been at a major medical institution in the Midwest for a month, and her insurance was billed about $3 million for medical evaluation without a definite diagnosis or the cause of her problems. The good news was that she was told she was not malingering, and she was not crazy with psychiatric problems. She only paid about $100 in co-payments. Her medical insurance covered the rest.

The $3 million woman suffered a stroke at 32 years old, and had since been diagnosed with asthma, autoimmune problems, bladder and cervical cancer, gallbladder and kidney problems, Lyme, mast-cell activation, postural orthostatic tachycardia syndrome (POTS), and more. Clearly, she was not healthy, and she had a lot going on. When chronic, complicated patients come to see me after extensive medical evaluations by academic institutions, they typically overlook hidden parasites/fungal/mycotoxins, EMF, and dental problems, including amalgams, root canals, TMJ, gum infections, and dental parasites. I call these medical and dental (MAD) complex problems.

My initial acupuncture meridian assessment (AMA) evaluation of my Kentucky patient showed 9 out of 40 meridians were out of balance, see Figure 63. Her physical exam was normal. For more detailed explanation of AMA, I recommend reading my books, *Accidental Cure* and *AcciDental Blow Up in Medicine*, my article, "JEDI Project: Exponential Healing by MAD JEDI," and related articles on my website.

Figure 63: Initial AMA Evaluation: 9 of 40 Meridians Out of Balance

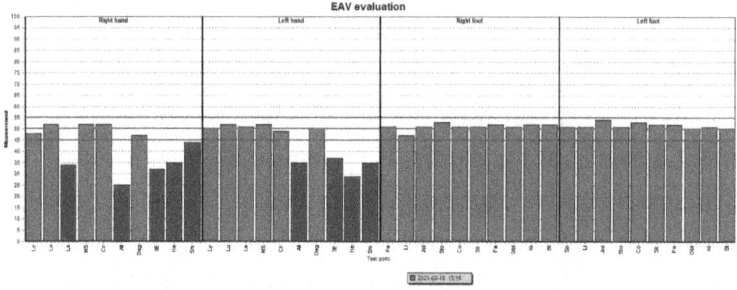

The middle bars mean normal range. The low bars mean chronic degeneration, out of balance. High bars mean acute inflammation. The evaluation indicated her large intestine and allergy-immunology systems as primary problems.

I then used a more advanced technique, stimulating five acupuncture points on her face and repeating the AMA evaluation to get more information. The first and second rounds of AMA were done less than ten minutes apart as a means of provoking deeper information on hidden problems. I have nicknamed this my "Enhanced Interrogation Technique."

My second evaluation revealed 22 out of 40 meridians were out of balance, see Figure 64. These included dental, pancreas, liver, and gallbladder as the major "hidden" deeper layer of problems affecting her nervous system. I prescribed ivermectin, mebendazole, praziquantel, tinidazole, and nystatin for multiple cycles, and I referred her for dental work to be done later as she begins to recover and rebuild her immune system. Dental work is the most unpredictable part of recovery, of which I have no direct control.

Figure 64: Second AMA with "Enhanced Interrogation" Technique: 22 of 40 Meridians Out of Balance

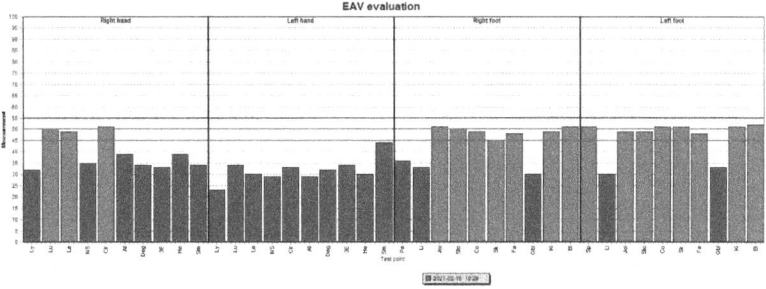

There are no guarantees that she will be cured – I never promise anyone a cure – I educated her that she will go through a process of gradual healing and fine tuning in the "right sequence." Dental problems are like a Death Trap to overcome. When she gets well, I may call it an "AcciDental Cure."

Recovery from adrenal burnout and multiple systems dysfunctions is analogous to tuning a fine musical instrument like a violin. It is a complex task which cannot be rushed and must be accomplished in orchestrated stages. The recovery process should include an understanding of the cause of underlying problems to eliminate continued burnout.

Many people feel that recovery is not worth the effort and look for a quick fix with medication. This attitude assures their sabotage and failure, especially on the dental part of medical and dental (MAD complex problems. This woman is motivated, and she is committed to finding the answers for her $3 million-dollar mysterious unsolved health problem. Dental is the big unknown. I plan to return to her case in a few months and write an update. Stay tuned.

Excerpt: RNA Based Nutrigenomic Therapy:
New Treatment for Autism and Neurodegenerative Disease

Here's an article I wrote nearly two decades ago, when people first started looking at genomic based nutritional therapy.

By the year 2000, the Human Genome Project mapped out about 30,000 genes in human DNA. DNA based genetic modulation therapy has become the new hope, the "magic bullet" for identifying genetic weak links and possible repair processes through genetic engineering.

I've been quite skeptical about DNA-based medical therapy. I've been waiting for the "miracle" to happen. Then I learned about RNA-based nutrigenomic therapy by Dr. Amy Yasko and the story of a four-year-old boy named Dillon and his struggle with autism. Dillon's genetic testing and the genomic information was the turning point for his gradual deconstruction of the neurological symptoms called "Autism." He began to communicate outside of his own world!

What is RNA based nutrigenomic therapy? Why use it with autistic children? Yasko identified environmental excitotoxins, heavy metal toxicity, chronic viral infection, inflammation, and genetic variations as the main culprits in autism. She has successfully treated many autistic children with RNA-based nucleotide extracts and nutritional supplements. She coined the term, "RNA-based Nutrigenomic Therapy."

For those of you not familiar with DNA and RNA, I'll provide a brief explanation. For your body to synthesize proteins and enzymes for growth and repair, information must be transcribed from DNA (the original blueprint) in the gene to specific messenger RNA (carbon copy of the specific duplicated DNA blueprint for that protein). The specific messenger RNA will then be translated by ribosomes to synthesize the specific proteins and enzymes for growth and repair.

Based on genetic profiling, the treatment plan includes: a) an intense nutritional program, b) bowel cleansing, c) heavy metal detoxification, d) excitotoxins elimination, e) the best means of blocking inflammation, and finally, f) using RNA-based nutritional support to bypass genetic mutations and correct the individual susceptible or weak genetic links.

Genetic profiling and RNA based nutritional therapy open new avenues for looking into all chronic and neurodegenerative disease including Autism, ADD, PDD, ALS, multiple sclerosis, and Parkinson's disease. For more information on RNA-based nutrients and nucleotides, go to Dr. Yasko's site, holisticheal.com. This is a rapidly evolving field.

Part 7
COVID and Post-COVID Syndrome

Chapter 11 COVID and Post-COVID Syndrome

What can we learn from the COVID-19 Pandemic and aftermath? There is COVID viral infection, genetically modified by the gain-of-function experiments, mRNA vaccination, and unexpected side effects from post-COVID syndrome.

There is a certain parallel with Lyme and Post-Lyme Syndrome, and with Chronic Fatigue Syndrome/Myalgic Encephalomyelitis (CFS/ME).

This chapter will discuss COVID-related problems without focusing on politically motivated conspiracies. COVID virus most likely reactivates dormant viral, fungal, mycotoxin, bacterial, and parasite infections, in addition to its own challenges.

Whatever we learn from COVID 19 can help guide how we prepare for future pandemics.

COVID-19: Hidden Coinfections and Chain Reactions Parasitic Infectious Relationships within Us

Viruses are technically parasites, a gray area between living and non-living: they cannot replicate on their own but do so in living cells. They have been evolving with us and some of them are encoded as a part of our genetic code from the point of evolution of biological life. They are unique and complex, composed of a protein coat surrounding RNA or DNA core genetic materials.

They can stay dormant for many years or be active seasonally and are capable of growth and multiplication only in living cells as unwanted guests, just like parasites. Parasites have their own parasites, fungus, mycoplasma, bacteria, and many types of viruses. Figures 65 and 66 are part of my lecture explaining the evolution of life and parasites, coinfections, and parasitic relationships from a universal, simplified perspective.

Figure 65: Evolutionary Tree of Universal Ancestors

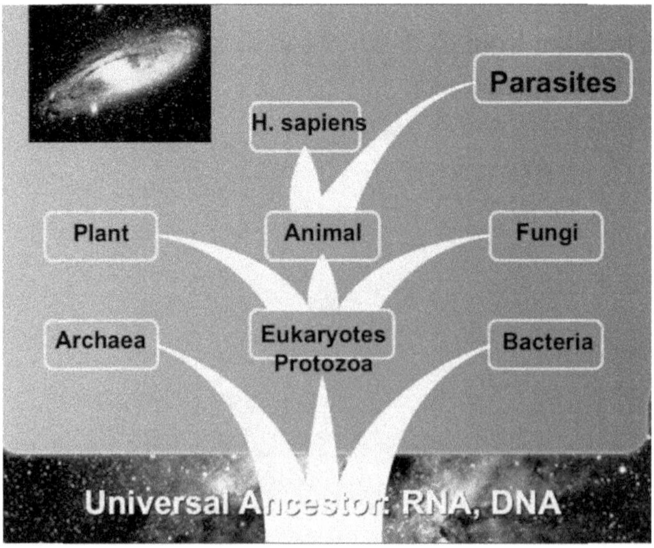

Figure 66: Parasitic Infectious Relationships: Concurrent Co-Infections

> **Parasitic Infectious Relationships: Concurrent Co-Infections**
>
> Virus
>
> Nanobacteria
>
> Intracellular Parasites
>
> Cell Wall Deficient Bacteria
>
> Mycoplasma
>
> Spirochetes and Lyme
>
> Prions
>
> Fungi related Molds, Yeasts and Candida
>
> Genetically Modified Biological Warfare Microbes
>
> Social, Political, Economical, Emotional, Spiritual

The virus is deceptive and creates a hidden chain reaction. COVID-19 will attack aggressively already vulnerable aging populations and immune-compromised, chronically ill patients, young or old. Many patients are nutritionally depleted and cannot support their immune system, so rapidly succumb to the viral infection.

By the time one develops pneumonia, COVID-19 may activate dormant, inactivated bacteria, fungi, mycobacteria, and parasites that were previously under the surveillance of the immune system.

COVID-19 pneumonia patients may be fighting more than viral infection but also bacterial, mycobacterium-TB like infection, fungi, and reactivated parasites, including dental infections. This might explain why some patients respond to chloroquine, a parasite medication, and azithromycin, an antibiotic for pneumonia.

My recent article covered hydroxychloroquine, an antimalarial parasite medication and losartan, an ACE inhibitor blood pressure medication provided by Dr. Helmut Retzek's findings as reported in his blog.

Hydroxychloroquine usage became a polarized hot potato for political-medical-scientific communities. You cannot get it anymore because of hoarding, inappropriate use, and controlled supply by higher powers. I do not recommend it for prophylactic use. It is also required by those on it for lupus and other serious medical conditions.

For prevention and prophylactic measures, use extra vitamin C up to 10,000mg/day, 10,000 IU of vitamin D3, vitamin K2, selenium, zinc, boron, and herbs and homeopathic remedies, such as elderberry and oscillococcinum. Also, glutathione can be taken for general immune support.

The good news is that coronavirus is seasonal and most active from January through April (see chart of seasonal activity in 2022, which is typical of annual patterns).

Spring is just around the corner. Let's get more sun and fresh air, keep social distancing for self-protection, practice good hygiene with frequent hand washing, supplement nutrients that support your immune system, and support your community. With luck, we will get a break from coronavirus season.

Figure 67: Seasonal COVID Activity

JAN	FEB	MAR	APR	MAY	JUN	JUL	AUG	SEP	OCT	NOV	DEC
		RHINOVIRUS									
CORONAVIRUS				ENTEROVIRUS							
	ADENOVIRUS										
			PIV-3					PIV2,3			
RSV										RSV	
INFLUENZA											
MPV											
	GROUP A STREPT										

Source: Medscape, Rhinovirus (RV) Infection (Common Cold): Practice Essentials, Background, Pathophysiology [35]

Don't let fears of COVID-19 paralyze you! We will also face Rhinovirus, Enterovirus, Adenovirus, Influenza and who knows what else lies ahead for the next pandemic.

To face all these challenges, we need to strengthen your ability to fight these invaders, and detect and treat coinfections of bacteria, mycobacterium, fungi, and parasites that cause acute, complex, concurrent diseases.

COVID-19, FUO and UFO Phenomenon:
Ivermectin to Treat Fever of Unknown Origin?

Coronavirus is a perfect storm pandemic virus – novel so unknown to the human immune system, easy to spread even when asymptomatic, sometimes hard to detect, unpredictable, and especially deadly in those with preexisting conditions. We lack sufficient testing capacity, and effective treatments. Some of the early ones proposed are not looking so rosy right now and are causing harm in some patients.

As a "Parasite Guy" - not by degree or training, but by US Army Reserve Medical Corps experience – I have learned to look more deeply into both evolutionary biology and how to repurpose medications. Ivermectin is a parasite medication I have used often in my practice over the last 25 years for many conditions seemingly not related to parasites by Western medical standards, including certain cancers, asthma, chronic fatigue, fibromyalgia, and TMJ. For an interesting case using ivermectin to treat fever of unknown origin (FUO) in military personnel, see my article, "Parasite Guy on UFO and FUO: Aliens and Parasites." A fever of unknown origin can be like a UFO, an "unidentified flying object" (or unidentified foreign object).

In the June 2020 issue of *Antiviral Research*, Leon Caly et al of Australia published, "The FDA-approved drug ivermectin inhibits the replication of SARS-CoV-2 in vitro."[36]

Highlights include:

- Ivermectin is an inhibitor of the COVID-19 causative virus (SARS-CoV-2) *in vitro*.
- A single treatment able to effect ~5000-fold reduction in virus at 48 h in cell culture.
- It is FDA-approved for parasitic infections and therefore has a potential for repurposing.
- It is widely available, due to its inclusion on the WHO Model List of Essential Medicines.

What about ivermectin use in COVID-19? Dr. Jean-Jacques Rajter, and his wife, Dr. Juliana Cepelowicz-Rajter, both pulmonologists at Broward Health Medical Center in Florida, are pioneering the use of ivermectin for COVID-19. She came up with the idea after reading the Australian research paper noted above. Dr. Rajter shared, "If we get to these people early… I've had nearly a 100 percent response rate, they all improve, if they're on more oxygen than that, then it becomes a little more varied, some people, they don't respond anymore because they are too far advanced." Dr. Cepelowicz-Rajter added, "More studies need to be conducted. We haven't had any ill effects from it and it's readily available, we have some patients who are pretty advanced, not yet intubated, and even those, in 12 hours, they showed a significant improvement."[37]

Here is some of my clinical experience in treating fever of unknown origin, parasites, and more with ivermectin. I first learned about treating parasites on a US Army Reserve Mission to Bolivia in 2001 and began to use it in my practice. In 2011, I received an email from a retired Air Force General asking to see me, he called me a "parasite guy." His physician was a U.N. tropical disease specialist and could not solve his parasite problems. The General had come to see me with a working diagnosis of Fever of Unknown Origin (FUO) for several years. He had been evaluated at Walter Reed Hospital, the best military hospital, and by an infectious disease specialist at the Centers for Disease Control and Prevention (CDC). He gave over 100 vials of blood, urine, and stool to the CDC for evaluation. There were no significant findings or improvement; he was officially diagnosed with FUO.

When he came to see me, he was still complaining of a 102–103-degree Fahrenheit fever, bone chills, elevated muscle enzymes, back cramps, lethargy, poor sleep, nocturnal urination, and muscle cramps. Acupuncture Meridian Assessment (AMA), an adjunct evaluation tool that I use, indicated his primary problems came from the Large Intestine, Gallbladder, Liver, and Spleen meridians. He was started on high doses of ivermectin and pyrantel pamoate (common dog parasite medications) for ten days. One year later, when I saw him in Washington DC, he said he was feeling well and his FUO had been resolved. I can only guess what type of parasites he had by his response to the medications. A hundred vials of stool, blood, and urine did not detect the specific infectious cause – a UFO, perhaps.

I have seen a few more cases of FUO. Another one came from a White House staff Air Force Colonel, who became deathly ill when he was in South America monitoring drug trafficking. He was air evacuated from La Paz, Bolivia and hospitalized at Walter Reed Army Hospital and also at Bethesda Naval Hospital. He had some improvement, but lots of residual medical problems. He had too many symptoms and diagnoses to mention but one of the diagnoses was FUO. Many of his symptoms responded to parasite medications. His dental problems were another nightmare, but that is a different story.

Over the years of my medical practice, prescribing ivermectin with different combinations of parasite and fungal medications based on acupuncture meridian assessment (AMA), I have seen dramatic responses by patients with tough diagnoses other than parasites: many neurologic disorders, cancers, FUO, and mystery diseases. I call their responses "Accidental Cure."

For descriptions of some cases, see these articles on my website: "Ivermectin Deficiency Syndrome," "Parasite Guy on UFO and FUO: Aliens and Parasites," "Parasites and a Mystery

Disease: Unusual Case from Sweden," and "Quarantine Iowa: Global Whining on Parasites." In addition, I have written articles on "COVID-19, Coronavirus and COVID-19: Good News from Abroad, ICIM and AMA," and "COVID-19: Hidden Coinfections and Chain Reactions," which have recommendations for general immune support and prophylactic measures.

Interestingly, patients on antiparasitic medications often report resolution of seemingly unrelated problems. Are parasites one of the coinfections that can lead to advanced respiratory distress syndrome (ARDS), hypercoagulation, systemic inflammation, and other bad outcomes? Or does ivermectin's method of action have an impact on virus entry, attachment, and replication due to biochemical factors.

> **If ivermectin can treat fevers of unknown origin, can it also treat fevers of known origin, COVID-19? It is one of the drugs worth a closer look in treatment, testing, and trials.**

If ivermectin can treat fevers of unknown origin, can it also treat fevers of known origin, COVID-19? It is one of the drugs worth a closer look in treatment, testing, and trials. UFO and FUO phenomena are in metaphorical parallel. But don't let the government and pharmaceutical giants figure that out, or it will become very costly to treat them.

Ivermectin Deficiency Syndrome, Part 2:
Staying Out of the COVID-19 Graveyard

Recently, a friend sent me a post by Dr. Richard Horowitz on work to advocate for US trials of ivermectin, GSH (glutathione), and nutraceuticals for COVID-19 viral infection. I want to share this vital information with my readers and to spread this important message to your friends and your doctors; it may save your life and your loved ones.

I have been advocating extensive usage of ivermectin, a common parasite medication, for many chronic, complex patients with asthma, pneumonia, bronchiectasis, IBS, IBD, migraine headache, chronic fatigue, fibromyalgia, diabetes, most neurological disorders including MS, Parkinson's, and ALS, cancer, and many more conditions. The selection of parasite medications is based on acupuncture meridian assessment (AMA).

How could a common heart deworming medication used in pets play such an important role in antiviral and COVID-19 viral infection? The idea is screening existing libraries of drugs already approved by the FDA in an effort to identify compounds that are effective in other diseases, called "drug repurposing." Ten years ago, I first wrote about using ivermectin for cancer patients.

Dr. Richard Horowitz includes extensive scientific documents and references in his post on using Ivermectin, glutathione, and nutritional supplements for preventive and active COVID-19 viral infection.

Here is Dr. Horowitz's COVID-19 Protocol from his post:

"Prevention: NAC 600 mg BID, Alpha lipoic acid 600 mg once to twice a day, glutathione 500 mg BID, curcumin 1000 mg twice a day, sulforaphane glucosinolate 100 mg twice a day (broccoli seed extract), zinc 40-50 mg/day, Vit C 1-gram TID, 3,6 Beta glucan 500 mg per day."

"For active infection: NAC is doubled to two capsules (1200 mg) twice a day, and glutathione dosing (oral or IV) increases to 2000 mg, 3 x per day, with an increase in Vit C to 2000 mg TID. The rest of the supplements listed above remain the same. Along with the nutraceuticals, we have been using ivermectin (0.2 mg/kg) once a day for 10-14 days based on multiple peer-reviewed articles on its efficacy for COVID-19. The above treatment protocol has worked well for approximately 30 active patients diagnosed with COVID. Not one patient has ended up in a hospital to date using this protocol, but due to low numbers, statistical significance is difficult to determine, which is why a RCT is essential. Ivermectin may also be useful in high-risk individuals as a preventative treatment, according to its pharmaceutical properties and published studies…" Many references are included in his post.

In my own practice, when indicated I use a much higher dosage and never use ivermectin alone to minimize resistance to the medications. I combine a couple of antiparasitic medications with antibiotics like doxycycline, and antifungal medications to address synergistic causes and effects of coinfections.

Dr. Helmut Retzek of Austria posted in his blog, "Ivermectin also great antiviral drug – useful even against Coronavirus." Dr. Atel Hemat of Germany has a blog post, "Is Ivermectin a therapy option for COVID?" He notes viruses are organic structures but strictly speaking not living creatures: "Without a host, viruses cannot replicate. Due to this big resemblance in their 'way of life' some scientists call viruses obligatory intracellular parasites."

Dr. Frederick T. Guilford, glutathione (GSH) expert, provided ample information on the importance of glutathione on virus COVID-19 triggers for the production of the cytokine IL-6. It turns out IL-6 depletes intracellular GSH. Many reports show that increased IL-6 is associated with the more severe forms of Covid-19 with cytokine storms. See Guloyan V, et al., "Glutathione Supplementation as an Adjunctive Therapy in COVID-19," in Antioxidants (Basel), September 2020.[38]

About ten years ago I wrote, "Ivermectin Deficiency Syndrome," as my frustration built up with the medical community for overlooking such an inexpensive parasite medication playing an important role in cancer therapy and antiaging medication. Ivermectin is also a promising antiviral and anti-COVID-19 agent. I highly recommend reading Dr. Richard Horowitz's post on COVID-19.

You can use much higher doses than 0.2 mg/kg of ivermectin, and Dr. Atel Hemat reports that you can use 10X higher than the recommended ivermectin dosage. So, you can help dig yourself out of your own graveyard if you know how to get and use parasite medications. Also, don't forget the basic recommendations in my article, "One Hundred Dollar Cure: Cure for Braves, Skeptics and El Cheapo."

Parasites Follow the Money: Disease Follows the Money

"Disease follows the money. Follow the Dollar bills." Can we predict the future of the world economy, finance, war, politics, and pandemic outbreaks based on global data in one big basket of information? Here is a prescient take on the origins of Artificial Intelligence.

According to David Weinberger, a senior researcher at Harvard University's Berkman Center for Internet and Society and co-director of the Harvard Library Innovation Laboratory at Harvard Law School, he thinks it is possible.

His article, "The Machine That Would Predict the Future,"[39] in *Scientific American*, December 2011, addressed the question:

> **"Is it possible as some of the most scientific minded scholars think that if you gather all the world's data into a black box, could it become a crystal ball that would let you see the future and even test what would happen if you choose A over B?"**

Imagine a novel in which a deadly flu virus emerges. Where will it spread? Physicists and epidemiologists have begun to tap enormous data streams to make predictions about how a pandemic might play out and what can be done to stop it. Scientists took data from the "Where's George project," which tracks the location of millions of dollar bills as they move across the US, to model how 2009's H1N1 flu virus would likely spread. Other researchers used air and land traffic patterns in the same way.

The studies demonstrated both the promise and problems of big data: they accurately predicted where the flu would spread, but they severely undercounted the number of people who would end up infected.

Weinberger's conclusion states that:

"The answer may come down to a disagreement about the nature of knowledge itself. We have for a couple of millennia in the West thought of knowledge as a system of settled, consistent truths. Perhaps that exhibits the limitations of knowledge's medium more than of knowledge itself: when knowledge is communicated and preserved by writing it in permanent ink on paper, it becomes that which makes it through institutional filters and that which does not change.

"Yet knowledge's new medium is not a publishing system so much as a networked public. We may get lots of knowledge out of our data commons, but the knowledge is more likely to be a continuous argument as it is tugged this way and that. Indeed, that is the face of knowledge in the age of the Net: never fully settled, never fully written, never entirely done..."

"Unless, of course, the messy contention of ideas-nerds arguing with nerds is a more fully true representation of the world."

David Weinberger, The Machine That Would Predict the Future[40]

After reading this *Scientific American* article, I could not help thinking that if disease follows money based on raw data following the movement of dollar bills, and if hidden parasite infections often precede the disease, parasites are disguised with a multitude of medical symptoms, and they are the ones going after the money. Parasites are followed by disease, disease follows money, and therefore, parasites follow money.

> **It is time to question the arrogant idea of the West's thought of knowledge as a system of settled, consistent truths. Big global data does not predict the individual expression of illness. We can vaccinate everybody and hope it will prevent the epidemic, or we can treat individually to strengthen each person's unique immune system and prevent the epidemic.**

I would rather treat people individually than support massive mRNA vaccination which benefits pharmaceutical giants and has dubious benefits with potential still unknown side effects for millions of vulnerable individuals.

There is also a big problem with the reliability of the testing for infectious parasites. Parasites are often carriers of bacteria and viruses. We have the ability to test stools for ova and parasites and also DNA testing, but most of the parasites are outside of the GI tract.

Follow the dollar and you will encounter disease and parasites. Parasites have their own parasitic relationship with environmental toxins, bacteria, fungi, and viruses. (It sounds more like our current American politics and finances as the money trail goes to politicians, lobbyists, and Wall Street.) Once the parasites have a stranglehold on you, they will drain your finances to treat whatever the name of the disease.

Name your disease and name your dollars. Current estimates:
- Kidney transplant: $300,000-$500,000.
- Coronary bypass: $30,000-$150,000.
- Heart transplant: $800,000-$1.5 million.
- Breast cancer treatment: $60,000-$135,000 (first year).
- Colon cancer treatment: $65,000 (first year).

Medical care and the burden of hospital expenses are one of the leading causes of personal bankruptcies in the United States. Sometimes, it's better not to know the name of the disease. Before you go to the hospital for an expensive mega workup, I would start with parasite cleansing and dental work, and you may notice your unexplainable medical symptoms disappear. Stop the money trail with parasite remedies. Watch CDC and WHO for pandemic forecasts. Follow the money.

Physician Perspective: Murat Isci, MD

During the Covid19 pandemic, I was approached by a woman diagnosed with advanced ovarian cancer. She had been referred to me through a mutual acquaintance after experiencing severe weight loss and debilitating diarrhea resulting from her chemotherapy treatments. Her quality of life had deteriorated dramatically, and she was desperate for help. I became personally involved in her care, working closely with her to manage her symptoms and help her regain strength and weight.

A former pharmaceutical industry professional, she was well-informed and proactive in exploring complementary treatment options. As our relationship deepened, she shared with me a treatment protocol she had received from the renowned holistic medicine expert, Dr. Thomas Lodi, following a consultation. The first two items on Dr. Lodi's protocol were as follows. First, you must have a 3D cone beam CT of the mouth and send me the scan so I can have it read by a biological dentist. Second, watch Dr. Simon Yu's video on Parasite Medications Targeting Cancer Cells (very important).[41] At first glance, I was puzzled. What relevance could a dental scan possibly have to cancer treatment? I moved on to the video.

It was just past midnight when I began watching—and I was so captivated that I ended up watching the 50-minute lecture three times in a row. What I didn't know at that moment was that this single video would radically alter the course of my medical thinking—and my life. I knew then that I had to meet Dr. Simon Yu. When I discovered he was hosting one of his annual training courses just a few months later, I booked a flight to St. Louis. I waited eagerly for the day I would finally step into his world.

The five-day training, followed by a week of clinical observation working alongside Dr. Yu, was intense, enlightening, and transformative. During this experience, a long-standing sense of incompleteness in my medical journey was finally resolved. After 35 years of medical education and clinical practice, something that had always eluded me—a missing link in modern medicine—was suddenly made clear.

Through Dr. Yu's teachings, I came to understand how quantum biology, dental and jaw health, persistent parasitic infections, latent viral burdens, heavy metal toxicity, and unresolved emotional trauma can profoundly influence human health—and how these critical factors often remain completely overlooked by conventional medical systems. More importantly, I learned how the failure to recognize and treat these underlying issues can leave patients suffering for years. This realization marked the beginning of a new paradigm in my medical practice—one rooted in integrative thinking, open-minded inquiry, and the courage to explore beyond the boundaries of traditional medicine.

Murat Isci, MD, Istanbul, Turkey

Part 8

How to Reboot Your Brain

Chapter 12 Brain, Bioresonance, Neuromodulation, Cyber, and More

There is no such thing as a brain meridian based on classical acupuncture. However, from the medical acupuncture based on Electro-Acupuncture according to Dr. Voll (EAV) from Germany, the two meridians that dominate regulating brain function are the gallbladder meridian and the dental meridian. The gallbladder meridian interacts and regulates the vagus nerve, and the dental meridian regulates the trigeminal nerve; the two dominant cranial nerves influencing brain activities. All meridians and organs are connected to teeth.

> **The gallbladder meridian interacts and regulates the vagus nerve, and the dental meridian regulates the trigeminal nerve, the two dominant cranial nerves influencing brain activities.**

Disturbance of the gallbladder meridian has been associated with microbiome problems and parasites. Disturbance of the dental/oral cavity meridian has been associated with periodontal disease, dental microbiomes, dental parasite infections, amalgams, root canals, implants, TMJ, bite issues, sleep apnea, etc. These two meridians can manifest thousands of unexplainable physical symptoms, creating hundreds of medical and neurological diagnoses. In this regard, the gallbladder meridian and the dental meridian are the equivalent of a "brain meridian" in my opinion.

If using Acupuncture Intelligence in the body as a diagnostic and treatment technique sounds too far out, think about physical therapy and the therapeutic treatments it now utilizes to stimulate blood flow, muscles, nerves, and more. Brain neuromodulation as a therapeutic treatment is also advancing. It is of great interest to me to complement and supplement AMA, which I use to detect and correct underlying problems. In combination, non-invasive brain neuromodulation and/or Transauricular stimulation can help reboot the brain.

Cognitive Decline to Dementia & Alzheimer's Disease: Unsuspected Parasite-Dental-Oral Infections

Do you have friends or family members suffering with dementia and Alzheimer's disease? They might have unsuspected dental-oral parasite infections, triggering chronic neuroinflammation, cognitive impairment, dementia, and Alzheimer's disease. My mother, a retired neurologist, passed away at age 90 with Alzheimer's disease at home in New York City in April 2020 and one month later, we will have a delayed bare-bones funeral service due to the COVID-19 pandemic.

I have been pondering if there is a better way to treat Alzheimer's disease (AD) for many years since my Internal Medicine training, including investigating qEEG brain mapping and neurofeedback therapy. Here is a short version of my "fact finding." I hope this short, condensed piece will be useful and help you take proactive action for any family members suffering from Alzheimer's disease.

Alzheimer's disease, a progressive neurodegenerative disorder, is the most common form of dementia. The cause of AD has been one of the great medical mysteries since Dr. Alois Alzheimer first described the disease in 1906.[42] Chronic neuroinflammation is a new catchphrase for the explanation of chronic inflammation in neurodegenerative diseases such as Amyotrophic lateral sclerosis (ALS), Multiple sclerosis (MS), Parkinson's disease, and Alzheimer's disease; I call it "Dementia Spectrum Disorder." At least 5.7 million Americans and 40-50 million people worldwide suffer from AD. It is the sixth (or higher) leading cause of death in the United States, and the incidence has been rapidly rising worldwide.

Identifying abnormal amyloid tau protein changes and tau protein disposal problems are only the tip of the iceberg. My position is that occult infections and coinfections from **viruses, bacteria, fungi, parasites, and dental infections** are the driving force for chronic neuroinflammation; exacerbated by lifestyle, diet and nutrition, occupational exposure, environmental toxins, heavy metals, and air pollution. Genetic variants help determine susceptibility and preexisting conditions exacerbate. As we have a deeper understanding of the modifiable individual risk factors, we can prevent and even reverse early stages of mild to moderate cognitive impairment and Alzheimer's disease.

A literature review identified many risk factors contributing to neurodegeneration in AD and has also identified several risk factors lesser known to academic medicine, such as heavy metals, toxins, parasites, bacterial infections, and hidden dental/oral bacteria, parasites, and fungi contributing to neuroinflammation. See Figure 68.

Figure 68: Risk Factors for Alzheimer's and Neurodegeneration

Demographic & Social	Genetic Variants	Diet/Nutrition & Lifestyle	Preexisting Conditions	Environment/ Toxins	Pathogens
Age	APOE4	Nutrition	Cancer	Air pollution	Bacteria
Gender	ABCA7	Alcohol	CVD/CHF	Water damage	Mycobacteria
Race/Ethnicity	CLU	Drugs	Diabetes	Workplace	Mycoplasma
Income	CR1	Smoking	Lipid disorder	Military	Fungi/Mold
Education	PICALM	Exercise	Obesity	Solvents	Lyme
Geography	PLD3	Activities	Stroke/TBI	Mercury	Parasites
Employment	TREM2	Learning	Anxiety/Dep	Lead, Copper	Viruses
Marital Status	SORLI1	Prescriptions	Stress/Trauma	Aluminum	Dental/Oral

Source: Author's research. For genetics, see Mayo Clinic, The Role of Genetics in Your Alzheimer's Risk.[43]

Due to the complexity of neurobiology, multiple risk factors, and social interactions of many interacting factors, my upcoming review article will focus on parasites and dental-oral infections. It will explore the cranial valveless vein, glymphatic (glia-lymphatic) drainage system of brain, and gut-brain connection which influence the cranial trigeminal nerve and cranial vagus nerve.

Acute and chronic parasite diseases of the central nervous system are associated with high morbidity and mortality, with lingering residual secondary neurological cognitive dysfunction. Many human parasites, such as Toxoplasma gondii, Entamoeba histolytica, Trypanosoma, Taenia solium, Echinococcus spp., Toxocara canis, Toxocara cati, Angiostrongylus cantonensis, and Trichinella spp., may involve the CNS.

Many believe parasite-related neurological and mental health problems are concentrated in tropical low-income third world countries. Parasite-related problems have been sadly ignored by Western medical communities. However, the frequent use of immune-suppressive medications, international travel, migration, and global warming have changed the landscape of geographic distribution of parasites.

Foreign unrecognized parasites are invading general populations and public health officials are unaware because no reliable parasites tests are available except for acute parasite infections showing in stool samples or blood tests. CNS symptoms include headache, dizziness, epileptic seizures, increased intracranial pressure, sensory disturbances, meningeal syndrome, cerebellar ataxia, behavioral changes, and cognitive decline in stages, sometimes sudden or gradual over a prolonged period. Early symptoms of CNS invasion are often nonspecific; therefore, diagnosis can be difficult.

The interaction of the trigeminal cranial nerve (CN V), vagus cranial nerve (CN X), and the glymph system are underappreciated significant contributors to epilepsy, multiple sclerosis, brain tumor, the development of neurologic disorders, and AD per Patrick Störtebecker, MD, Ph.D. from Sweden.[44]

> **The interaction of the trigeminal cranial nerve (CN V), vagus cranial nerve (CN X), and the glymph system are underappreciated significant contributors...**

More recently, there has been an explosion of studies investigating the connections among bacteria, oral parasites, periodontitis, and the onset and progression of neurodegenerative diseases like AD. Oral mucosal dendritic cells activate Th17-mediated inflammatory response when they encounter microorganisms. This triggers local and systemic inflammation and spread at distant peripheral sites, initiating comorbid diseases including atherosclerosis, AD, macular degeneration, chronic kidney disease, rheumatism, and others.

> **More recently, there has been an explosion of studies investigating the connections among bacteria, oral parasites, periodontitis, and the onset and progression of neurodegenerative diseases like AD.**

Migration of oral-dental bacteria and parasites to the CNS and brain can be explained by cranial valveless veins and the glymphatic drainage system once the endothelium mucosal barrier is interrupted at the site of periodontal and deep apical dental/jaw infections.

With this knowledge, neurodegeneration may be delayed by early intervention of chronic bacterial, fungal and parasite infection in the dental/oral cavity and gut, influencing the trigeminal cranial nerve (CN V) and vagus cranial nerve (CN X), thereby reducing infection and endotoxin-induced neuroinflammation.

Two Case Studies

Early-stage mild cognitive impairment: 53-year-old nurse with multiple complaints including Lyme, ADHD, job stress, memory loss, brain fog, insomnia, concentration and focus problems, Hashimoto's thyroid, and abscessed teeth was on multiple rounds of antibiotics. Her children were making fun of her because she was so forgetful.

Treatment plan: Stress management, diet, and nutritional support, two root canaled tooth extractions, and antiparasitic and antifungal meds azithromycin, tinidazole, and nystatin for chronic infections based on her dental DNA test indicating multiple infections including Treponema denticola and Entamoeba gingivalis. The patient feels and sleeps better, has less brain fog, and sees the treatment as a true prevention to progress from early dementia to Alzheimer's disease.

Mild to moderate AD: 63-year-old businessman, chief financial officer of a billion-dollar company, was forced to retire because of memory loss and inability to function as a CFO. His memory loss started after receiving a cochlear implant to treat sudden hearing loss three years earlier. He was losing weight, suffered from severe environmental allergies, and was previously treated for Lyme with antibiotics. He had been extensively evaluated and treated by major academic institutions and an AD clinic in the Midwest without significant improvement. Is it possible that he got an occult infection post-cochlear implant?

In my evaluation, the patient had extensive dental infections including a jawbone infection that was corrected by referral to an oral surgeon. He was treated for parasite and fungal infections, received hormonal support and IV chelation therapy for mercury and lead toxicity, and daily oral chelation therapy and hyperbaric oxygen therapy (HBOT) at home. Overall, his memory decline has stabilized, he is still driving, his sense of humor is coming back, and he is reading his favorite books, but he still cannot use an Excel spreadsheet like before. Consider this case as a moderate success to slow down the progression of moderately advanced AD.

A literature search identified a number of studies which support the use of parasite medications, and aggressive detoxification of identified environmental toxicity, heavy metals, and dental infections. Think of Alzheimer's disease as both an infectious disease and metabolic disease. Consider using antibacterial, antifungal, and antiparasitic medications as part of a treatment plan for early AD under a new understanding of the role of inflammation, infection and mitochondrial dysfunction in the development of Dementia Spectrum Disorder and progression of Alzheimer's disease.

> **Think of Alzheimer's disease as both an infectious disease and metabolic disease.**

The existing drugs used to treat AD based on the amyloid hypothesis have been disappointing. If we can address unsuspected multiple sources of infections, remove heavy metals and environmental toxins, and provide nutritional support, these drugs may become more effective and achieve a desirable response even in moderately advanced AD.

First, we should screen for and treat infectious pathogens, dental/oral infections, parasites, and environmental toxins, and develop a battle plan staging therapeutic trials and medications.

We can reexamine the application of medications: acetyl cholinesterase inhibitors donepezil (Aricept: 1996), galantamine (Razadyne: 2001), rivastigmine (Exelon: 2002), and NMDA receptor antagonist memantine (Namenda: 2003).

Natural remedies include phospholipids like phosphatidyl serine, phosphatidyl choline, omega 3 fatty acids, antioxidants like blueberries, dark chocolate, green tea and turmeric, nuts and seeds, and leafy greens, and herbal remedies like gingko biloba, bacopa, lion's mane, rhodiola, and ashwagandha.

Exercise, sleep, hydration, sun, puzzles and games, and social interaction are also important.

These should be part of our multipronged, multimodal approach to the worldwide pandemic phenomenon of dementia and Alzheimer's disease.

Noninvasive brain neuromodulation can help, as outlined in my next article.

Brain Neuromodulation Therapy from Cyprus: Transcranial Direct Current Stimulation

This is a report on my new experience at the SOZO Brain Center at AIMIS Clinic in Cyprus for treating neurological conditions. At my advanced Acupuncture Meridian Assessment (AMA) training in Saint Louis in August 2023, we had a case study of a Parkinson's disease patient who was not responding to the current regiment of standard medical care with other alternative treatments.

Together as a group of 15 physicians, dentists, and other medical professionals, we brainstormed how to evaluate based on AMA and treat an advanced Parkinson's disease case with significant tremors. The patient happened to be a physician from out of state. He had some improvement with stem cell injections and dental TMJ/bite revision, but the benefits did not last long enough to correct his tremors, and his condition regressed after he had additional dental work (eight dental implants) done.

One of the physicians from Germany, Dr. Atel Hemat, mentioned hearing of some promising success cases of movement disorders including Parkinson's disease in Europe, as reported by Dr. Helmut Retzek of Austria.

Dr. Retzek had been in Cyprus for Neuromodulation Therapy training conducted by Dr. Petros Kattou earlier in the summer. Some of the responses were almost miraculous. He thought it might have been staged by actors pretending to be patients with Parkinson's disease. We had a Zoom video conference with Dr. Retzek and Dr. Kattou and reviewed a case study of a severe Parkinson's disease patient who responded within a few hours to Transcranial Direct Current Stimulation (tDCS) and

Transcutaneous Auricular Vagus Nerve Stimulation (taVNS), two medical devices.

To make a long story short, I signed up for two days of training with Dr. Kattou, along with Dr. Hemat and eight other physicians from Europe in December 2023. I wanted to believe what I saw in the video was possible, but witnessing the video was not good enough for me. Could it be fake or too good to be true? I needed to see it in person. We had ten new cases of a variety of psychological and neurological patients during two days of training. Dr. Kattou did a quick neurologic examination, reviewed MRI scans when available, and started tDCS and taVNS treatment on some patients.

On the first day, a Swiss physician in his 50's came with a working diagnosis of Parkinson's disease and chronic pain. He had rigidity of extremities and chorea-like limb movement, unsteady gait, and speech. An MRI was done at the clinic which showed significant atrophy of the cerebellum. He most likely had a stroke with Parkinsonian-like features but not necessarily Parkinson's disease. He got treatment with taVNS on the first day and tDCS on the second.

That afternoon, to my surprise, he was running around the clinic front desk in the lobby. If I had not eye-witnessed him running around, I would never have believed that it was possible. I also had the opportunity to evaluate him using acupuncture meridian assessment (AMA) earlier and found he had significant dental infections and a gallbladder meridian disturbance. Dental and gallbladder are paired meridians.

One of my big questions is how long will functional improvement last from brain neuromodulation using tDCS and taVNS, especially when the patient has active dental and parasite infections influencing gallbladder and dental meridians? I have investigated many different modalities including Frequency Specific Microcurrent (FSM) developed by Carolyn McMakin, DC, qEEG, transcranial neurofeedback, IASIS, Alpha-Stim and more. This device seems safer, simpler, cheaper, and easier to use. The Air Force has been using tDCS as a part of pilot training.

Research using microcurrent for neuromodulation has been growing exponentially. There are over 4,000 published papers on tDCS, which is separate from transcranial magnetic therapy. There are many tDCS and taVNS devices on the market. Dr. Petros Kattou's training is highly informative, creative, entertaining, and takes you to another level of what is possible. He did not invent tDCS or taVNS but figured out how to apply it effectively using existing technologies based on his understanding of neurobiology, a quick neurologic examination, and neuromodulation. Any further details are considered confidential information and cannot be shared.

Some of the medical conditions which benefit include:

- Chronic, post-operative, and oncology pain
- Migraine and fibromyalgia
- Multiple sclerosis and Parkinson's Disease
- Depression, Bipolar Disorder
- Stress anxiety disorder and PTSD
- Mild cognitive impairment, memory issues
- Cerebral learning disabilities
- Addiction, Fatigue, and Insomnia

Research using microcurrent for neuromodulation has been growing exponentially.

Combining new ideas from international medical communities, such as brain neuromodulation therapy by Dr. Petros Kattou of Cyprus, can be an exciting new way of restoring brain function and treating neurological disorders. Medical professionals can travel to training with Dr. Kattou at www.sozubraincenter.com and explore what is possible. Dr. Helmut Retzek from Austria has extensive information and videos at www.ganzemedizin.at, including many case studies. I co-teach training sessions with Dr. Kattou at Prevention and Healing that combine Advanced AMA and Brain Neuromodulation.

For patients suffering with these medical problems, you may explore on your own or with a physician familiar with tDCS and taVNS. Although these devices have been researched for many years in academic and military institutions, they are not FDA approved as medical devices yet and not covered by insurance. There are self-help guides available. I found tDCS and taVNS to be new eye-opening therapies and will try them with one patient at a time - starting with restoring the brain meridian by correcting dental and parasite infections - as part of my brain neuromodulation therapy.

Dr. Simon Yu

Five Seconds Saves Ten Years of Suffering:
Quantum Random Non-Sense AI

Think the impossible possible. Earlier I wrote, Brain Neuromodulation Therapy from Cyprus: Transcranial Direct Current Stimulation (tDCS) for Parkinson's, Depression, Mild Cognitive Impairment, etc., based on the training by Dr. Petros Kattou from Cyprus. In medical training we are taught that damaged neurons do not regenerate. Until you see and witness what you thought was impossible, many physicians are stuck in that mindset despite overwhelming evidence of neuroplasticity.

The paradigm is shifting. In June 2024, we each presented at IGMEDT Austrian alternative medical conference in Vienna. Dr. Kattou's brain neuromodulation therapy lecture has been a highlight in the European medical community. I spoke on parasite and cancer connections and how to use Insulin potentiation therapy (IPT) to deliver lower doses of medications with high efficacy and fewer side effects.

Dr. Kattou came to St. Louis in August to co-lead my joint advanced acupuncture meridian assessment (AMA) training and his brain neuromodulation therapy for neurologic disorders – the first time in America. The response has been overwhelmingly positive; it was well attended by physicians and dentists from all over the USA and Europe. Time will tell the impacts of his new ideas on the American medical system: to embrace, or ridicule and resist (the "American way").

One of the audience members in Vienna asked a question: How long does it take to detect hidden dental problems that did not show on dental X-ray or CBCT? I said, "Five seconds." I was surprised to hear myself speak quickly without thinking. Five seconds to detect dental problems? It seemed far-fetched that it would take only five seconds. I could not believe what I had said. It took me over ten years of acupuncture meridian assessment (AMA) training and practice, trial and error, to feel comfortable picking up hidden dental infections not visible on dental X-ray or CBCT with strong probability. After thirty years of practice, I can say this with some degree of certainty.

> **How long does it take to detect hidden dental problems that did not show on dental X-ray or CBCT? I said, "Five seconds."**

Was I making things up to impress the audience? Time for me to question myself. Typically, I measure forty main acupuncture meridians as a system, somewhat like inspecting or tuning a violin. Each individual measurement may take up to five seconds for forty meridians, a total of two hundred seconds. Each five seconds has an interval with a long or short pause depending on the patient when I interact and ask questions. The whole evaluation may take 10-15 minutes, followed by enhanced interrogation that may take another 10-15 minutes. The whole process takes about 30 minutes.

These five-second intervals of one meridian measurement can tell a patient's story of many years of suffering. It can be one year, a decade, or more. It often comes down to dental, parasite, and/or fungal problems that have been overlooked by physicians and academic medical institutions. We live in a narrow spectrum of frequency based on our senses to see, feel, and measure. AMA evaluation is based on ancient, acupuncture intelligence that seems unpredictable, random, non-physical, even non-sense (does not always correspond to western lab test measurements) called Chi, Prana, or Life Force.

At the joint AMA/Brain Neuromodulation seminar, 12 advanced neurologic patients were evaluated by Dr. Kattou with his unique brain neuromodulation program using a Plato headset from PlatoScience in Denmark. We did not have the auricular Vagus Nerve stimulation device available at the time of the training. It is too early to tell how they will respond to Plato brain neuromodulation alone. Some of the cases included Parkinson's disease, cerebellum ataxia from traumatic brain injuries, ALS, glioblastoma multiforme with neuropathy, hemorrhagic stroke in a wheelchair, myalgic-encephalomyelitis (ME) and chronic fatigue syndrome, head dystonia, etc.

On further thought, I should have invited mild to moderate neurologic cases for the training rather than advanced cases. I was hoping for a dramatic miraculous response in our training and that may not be realistic. I wrote about a limping Parkinson's patient leaping and running after a two-day training in Cyprus. He received combined synergistic tDCS and auricular vagus stimulation together. It may take many weeks, months, or years of treatment to see a response in advanced cases.

Dr. Helmut Retzek of Austria, who introduced me to Dr. Kattou last year, sent a post on the importance of vagus nerve stimulation (VNS) for the overall survival of cancer patients. He referenced, "The Role of the Vagus Nerve in Cancer Prognosis: A Systematic and a Comprehensive Review," from the Journal of Oncology (2018), which reported that VNS increased survival rates by 30 percent.[45] Vagus nerve stimulation is an important part of brain neuromodulation.

> **"Vagal nerve activation improves cancer prognosis."**
> Marijke De Couck and Ralf Caers

Here is a summary from Dr. Retzek's website, ganzemedizin.at.[46]

Vagus stimulation improves cancer prognosis through these mechanisms:

- Increase in heart rate variability (HRV): Studies show that high HRV, which reflects the activity of the vagus nerve, is associated with better cancer prognosis. Patients with higher HRV have lower mortality rates and better survival rates

- Reduction of inflammation: The vagus nerve activates the cholinergic anti-inflammatory pathway, which reduces the release of proinflammatory cytokines. This anti-inflammatory effect can slow tumor growth and metastasis

- Reduction of oxidative stress: Vagal stimulation can reduce the oxidative stress associated with DNA damage and tumor development

- Influence on tumor immunology: Recent evidence suggests that vagus nerve activity can enhance immune response against tumors by influencing certain immune cells involved in fighting cancer.

In summary, high vagus nerve activity improves cancer prognosis through a combination of neurological, immunological, and anti-inflammatory effects. There are other means to activate vagus stimulation by meditation, prayer, breathing exercise, yoga exercise, and even the beta-blocker propranolol by blocking the action of adrenaline and downregulating the sympathetic nerve system, and upregulating the vagus parasympathetic nervous system.

A retired 45-year-old Air Force pilot had a 4+ year history of muscle fasciculations throughout the body. He had seen five neurologists, had every known test, and was told he had autoimmune disease caused by voltage-gated calcium channel (VGCC) antibodies which have been associated with Lambert-Eaton myasthenic syndrome (LEMS): an autoimmune disease that affects neuromuscular junctions. The causes are unknown. Symptoms include proximal muscle weakness, areflexia, and autonomic dysfunction. About 85 percent of LEMS patients test positive for VGCC antibodies. No lab tests were available to verify his medical diagnosis on his visit.

In his AMA evaluation (Figure 69), his main problems were in his dental-oral cavity with two impacted wisdom teeth pressing on his trigeminal nerve, low-grade infections surrounding the impacted teeth, and environmental toxins from heavy metals, petrochemicals, and possible fungal mycotoxins. Otherwise, he was physically fit and could expect to fly for many years to come as a commercial airline pilot. He had subtle muscle fatigue with a simple rapid forced fist closure test.

In my experience, if his underlying conditions are not corrected, he will have many different manifestations of medical and neurological conditions, and perhaps eventual diagnosis of ALS ten years later. Here is his AMA Evaluation chart. Ly stands for dental, Al for allergy-immunology, and 3E for hormonal imbalance; the low bars show chronic degeneration; the middle bars are in normal range.

Figure 69: AMA Evaluation of Retired Air Force Pilot

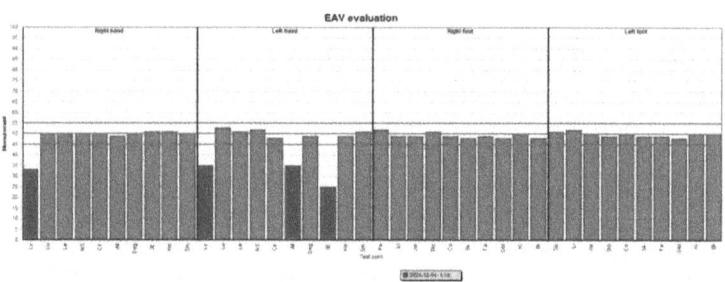

My 5-second interval 40-point AMA evaluation picked up dental, allergy-immunology, and hormone disturbances. I referred him to an oral surgeon, with brain neuromodulation as a recommended preventative measure. Oral surgeons often decline to extract impacted wisdom teeth as a risky operation, possibly damaging the nerve, but at what cost? AMA, oral surgery, and brain neuromodulation may change the course of this pilot's life by tapping into the ancient intelligence of acupuncture intelligence (AI 2.0). This is my deep dive into 5-second Quantum Random Non-Sense AI.

Part 9
Biohacking Basics to Advanced Therapies

Chapter 13 Blending AMA, AI, and Biohacking for Health

In my view, Acupuncture Meridian Assessment is a great adjunct tool for physicians, dentists, and patients to hack and improve their disease challenges and health outcomes. By definition and by design, AMA is AI applied to the domain of the body. What better source than the patient's own meridian strings and bioresonance to indicate health and disease?

Many factors fuel the growth of self-help, self-improvement, healthy eating, natural healing, optimizing health, functional or precision medicine, biohacking, antiaging, and more. When patients reach the limits of conventional medicine and are not satisfied with lifelong medication to manage chronic health problems or slow disease progression, they seek new ways to get better and embark upon a quest for health. When physicians, dentists, and other health professionals get tired of naming diagnoses and medicating symptoms, they seek new ways to identify and treat root causes.

The growth of AI has opened up new ways to search for and sort medical and scientific knowledge. Growth of social media has fueled extensive peer-to-peer sharing. Today's medical, dental, and health fields are a battle royale between pharma, device companies, government regulators, insurance companies, medical/dental specialty groups, and private equity. Doctors, dentists, and patients are increasingly on their own to sort through self-interest and conflicts, solid information, disinformation, grift, scams, and help.

What is Biohacking?

Biohacking has many dimensions. According to AI, "Biohacking refers to the practice of using science, technology, and self-experimentation to improve one's biology and performance. Essentially, it's a way of optimizing the human body and mind through various methods." It includes nutrition, sleep optimization, exercise, mindfulness and meditation, wearables, and epigenetic modification.

You will find many resources for biohacking in the Appendix. Unifying and integrating these complementary ways to help heal and strengthen, I will add another dimension: Use acupuncture meridian assessment on the domain of the whole body. AMA will help gather and translate intelligence via the bio-frequency scale for optimizing nutrition and metabolism, identifying and treating infectious pathogens, detoxing heavy metals and chemicals, and restoring and supporting healthy functioning. One might also call it "balancing meridians" or "enhancing epigenetics."

Color Me Red, Color Me Blue: Red Light and Methylene Blue Therapy May Save Your Life

The Color Spectrum Therapy has been known since ancient times for medical incurables but not well known in the chemistry based, pharmaceutical dominant Western Medicine. When in doubt, let the patients get out of the cave or out of the dark room and expose them to sunlight (simply called Sunlight Therapy), or Heliotherapy and cosmic rays. Miracle cures can happen. The average healthy person needs full spectrum sunlight plus cosmic rays. An unhealthy person needs additional specific color spectrum light to promote healing. I wrote an article on this subject in 2010, "Color Me Blue, Color Me Red: Biocybernetics and Color Medicine Conference in St. Louis."

Colors have been used for medical therapeutic purposes over the ages since ancient times. There are assignments of colors to certain organs, functions or conditions in the teaching of Ayurvedic Medicine with the Chakra system, and in Traditional Chinese Medicine (TCM) with acupuncture meridians. Each color spectrum has its own frequency, wavelength, and pitch; and each organ responds to certain wavelength, chakra and color frequency. See Figure 70.

Figure 70: Color Spectrum, Wavelength, Notes, Pitch

	Wavelength Angstrom Units	1 A = 10*-10th Meters	Converted to Hertz	Note	Orchestra Pitch	Physical Pitch
Infra Red Begins	7653A	to 7813A	392X10*12thHz	~~ G	392 Hz	384 Hz
Red	7228A	to 7317A	415X10*12thHz	~~ G#	415 Hz	410 Hz
Red-Orange	6818A	to 7042A	440X10*12thHz	~~ A	440 Hz	426 Hz
Orange	6438A	to 6522A	466X10*12thHz	~~ A#	466 Hz	460Hz
Orange-Yellow	6058A	to 6250A	493X10*12thHz	~~ B	493 Hz	480 Hz
	5736A	to 5859A	523X10*12thHz	~~ C	523 Hz	512 Hz
	5415A	to 5474A	554X10*12thHz	~~ C#	554 Hz	548 Hz
Green	5110A	to 5208A	587X10*12thHz	~~ D	587 Hz	576 Hz
Green-Blue	4823A	to 4878A	622X10*12thHz	~~ D#	622 Hz	615 Hz
Blue	4552A	to 4688A	659X10*12thHz	~~ E	659 Hz	640 Hz
Indigo	4298A	to 4392A	697X10*12thHz	~~ F	698 Hz	683 Hz
Violet	4054A	to 4098A	740X10*12thHz	~~ F#	740 Hz	732 Hz
Ultra-Violet Begins	3827A	to 3906A	784X10*12thHz			

Frequency X Wavelength = Speed Of Light
Speed Of Light = 300,000,000 Meters Per Second

These wavelengths and color spectra correspond to different chakras in the body; see Figure 71.

Figure 71: Color Spectrum, Wavelength and Chakras

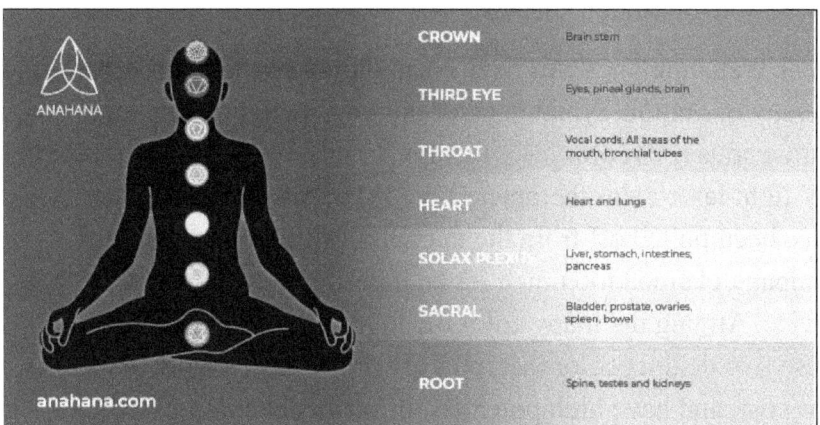

According to Franz Morell, MD from Germany, who wrote, *The MORA Concept*, it is less well known in Western Medicine that colored light is of vital importance to life. Small animals, which were kept in total exclusion from light, became ill or died, although they had been fed well and had sufficient space to move around. Fritz-Albert Popp, PhD, prominent German biophysicist, found that every living organism has photon emissions which cannot be suppressed. Cell-to-cell communication through biophotons before, during and after billions of biochemical interactions in the body at the cellular level. Even blind children respond to color therapy. They respond to the frequency of the color spectrum.

Color frequency can be amplified. Dr. Zenon Gruba of Australia was able to amplify 400,000 times to achieve a dramatic response to pain. 90% of people responded to the color Red, and 10% responded to the color Blue for pain, according to Dr. Gruba. His lecture in November 2006 stunned the audience at the International Symposium of Biocybernetic Medicine in Germany. I was there and witnessed it, and since then have been using Biophoton Laser Therapy and Color Therapy with limited success.

Since then, many articles have been published on biophoton therapy or photon-dynamic color therapy, including low level intravenous (IV) color laser therapy. I had two IV intravenous UV light laser color therapies (UVLrx) in my clinic, but they have been pulled off from the market, most likely because the company claimed too much for an investigational medical device. Among the many color therapies on the market today, these two distinct color therapies are promising, simple to use, low cost, and have high potential for medical benefits: Red Light Therapy and Methylene Blue dye.

Red Light therapy works by activating mitochondria cytochrome c oxidase (Complex IV) and turning on mitochondrial oxidative phosphorylation respiration. This is the fourth step of cellular respiration, the metabolic pathway that uses glucose to produce adenosine triphosphate (ATP), an organic compound which the body uses to produce energy. Another mechanism is through the concept of "Hormesis" and red-light stimulation by creating a transient metabolic stress-like exercise. The red-light color spectrum goes from about 600 to 700 nm; the near infrared spectrum goes about 700 to 1,100 nm. Red and near infrared light therapy devices have been FDA-approved for several purposes to date, including pain relief, wound healing, anti-aging, hair loss reversal, acne treatment, fat loss, etc.

Benefits of red and near-infrared light therapy from Ari Whitten's book, *The Ultimate Guide to Red Light Therapy*.[47]

- Increase overall energy
- Combat skin aging, wrinkles, cellulite

- Speed up fat loss
- Improve muscle recovery and athletic performance
- Improve mood and cognitive function
- Speed healing from injury
- Improve metabolism and hormonal health

Methylene Blue (Methylthionium chloride) was first synthesized in 1876 by German chemist Heinrich Caro to stain wool for the textile industry. In 1880, microbiologist Robert Koch pioneered the use of methylene blue for staining cells and microbes. The application of methylene blue has been expanded for Malaria-causing intracellular parasites called Plasmodium vivax, and during the Second World War, methylene blue was given to soldiers as an antimalarial drug, until it was replaced with the patented drug, hydroxychloroquine, which is based on methylene blue dye.

The primary way that methylene blue benefits the body is its role as a nitric oxide inhibitor and estrogen antagonist. By reducing nitric oxide and estrogen, thyroid function is increased, and the body benefits from increased metabolic rate and overall energy production. Methylene blue acts on the mitochondria respiration chain I-IV complex. For more information, see Gonzalez-Lima and Auchter's 2015 article in *Frontiers in Cellular Neuroscience*.[48]

Combining Red Light therapy and Methylene Blue dye color therapy are relatively cheap, synergistic adjunct therapies to IV UV light/Ozone therapy. The benefits and side effects of methylene blue are reviewed in a 2010 article by Ginimuge and Jyothi, "Methylene Blue Revisited."[49] It has many benefits but is contraindicated in patients with renal insufficiency. It is an MAO inhibitor and can interact with selective serotonin reuptake inhibitors (SSRI) and MAO inhibitors. It interacts with dapsone and forms hydroxylamine which oxidizes hemoglobin causing hemolysis – destruction of red blood cells.

Interestingly, heavily promoted Nitric Oxide (NO) may do more harm than good in the long run. Sildenafil (Viagra), the new wonder drug for erection, works by blocking what's called PDE5 (phosphodiesterase type 5), an enzyme in the body that breaks down chemicals responsible for reactions and raises nitric oxide. As a result, penile tissues stay relaxed and engorged with blood.

Pharmaceutical industries have sold to the unsuspecting public the virtues of raising Nitric Oxide with sildenafil (Viagra) or tadalafil (Cialis) as a new generation of molecular medicine for Erectile Dysfunction, and additional hypes include reducing risk of Alzheimer's disease and pulmonary hypertension. Robert F. Furchgott, Louis J. Ignarro, and Ferid Murad shared the Noble Prize in 1998 for their discoveries concerning nitric oxide as a signaling molecule in the cardiovascular system for the vasodilation.[50]

However, basic science indicates raising nitric oxide may also be a concern as it acts as a free radical, is highly reactive, and can add oxidative stress that increases in the body with age. The body's primary vasodilator is carbon dioxide (CO_2). Nitric oxide acts as a stress signaling molecule for short-term benefit and contradicts long-term benefit claims.

The top 10 benefits and potential indications for Methylene Blue, from Mark Sloan's book, *The Ultimate Guide to Methylene Blue*:[51]

- Chemical Poisoning and Overdose
- Anti-Malarial Drug
- Virus Warrior

- Dementia: Alzheimer's and Parkinson's
- Cognitive Enhancement
- Depression
- Autism
- Pain Reliever
- Heart Health
- Cancer

It is also now being used for Lyme and coinfections.

Prevention and Healing added a Nordic Health Solutions Red Light Therapy Bed. It has two pulsing red-light frequencies and two near infrared light frequencies. This light bed has the most scientifically proven health benefits of red-light therapy with 635nm and 660nm red light frequencies. In addition, it has near infrared light frequencies of 850 nm and 940nm.

One caution: Application of Red Light and Methylene Blue Therapies may sound too good to be true. These therapies can be done at home but are not as simple as you may think. Be informed. If you have active dental infections, parasite/fungal infections, nutritional deficiency, heavy metals, environmental toxin exposure, or trauma, these problems must be addressed first, or concurrently; otherwise, you may have a disappointing response, another hype and another disappointment.

I highly recommend the two books noted above, *The Ultimate Guide to Red Light Therapy* by Ari Whitten and *The Ultimate Guide to Methylene Blue* by Mark Sloan. These two therapies may save your life, or the life of a loved one.

Here is my favorite article on Biohacking, about a former patient, an MIT engineer who helped heal her family and developed her own website, Debug Your Health, to help others.

Excerpt: Parasite Treatment Hacked by an MIT Engineer: Think Small, Dream Big for Pandemic

What would you do if I told you that you can treat parasite problems by yourself, and treat your family without visiting a medical doctor? It may seem a daunting task, but would you like to know? It is not simple, but it can be done. I just found out from one of my patients, whom I will call Bible Man.

I was driving with my wife, Kate, on my way to the West Coast in January 2017 in my convertible and became snowbound when several feet of snow fell in Northern Arizona. I did not expect nor prepare for a snowstorm on this trip. My wife was not happy with my lack of planning, driving through a snowstorm with summer tires. Luckily, Bible Man knew we were driving through and offered us an invitation to stay at his house for temporary shelter from the storm. My wife said yes, and I did not dare to say no.

We stayed at his house for two nights until we could drive again. Bible Man and his wife were gracious hosts, and we had many interesting conversations on worldly topics of medicine, politics, science, religion, etc. During our evening talk, he got an urgent message from his friend to check out a website on how to treat parasites developed by an MIT engineer. We found *Debug Your Health* at debugyourhealth.com, developed by Susan L., PhD, from MIT, living in Silicon Valley.

I almost fell off my chair. She has been a patient; I had taken care of her and her family a few years ago. Her website covered how to detect hidden parasites and dental related problems. She is an MIT engineer who cracked the secret of hidden parasites and dental problems based on her experiences as my patient, observing my acupuncture meridian assessment

(AMA) testing, and from her work with other practitioners. She refined my technique with some form of self-muscle testing.

It took me many years of training in medical school, Internal Medicine training, US Army medical doctor experiences, and years of trial and error in the clinic to figure out hidden parasites and dental problems. Most medical professionals miss the connections between hidden parasites and dental problems that can impact chronically ill patients. In a few years, an MIT engineer figured out how to test for hidden parasites and dental problems based on her personal experiences as my patient, and she was able to "hack" the medical system.

She cracked the code like a good engineer. I have been pondering about her audacity to put this information on the internet while most physicians are in denial about the existence of parasite and dental problems. There is always the danger of people self-treating with the wrong medications, and most medical doctors are not familiar with parasite medications to help guide these desperate patients.

I like to think small. I treat one patient at a time based on acupuncture meridian assessment. From now on, I can think small and still dream big. I will let engineers think big, dream big, and solve the mystery of pandemic parasite problems: a global environmental health threat. The pandemic is here. The CDC and medical communities are not ready to crack the hidden code for detecting hidden parasites and dental problems. The paradigm is shifting. Dream big and you can hack the medical system by navigating sites like debugyourhealth.com. You may stumble onto an accidental cure but be mindful of your limitations.

Patient Story: Chronic Illness from Parasites

Here is a patient testimonial Dr. Retzek shared with Dr. Yu. After working for months in Egypt, this woman and all her colleagues got sick. When she visited Dr. Helmut Retzek of Austria, the first time she brought pictures of Ascaris (roundworm larvae creeping out of her eye. She also had a cyst in her face where she felt them moving. He found typical Ascaris larvae in her darkfield blood analysis.

Upon starting parasite treatment by Dr. Retzek per Dr. Yu's protocol, she had a huge Herxheimer reaction,[52] including epileptic fits and swelling of her entire body, for which she was hospitalized. Since then, she has had tremendous improvement.

In a video, she thanks Dr. Simon Yu of St. Louis, an integrative MD who developed this form of treatment. Dr. Yu discovered parasites are an underestimated source of many diseases after serving as a US Army Reserve Medical Corps Officer in South America doing parasite treatment for large numbers of people.

This patient testimonial video was submitted with permission by the patient and Dr. med Helmut Retzek who has a practice for integrative and biological medicine in Voecklabruck, Austria, you can watch it on YouTube.[53]

Excerpt: Insulin Potentiation Therapy (IPT) for All Chronic Disease: Can Old Cranky Physicians Try New Approaches?

Let me reintroduce an old forgotten and neglected medical therapy called Insulin Potentiation Therapy (IPT) developed by Mexican military surgeon, Donato Perez Garcia, Sr., MD in

1932. He was able to cure many medical conditions from asthma, psoriasis, migraine headache, neurosyphilis, lupus, multiple sclerosis and even some cancers. *Time* magazine covered Dr. Garcia's therapy as Insulin Shock Therapy in 1944. Despite media coverage, his ideas were never fully accepted in the United States.

Most young physicians follow prevailing medical policies and guidelines. There is too much risk of losing everything and their livelihoods. Is there room for older, independent, solo-practice established physicians who refuse to accept insurance-driven models so they can apply their experience in clinical decisions – rather than using cookie-cutter insurance, pharma, and algorithm driven protocols?

They can be uncompromising contrarians, raising hell for their patients' welfare, truly a rare, dying breed of independent, cranky old practitioners. The crankier the better. These physicians are far less likely burned out and depressed than those employed by a hospital or large healthcare organization.

Consider all the modern chronic diseases such as cardiovascular disease, hypertension, diabetes, Lyme, obesity, neurologic disorders, Alzheimer's disease, many forms of cancer, and more. These chronic diseases have become a very promising growth industry for the medical-industrial complex, bigger than the military-industrial complex. Medical science, Pharma and Big Money investors are betting on advances in Molecular and Gene Therapy, CRISPR technology, and Artificial Intelligence (AI) for breakthroughs in managing chronic diseases – not necessarily in finding the cures. The magic word is disease management. IPT may change the playing field from managing diseases to the possibility of cures if you incorporate dental, fungal, and parasite infections as an integral part of medical therapy – three commonly overlooked underlying causes.

Most chronic diseases are not driven by genetics but by epigenetic changes resulting from underlying infections, environmental toxins, endotoxins, nutritional deficiencies, excessive calories, and overloading our main detox organ systems. Our current medical model rarely addresses dental-related medical issues and parasite infestations.

Ask old timer physicians who do not take insurance, are independent, and not employed by hospitals. One of the neglected therapies is IPT, brought to the United States by a Canadian American physician, Steven Ayer, MD in collaboration with Donato Perez Garcia, MD.

IPT has been combined with low dose chemotherapy (typically 10 percent of the standard dose for cancer treatment as a safer, cheaper alternative to high dose chemotherapy. IPT can be also used as an independent Immune Support Therapy without using low-dose chemo by adding antiviral, antibacterial, antifungal, and antiprotozoal medications, and anti-inflammatory agents, to reduce the total body burden of infectious loads and reduce inflammation. I have used IPT on numerous patients over the years and have been quite satisfied with the results. For more, see the full article on my website.

Excerpt: EBOO – Ozone Dialysis Therapy for Veterans, Firefighters, Farmers and Others Exposed to Toxins

Let me introduce you to a new extraordinary therapy called ozone dialysis therapy, short for **extracorporeal blood oxygenation and ozonation (EBOO)**. Another name for

EBOO is Recirculatory Hemoperfusion (RHP) therapy. I have been searching for medical facilities that can do dialysis to remove environmental toxins like pesticides or organic compounds for some of my patients without much success. One patient, diagnosed with ALS, had exposure to massive amounts of petrochemicals and organophosphate compounds.

Regular IV ozone/UV light therapy (each treatment is called a pass) is too slow to remove environmental toxins when there have been massive exposures. Ozone dialysis therapy or EBOO, relatively unknown, may be a game changer for many chronically ill patients who have environmental toxin exposures, and are not responding to traditional or alternative, integrative medicine. Farmers, firefighters, soldiers, and unsuspecting members of the general population may benefit given their exposures.

Academic institutions and military/VA medicine need to explore this exciting technology that is available and already used overseas in Europe and Asia. EBOO does not use any new technology or medications and hopefully it will not be sabotaged by Big Pharma or entangled with FDA regulations. I have used EBOO on several patients who were quite satisfied with its results. For more, see the full article on my website.

Part 10
Biology of Belief

Chapter 14 Looking Back, Looking Ahead

To move ahead in medicine, we need to go back and rediscover ancient, authentic intelligence from the domain of the body. Acupuncture meridians reveal subtle microcurrents or bioelectrical frequencies that are in tune when physiological systems are in harmony and disrupted when they are not.

Here are a few of my favorite articles to help summarize what I have learned, and you can apply in your practice, and for patients, in your healing. They can also help us look forward to new discoveries and ways of healing if we can embrace the new biology of ancient, authentic belief.

Bruce Lipton's Biology of Belief and Epigenetics: Quantum Entanglement of Parasites?

Quantum Entanglement and Epigenetics were a part of Bruce Lipton's keynote lecture at the September 2024 International College of Integrative Medicine (ICIM) Conference in Indianapolis, which drew on his landmark book, *The Biology of Belief: Unleashing the Power of Consciousness, Matter & Miracles*.[54] Now about ten years after his updated 10th anniversary edition, he shared his revolutionary point of view on how individual cells interact with their environment, and how the principles of cellular biology also need to be rewritten in evolutionary biology. Darwinian genetic determinism and survival of the fittest is an outdated and incomplete evolutionary paradigm – communication and cooperation are essential.

I am familiar with Lipton's work in what he calls the field of New Biology… New Medicine. He describes the power of consciousness, Quantum Mechanics, Quantum Biology, Quantum Entanglement, and how epigenetics (environment, emotion, belief and spirituality) is the driving force for gene expression. He reminds us that modern medical care is the third leading cause of death after cardiovascular disease and cancer. He calls to reexamine pharmaceutical and biochemistry-based medicine and challenge the dogma of gene theory.

I agree with Lipton that healing must come from within. We are living in Quantum Fields beyond Newtonian's mechanical material world, where belief, bioenergetics, emotions, environment, and spirituality are key. Genes are merely a blueprint. The master architect is you. The master of the master architect is the Universe, the Creator. Anything is possible and *The Biology of Belief* is a must read.

I like to ask simple questions. Is it possible that "parasite entities" – physical and non-physical forms of parasites – are entangled in the Quantum Fields?

We live in a quantum field of weirdness. At least, that is my understanding of quantum physics based on Schrödinger's experiment. Schrödinger's Cat, dead and/or alive at the same time, is a famous **"thought experiment"** that demonstrates the idea in quantum physics that tiny particles can be in two states superimposed at once until they are observed, both a particle and/or a wave.

In a quantum torsion field, left can be left and/or right, up can be up and/or down. At least, that is my observation based on acupuncture meridian assessment (AMA) evaluation of my patients, and in my learning and teaching on how we interact with the Universe and the human body.

My experience of diagnosing and treating parasites based on AMA has been a strange, accidental journey, as described in my first book, *Accidental Cure*, from my work in the US Army Medical Reserve Corps targeting parasite infections in Bolivia.

When using parasite medications for officially documented parasites or for suspected (or perhaps imaginary or non-physical) parasites based only on AMA, there is often a random, unpredictable "accidental" cure for medical problems such as asthma, pneumonia, COVID-19, multiple sclerosis, brain tumor, cancer, chronic fatigue, fibromyalgia, seizure, migraine headache, anxiety and depression, etc. How can we explain this based on science and evidence-based medicine when there is no physical proof of the parasite infection based on current medical technology which focuses on stool samples, but the patient responds to parasite medications anyway? What are we missing?

Is it possible that imaginary non-physical parasitic entities respond to parasite medications based on the Biology of Belief of patients by placebo effects and/or parasites themselves having nocebo effects? Do parasites have consciousness? Nocebo is the opposite of a placebo: when negative expectations about treatment cause a worse outcome than would otherwise have occurred. Or is there an earlier evolutionary link with a primitive parasitic cell or organism that responds to the same medication?

Parasites have their own parasites which carry bacteria, fungi, and viruses. Parasites live in a complex ecosystem with complex life cycles and are a driving force of evolution. In one sense, parasites are at the top of the food chain, the master of Evolutionary Force, living within us. Homo sapiens struggled and evolved with parasites, along with many other microorganisms in our oral, gut, and other microbiomes: the trillions of symbiotic microbial cells residing within us, including viruses, bacteria, and fungi.

And then, there is the **shadowy parasitic Homo sapiens**, see Figure 72. They are the elites, billionaires, big pharma, big insurance, big tech and big science, and private equity. They are the top of their game in evolution. For them, the belief of "creation" is just a matter of inconvenient theory. They do not want you to know the other superimposed theory of quantum entanglement of the evolution of Life, the creation of Life.

Figure 72: Universal Ancestors: RNA, DNA – Evolution via Cooperation vs. Competition

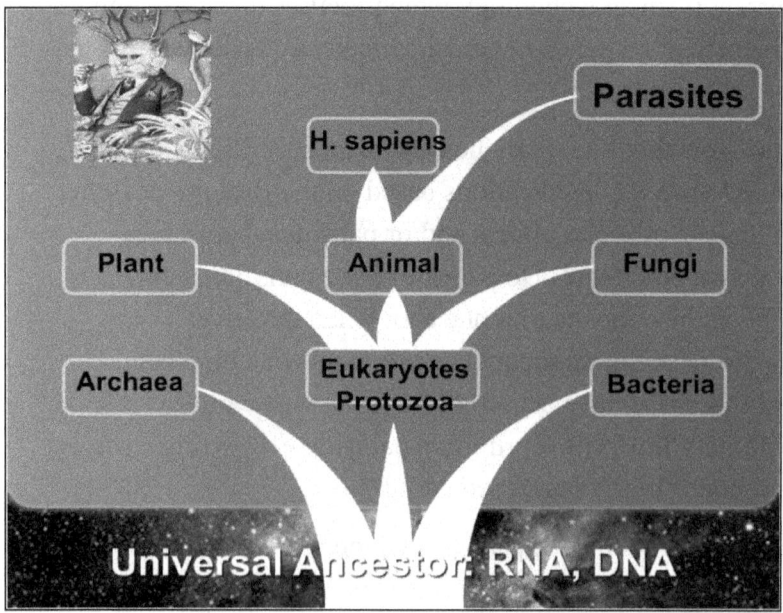

Figure 73: Multiple Signs of Parasite Infections

Multiple Signs of Parasites:

- Gas/Bloating
- Grinding teeth
- Coughing at night
- Weight loss/gain
- Obesity/under-weight
- Lethargy/chronic fatigue
- Sexual dysfunction
- Migraine headache
- Vision problems
- Brain fog
- Craving for foods
- Anemia/eosinophilia
- Bruxism
- Allergies
- Suppress allergies
- Immune deficiency syndrome
- Mental/behavior problems
- Constipation/diarrhea
- Psoriasis/eczema
- Food allergies
- Knee/hip pain/fibromyalgia
- Abdominal pain
- IBS/Colitis
- Waking up at night/bed wetting
- Night sweats/nightmares
- Rectal itching
- Muscle/joint pain
- Cyst/tumor

When you have multiple signs of parasites (Figure 73), it is worth trying parasite meds based on AMA or other energetic testing. Miracles happen randomly (or not). It is no accident that so many medical problems disappear with appropriate parasite medications. Medical science has long focused on viruses, bacterial, and fungal infections and overlooked the importance of parasite infections from an evolutionary point of view. Millions of people suffer or even die from complications of parasite infections and other unrecognized chronic illnesses, like cancer, asthma, pneumonia, possibly COVID-19, etc.

I have written many articles on parasites to share my perspective and reflections as an Internal Medicine physician, not a parasitologist, on parasites as an accidental discovery. Go to the articles page on my website and select the Parasites/Fungi category, and it will bring you to over 60 articles.

Scan for titles that take you to the subject of your interests. Some of my favorites are:

- Parasites and Allergies: Paradise Lost in the Parallel Universe,
- Parasites and Allergy Related Symptoms,
- Parasites and Meat Allergy,
- Parasites and Mental Illness: Delusions of Parasitosis,
- Parasites and Mind Control: Evolution of Social Parasites,
- Parasite as a New Emerging Global Environmental Threat,
- Parasites Follow Money: Disease Follows Money,
- Parasites Without the Borders,
- Parasites, Inflammation and Cancer: Ring of Fire Feeding Tumor Cells,
- Parasite Infections are Leading to Undiagnosed Health Problems for Veterans,
- Parasites Speak Many Languages
- Parasitic Human Called Para-sapiens: Forgiveness for Nobel Prize Winners Gone Bad, and
- Ivermectin Deficiency Syndrome (Parts 1 and 2).

In summary, my journey of encountering unexpected global parasite problems, developing treatment plans based on my experience in my US Army Medical Corps Reserve deployment to Bolivia, and use of acupuncture meridian assessment (AMA) to detect and guide treatment of underlying health problems via measuring disturbances in meridians pathways and medication testing to rebalance their bioenergetic frequencies, has been a somewhat strange pathway. My treatment plans have continued to evolve as I have gained more experience from the successes, failures, refinements, and input of my patients.

Hidden dental problems and dental parasites and fungal infections add another dimension to the body burden for oral/gut microbiome dysbiosis and help explain why it is difficult to break the cycle of parasite infestation. Once the public and the medical professions acknowledge that hidden parasite problems are real, on a global scale, we have a better chance to fight parasites and parasitic entities.

In my practice, I find many health problems – as indicated via meridian disturbances – respond best to parasite medications (which are poison to parasites), but they may evade natural parasite remedies (which can drive them deeper and provide false security). My treatments and recommendations are paired with dental work, detoxification, and other supports to improve the patient's biological terrain, circulation, diet, elimination, and immune system; and to restore harmony and cellular homeostasis.

You may begin to see the complexity of intracellular, intercellular, and evolutionary ecosystems; we are only at the beginning of understanding parasite-related medical problems. You may discover quantum entanglement of parasites and other parasitic entities. It gets a little weird. Enjoy reading Bruce Lipton's *The Biology of Belief*.

Unresolved Feelings and Their Target Organs

As you can tell by reading this book, everything is connected in Acupuncture Intelligence in the domain of the body, which includes the mind, spirit, soul, consciousness, unconsciousness, thoughts, emotions, feelings, and more. Traditional Chinese Medicine included emotions and feelings in its mapping of the meridians, elements, and target organs. See the Chart on the next page, which I have referenced throughout the book.

How did or does being ill make you feel? Which of these have you experienced? Did treatment and recovery change your emotions and feelings?

Figure 74: Unresolved Emotions and Target Organs

FIRE

Small Intestine	Emotional Heart	Physical Heart	Thyroid
Loneliness	Acute Grief	Unlived Joy	Humiliated
Abandoned	Shock	Self-Protection	Indecisive
Unreceptive	Broken Trust	Feeling Used	Left Out
Lost	Remorse	Rigid	Denial

WOOD / EARTH

Liver	Gallbladder	Spleen/Pancreas	Stomach
Anger	Resentment	Inadequacy	Anxiety
Frustration	Victimhood	Inferiority	Dislike
Toxic	Bitter	Oversensitive	Stressed
Unyielding	Blaming		Obsessed

WATER / METAL

Kidney	Bladder/Sex Organs	Lung	Large Intestine
Fear	Shame	Chronic Grief	Overcritical
Guilt	Dependency	Sadness	Controlling
Disappointment	Helpless	Longing	Dogmatic
Exhaustion	Yearning	Loss of zest	Uptight

Source: Traditional Chinese Medicine

Patient Story: Dr. Yu Saved my Life

2025: I was sick for eight years with interstitial cystitis, chronic fatigue, and pelvic inflammatory disease. After years of research and trial and error, I managed to cure my interstitial cystitis on my own, but I couldn't overcome the other two conditions. Through Jesus' guidance, I realized the root cause was parasitic. I started my own protocol based on information I found online (don't do this!), and while I saw some improvement — especially with the pelvic inflammation — things took a sudden and severe turn for the worse.

I collapsed. I couldn't eat, drink, or sleep for six weeks and was on the edge of death. I went to the ER twice and was even admitted to the hospital, but because conventional medicine doesn't acknowledge parasites as a cause, I was repeatedly discharged in worse condition than when I arrived. I live in Tulsa, OK, and not a single doctor — whether holistic, alternative, or conventional — could help me. I was slowly and painfully dying. The pain in my colon was unbearable — perhaps the worst pain of all.

By the grace of God, I heard about Dr. Yu on Facebook. In the middle of the night, we left Tulsa and drove straight to him because I knew I was out of time. Dr. Yu believed me. He quickly identified the problem and treated me accordingly. I am alive today because of Jesus and because of him!

I've seen so many happy, cured patients in his office. The reviews you read don't fully capture his impact in people's lives. It reminds me of when Jesus healed ten lepers, but only one returned to give thanks: "Were not all ten cleansed? Where are the other nine?" Dr. Yu is truly a gift from God, and I am forever grateful.

Igor, my Bad Patient: Deworming as a New Uncertain Preventive Medicine

Igor, a 60-year-old, noncompliant patient returned to my clinic recently. He was having abdominal pain and rectal bleeding with bowel movement. He had been evaluated by another physician and told his CT scan was consistent with liver problems including fatty liver. He was warned that he may have other serious medical problems and required further evaluation including colonoscopy.

He was scared he might have cancer and wanted my opinion. I reviewed his medical record; he had episodes of abdominal discomfort from time to time. I saw him twice during the last two years; my acupuncture meridian assessment (AMA) picked up disturbances on his large intestine, spleen/pancreas, and liver meridians. I prescribed parasite medications, but he said he did not take them.

I told him he was a noncompliant, bad patient. He sheepishly smiled, agreed he was a "bad patient," and promised he would take his parasite medications now. He had been afraid to take them and was hoping his abdominal pain would go away on its own as it had before. I told him his colonoscopy can wait until he finished his parasite medications, but to take the blood screening test for cancer now.

Fear of the Known and Unknown

When the possibility of cancer enters the patient's mind, fear takes over, thinking of the horrors of chemotherapy, radiation, surgery, financial burdens on the family, death and dying, and the end time.

The End Time and Existential Threat are catchwords to provoke fear from climate change, pandemics, overpopulation or depopulation, environmental pollution, and nuclear war. On a personal level, we all share a universal fear of dying from cancer, going blind, losing our minds with Alzheimer's disease, or dying alone. A common denominator: fear of the unknown.

Global Whining

Uncertainty promotes more fear. Global warming, nuclear war, compromised science, changes in lifestyle and moral values, and increasing environmental pollution have contributed to weakening our immune response and make us more susceptible to parasite, fungal, bacterial and viral infections, including global pandemics. All these fears turn into a media-promoted Global Whining, some real and imaginary. Who benefits from Global Whining? You can decide.

Social Parasites and Parasitic Relationships

Let me introduce an additional concept of social parasites and parasitic relationships triggering the end-game and existential threats on a global scale. I have been writing about parasites and dental problems as major overlooked medical problems for many years. There has been a general increase in public awareness of parasite-related chronic modern illness in many levels from viral infections and cancer.

Thanks to the COVID-19 pandemic and Joe Tippens describing a complete recovery from lung cancer by using fenbendazole, animal grade parasite medications went viral on the internet. People have been self-medicating with OTC parasite medications. Some are designed only for animals at a fraction of the cost of prescribed medications.

At the same time pharmaceutical companies have been shamelessly, aggressively raising the prices of parasite meds. At times, I get panicked phone calls from my patients that it will cost them $5,000-$10,000 from a regular pharmacy. The multiple doses I use for a prolonged time are not covered by the insurance. Is it possible that the pharmaceutical companies are social parasites, taking advantage of the unsuspecting public? See my article, "Medical Acupuncture on Large Intestine Meridian: Ancient Romans and US Army Targets Demons."

How do we solve the dilemma of global pandemic parasite problems when pharmaceutical companies reap massive profits and behave like financial parasites at the top of the food chain? Parasites infections can engage in mind-control and manifest as mental illness. Deworming is not a dirty word. All my patients from Iowa who went to the Mayo Clinic for chronic mysterious illnesses without success, have since been dewormed, and most of them seem to respond and feel better (if they do not have concurrent dental problems that need to be addressed). Read my articles on my website, "Quarantine Iowa: Global Whining on Parasites," and "Medical Acupuncture on Stomach Meridian: Global Whining and Fearmongering to Global Healing Rebellious Stomach Nobel Prize."

There is no promise or guarantee, but deworming the entire population might be one of the best public health policies for the prevention of modern chronic diseases. It might also break the vicious cycle of money grabbing by pharmaceutical industries for new expensive patented medications, but I doubt there will be strong political will or broad public support. Fake news, false flags, and propaganda sought to kill ivermectin as a horse dewormer, crude, unscientific, and even dangerous. Let's start with deworming people with ivermectin, pyrantel pamoate, and praziquantel; these triple parasite medications are best for tapeworms, flukes, and common nematodes like Ascaris, pinworms, and Strongyloides.

For Igor, I told him the ivermectin, pyrantel pamoate, praziquantel, and nystatin (for fungal infections) which I had prescribed two years ago were still good after two years at room temperature and he did not have to buy new medications. Most of the stockpiled medications after the Gulf War were still good for at least 15 years stored at room temperature per a US Army study, with some caveats.[55]

From practicing AMA evaluation on patients for three decades, I know there is an increased risk of cancer when I see disturbances on the spleen/pancreas, liver, and large intestine meridians. Igor will be on triple parasite meds and one fungal med for a long time not only for parasites, but for prevention in developing more serious medical conditions. Tolerate the uncertainty in medicine – the art of medicine – and rely less on random, double-blind control studies. Deworming is a New Uncertain Preventive Medicine.

Patient Story: Understanding Dr. Yu's Approach

I decided to write a review because I see that most people in these reviews seem to not understand the process. Our society has been tricked into believing that you can just take a pill and that everything will be all good... Well, real healing, and actual reversal of conditions takes time - a long time in some circumstances.

Dr. Yu saved my life about a year and a half ago. Additionally, he taught me wisdom that you couldn't buy if your life depended on it. Because of him I've changed the entire trajectory of my life... I've been able to reverse SEVERAL conditions deemed "permanent" through the understanding I've obtained from him...

It's unfortunate that we've all been conditioned to believe western medicine indoctrination of asymptomatic suppression. So therefore most won't understand why they aren't healing. It takes time. No condition happens overnight and no reversal happens overnight.

Moreover, I expect it to take me between 3 and 5 more years until I get to a baseline to healing... It took 30 years to get sick - it'll take at least 6 to 8 to get anywhere. Thank you, Simon Yu, for practicing real medicine.

Emotional Response to Stress, and Your Response? Mark Twain's Way of Looking at Things

> "The more I learn about people, the more I like my dog."
> often attributed to Mark Twain

Stress may kill you or make you stronger: Fight, Flight or play Dead. It is not stress itself but how we respond to the stress that can kill us or make us stronger. We have a new pandemic of "psychological warfare" as a society with anxiety, depression and PTSD. What is going on? The quotes in this article are from Mark Twain, the great writer and humorist. Whenever I see his quotes in the newspaper, a book or on the internet, I cannot help laughing at his get-to-the-point humor with inspirational sarcasm.

I decided to take a long view and look back at what I have learned and written about the emotional aspects of healing and how they are essential to recovery: the burdens of stress and negativity, how they impact health over time, and the range of emotional and cognitive healing practice. These include a range of therapeutic approaches and new technologies that can help refresh and reboot our emotions, feelings, thinking, behavior, brains, and physical health.

Here are some examples from my work over the past 15-20 years. I hope we can indulge in Mark Twain's popular quotes in bold throughout this essay.

What has changed over this period? We have gone from the gifted village idiot in the holistic medical community to the gifted internet idiot. We have added stress from COVID and post-COVID, the pandemic shutdown causing fear and isolation, the polarization of politics and polemics of fake news and false election claims, the rise of Big Pharma, insurance-driven health care, and of private equity hospitals, heightened income inequality, etc.

> *"If you don't read the newspaper, you are uninformed. If you read the newspaper, you're misinformed."* – Mark Twain

What is the next rigged event? World War III? Bird flu or hemorrhagic fever? The Internet and social media amplify this on steroids.

My 2008 article, "Stress? What Stress? Psychological Warfare and Bio-feedback Therapy," focused on medical-related psychological stress. It discussed how unresolved stress and emotional conflict feed each other and escalate into medical illnesses.

Your anger and resentment may manifest as liver and gallbladder dysfunction. Emotional shock may trigger a heart attack. Fear and grief may suppress your immune system. Anxiety and loneliness may affect your digestive function.

> *"If voting made any difference, they wouldn't let us do it."* – Mark Twain.

There is psychological warfare going on in America today. Do you know who's engaged in psychological warfare on people? It is not who you may think it is. However, not voting does make a difference.

Dealing with a patient's fear, anxiety and depression and managing their stress has been the most challenging part of my practice. It is not so much how much stress you have, but rather how you deal with it. We age not by years but by events and our emotional reactions, paraphrasing Dr. Arnold Hutschnecker.

> *"Ignorance is not, not knowing something. It is knowing what isn't so."* – Mark Twain.

This is true for patients, physicians, and dentists. We need deeper ancient intelligence, which is why I use Acupuncture Intelligence (AI), via Acupuncture Meridian Assessment.

My 2010 article, "Original Incurable: The Gifted Village Idiot in the Holistic Medical Community," told the story of Dandy PouPou, one of the more challenging of many incurables I have encountered over many years. Every village seems to have their village idiot. Dandy Poupou was the gifted village idiot in the holistic medical community. He challenged everything and wanted cold hard proof and guarantees before taking the first step. I wished him well; however, it was up to him to choose to be truly gifted or simply the gifted village idiot.

> *"The truth hurts, but silence kills." – Mark Twain.*

My 2015 article, "Rip-off Report on Stress and Negativity," noted how we live in a society perpetually engineered by an artificially generated fear, stress, and negativity. Many people are unfortunately naturally attracted to negative publicity.

Sensationalism and fear mean making a fortune for those who can benefit from it and stealing fortunes from the fearful and gullible. There are many professionals, including physicians, who are afraid of negative reviews on the Internet, and, therefore, are willing to spend money to attempt to remove any real or unfair malicious reviews.

I find that even though a patient has decided to see me, the more that he/she is attracted to negativity from the Internet, social media, or other sources, the less likely they are to respond to any therapies no matter what I do. These negative thoughts and emotions are often based on Fear, Blame, Anger, Shame, Guilt, Insecurity, or Victimhood.

My message to you is, Do Not Surrender to Negativity! Negativity is an unseen force, like whispering gossip or Internet bullying, that damages our lives and poisons our dreams. Try this: trust your instinct and gut feeling.

> *Just because you're taught that something's right and everyone believes it's right, it doesn't make it right. – Mark Twain.*

From the political point of view:

- *No man's life, liberty, or property are safe while the legislature is in session.*
- *It could probably be shown by facts and figures that there is no distinctly American criminal class except Congress.*
- *God created war so that Americans would learn geography.*
- *The nation is divided, half patriots and half traitors, and no man can tell which is which.*

On eating and lifestyle:

- *Part of the secret of success in life is to eat what you like and let the food fight it out inside.*
- *The worst loneliness is to not be comfortable with yourself. The more things are forbidden, the more popular they become.*
- *Quitting smoking is easy, I've done it hundreds of times.*
- *Too much of anything is bad, but too much good whiskey is barely enough.*
- *Respect food allergies but enjoy what you eat.*

On general topics:

- *Work is a necessary evil to be avoided.*
- *Kindness is the language which the deaf can hear and the blind can see.*
- *Truth is stranger than fiction.*
- *I have never let my schooling interfere with my education.*
- *God cures and the doctor sends the bill.*
- *Good judgment comes from experience, and experience comes from bad judgement.*

> - *A gentleman is someone who knows how to play the banjo and chooses not to.*
> - *The lack of money is the root of all evil.*
> - *To succeed in life, you need two things: ignorance and confidence.*

I hope you enjoyed these quotes from Mark Twain! When you are under stress, triggering anxiety, depression or PTSD, and cannot break the cycle by yourself, read my recent articles including "Brain Neuromodulation and Vagus Nerve Stimulation" rather than just relying on medications.

When you are under stress, read Mark Twain's quotes or watch your favorite comedies, relax, practice mindfulness, enjoy nature, fight, run, play dead, and remember:

Humor is mankind's greatest blessing – Mark Twain

Placebo Effects on the Brain's Inner Pharmacy: Quantum Uncertainty of Matching Reality with Expectation

A placebo (Latin for "I shall please") treatment is considered a medically ineffectual treatment for a disease or medical condition intended to deceive the patient while professing to help the patient. According to the British Medical Journal published in 2004, 60 percent of the physicians in Israel used placebos in their medical practice, most commonly to "fend off" requests for unjustified medications or to calm the patient.

A study of Danish general practitioners found 48 percent had prescribed a placebo at least 10 times in the past year. The most frequently prescribed placebos were the use of antibiotics for viral infections and vitamins for fatigue.

Placebo effects have been a major controversial subject for the doctor-patient relationship and treatments based on calculated measured suggestions with sugar pills or sham surgery. The effects of placebos are a pervasive phenomenon known since ancient times. Some physicians advocate proper usage of placebo should be encouraged for patients. Other physicians consider placebo treatments to be ethically problematic as they introduce deception and dishonesty into the doctor-patient relationship.

The placebo effect is related to the perceptions, beliefs, conditioning, and expectations of the patient. If the substance is viewed as helpful, it can promote healing even if the remedy is a sugar pill. However, if it is viewed as harmful, it can cause negative effects, known as the Nocebo effect.

Because the placebo effect is based upon expectations and conditioning, the effect rapidly disappears if the patient is told that their placebo intervention is a sham and is ineffective. Cultural background, quantity of pills, brand names, past experiences, and high prices, may all impact placebo effects. Injections and acupuncture have been known to have higher, larger placebo effects than pills.

The latest study showed the brain can be manipulated by placebo. The brain controls the body process as documented by a high-resolution positron emission tomography (PET) scanner. Once dismissed as a psychological phenomenon, new evidence has established that a placebo triggers the brain's "inner pharmacy," that, in essence, is a warehouse perpetually stocked to deliver active drugs to itself. It can improve Parkinson's symptoms, pain, depression, irritable bowel syndrome, anxiety, schizophrenia, and more. It is as though the brain goes out of its way to ensure "reality matches expectation;" see *Discover Magazine* July/August 2014 article by Erik Vance.[56]

The placebo effects are hard wired into our brain through the prefrontal cortex, anterior cingulate cortex, and thalamus insula regions of the brain. These areas try to match the expectation with reality. We are entering into the Quantum Uncertainty of Matching Reality with Expectation: Placebo or Nocebo effects which are also influenced by our intention and attention.

A placebo does not work for everyone. Placebo effects occur in about 35 percent of the general population. In my opinion, alternative natural medicine and homeopathy tend to attract people who had Nocebo effects (expecting bad side effects) of standard orthodox medical care. They are attracted to the milder, gentler therapies with higher expectations, beliefs, perceptions, and conditioning of what we call the placebo effects by my medical colleagues.

Every day, I evaluate and treat my patients based on mapping out their bodies' acupuncture meridian systems, which have been known for several thousand years. Often, I find allergies, heavy metals, hidden dental infections, and parasite problems that have been overlooked by conventional and alternative medical doctors. Those patients who read my articles or my book, *Accidental Cure*, and know what I do, get excited to follow my recommendations. As a rule, they do very well with faster, better responses.

The patients who were dragged to my office by family members, and came with lots of hesitation and skepticism, usually take much longer to respond, or don't respond at all, despite identifying problems similar to the patients who came to me willingly. Hesitant and skeptical patients often focus on the Nocebo Effects of all potential side effects of parasite medications and use excuses of the expense of dental work or the hardship of avoiding their favorite foods or drinks, in order to avoid complying with treatments. They want a guarantee that my therapies will help them. The more they demand some form of guarantee, the harder it seems for them to respond.

Your medical problems may not be what you think, what you have been told, or what has been diagnosed. For that matter, I do not dwell on your symptoms or diagnosis. A diagnosis only helps the insurance companies to categorize you into a profile for medical treatment and payment. The shortcoming of categorizing and profiling, with branding a diagnosis, is that it never addresses the underlying problems.

- **Your medical problems may not be what you think, what you have been told, or what has been diagnosed. For that matter, I do not dwell on your symptoms or diagnosis.**
- **A diagnosis only helps the insurance companies to categorize you into a profile for medical treatment and payment.**
- **The shortcoming of categorizing and profiling, with branding a diagnosis, is that it never addresses the underlying problems.**

Placebo effects are a real phenomenon, hard wired into our brain by belief, intention, attention, expectation, conditioning, and perception. Understanding and maximizing the placebo effects on the brain's inner pharmacy and minimizing the nocebo effects can make a difference as to why some people respond and some people do not respond.

You as a patient, not the physician, choose Placebo effects or Nocebo effects. Placebo or Nocebo, choose wisely. That is the quantum uncertainty of matching reality with expectation.

Seventh Sense for Your Health

What is the seventh sense? Dr. Jonathan Kipnis, PhD, Professor of Neurology, Neuroscience, and Neurosurgery at the Washington University School of Medicine, wrote "The Seventh Sense" in the *Journal of Experimental Medicine*.[57] I was excited reading his article on the central nervous-immune system connection. I will share my thoughts on the brain, immune cells, and the interconnectivity of the acupuncture meridian matrix and beyond.

Energy Medicine embraces biophysics as a new generation of physics connecting the energy medicine described by ancient civilizations, called Chi or Prana. Subtle energy frequencies and biophotons are ways that trillion cells are communicating in synchrony. When there is miscommunication, disconnection, or distortion, it can be detected by our senses and meridians.

The Brain-Gut-Immune Connection

The five senses have long been known to us: smell, touch, taste, sight, and hearing. The sense of position and movement, "proprioception," is often referred to as the sixth sense. The "Brain-Gut-Immune Connection" is emerging as a new unrecognized seventh sense. Neuroscience textbooks describe the brain focusing on the business of operating the body, including all six senses, and the immune system defending it.

Mounting evidence indicates that the brain and the immune system interact routinely as a surveillance organ that detects and senses foreign invaders in and around the body and informs the brain about them by means of cytokines, chemokines, and other "unknown" signals. *One of the lesser-known communication signals may be the acupuncture meridian matrix described by ancient civilizations.*

The healthy brain was long thought to be off-limits to the peripheral immune system. Although the brain harbors native immune cells known as microglia, common immune cells that originate elsewhere in the body are not normally found in the brain. The so-called blood-brain barrier keeps these peripheral immune cells from entering.

Recent findings show highly interactive communication between the brain and the entire immune system. You may experience sense of uneasiness or feel "dis-easy" before you get sick with a sense of impending doom and malaise, which is then followed by a cascade of symptoms including fever, pain, and full activation of your immune system to fight foreign invaders: virus, bacteria, fungi, and parasites.

> **One of the lesser-known communication signals may be the acupuncture meridian matrix described by ancient civilizations.**

Cytokines released by peripheral immune cells can affect the brain. They presumably gain entrance through brain areas that lack the regular blood-brain barrier and could directly impact the brain through the Vagus nerve which runs from the gut to brain: the Brain-Gut Connection. From the teaching of Electro-acupuncture according to Voll, the Gallbladder meridian is the main meridian system that regulates the Vagus nerve. See my earlier article, Medical Acupuncture on Gallbladder Meridian.

Our immune system, innate immunity, and adaptive immunity are hardwired into the brain. That would make it a seventh sense according to Professor Kipnis. Cytokine IL-17 can interact with neurons in the brain cortex and can alter behaviors related to autism spectrum disorder per Kipnis.[58]

When I describe acupuncture meridian assessment (AMA), parasites, meridians, and brain, gut, and immune system connectivity to an audience at a conference, I feel like I am talking to a Wall of Skeptics for good reason. There is insufficient hard evidence and literature of finding ova, parasites, or mycotoxins in the stool or blood test. I am speaking a foreign language called acupuncture meridians, part of the language of nature.

When some patients complain parasites are crawling under their skin, rather than dismissing them as suffering from Delusional Parasitosis, it will be worthwhile to treat them with parasite medications based on empirical guidance from AMA or some other form of energy testing, such as muscle testing or Autonomic Response Testing (ART) developed by Dietrich Klinghardt, MD, PhD. What they are sensing is not a delusion, but an immune system alarmed and screaming – via cytokine release or cytokine storms - to tell their brain to take action.

> **What they are sensing is not a delusion, but an immune system alarmed and screaming – via cytokine release or cytokine storms - to tell their brain to take action.**

What does all that mean to you? The seventh sense monitors the brain-gut-immune connection. It may detect parasites, pathogens, or other problems and send signals to the allergy-immune surveillance system. Your sympathetic nervous system upregulates, your body is highly alert, releases cytokines and adrenal hormones, and looks for the invaders, filtering through the ancient meridians matrix system. Muons (fat or heavy electrons and meridians are a part of Nature that needs to be better understood. Beyond our perceptions, our intuitions and gut feelings are a real phenomenon and are a part of your seventh sense, that can be measured.

Seventh sense alone is not good enough to overcome the pitfall of chronic illness and premature death. Here is my unscientific basis of a longevity/anti-aging program, a cure based on personalized, individualized medicine: Power of N-of-1.

Unscientific Basis of Anti-Aging Program:
Power of N-of-1

Millions of people are taking prescribed medications that will not help them with potential life-threatening side effects However, based on clinical trials and scientific statistical analysis, funded by pharmaceutical companies, physicians keep pushing specific drugs. They explain to patients that the latest medical science proves the need to take the medications for whatever their conditions or ailments and may extend their life.

> **The Precision Medicine Initiative is trying to design a true single person "Individualized Medicine" approach to healing.**

Nature, the International Weekly Journal of Science, April 2015, published an article, "Time for One-person Trials."[59] Nicholas J. Schork explained that precision medicine requires a different type of clinical trial that focuses on the individual, not the average, response to therapy. For some drugs, such as statin drugs routinely used to lower cholesterol, as few as 1 in 50 people may actually benefit from their use.

There are many drugs that are harmful to certain ethnic groups because of the bias towards white Western participants in the classical trials. Physicians need to take individual variability into account. Therefore, the Precision Medicine Initiative was announced in 2015. This initiative includes, among other actions, the establishment of a national database of genetic and other data of one million people and focuses on a single person, known as N-of-1 trials.

To create N-of-1 trials, according to the article, all sorts of relevant data need to be collected for one person over a prolonged period. The article also addresses the difficulty in designing a control study and the enormous cost of creating databases which include genomic DNA, RNA, microbiome data, metabolomes, and more.

The Precision Medicine Initiative is trying to design a true single person "Individualized Medicine" approach to healing. Its methodology is based on mega databases, an example of which is matching drugs to specific tumor profiles for a better clinical outcome. A major advantage of the N-of-1 approach over classical trials is that patients are no longer guinea pigs. At least, that is the main goal, with physicians being aware of the unique circumstance of each patient, that is, the unique individuality of the illness as it pertains to a single person.

From my point of view, one of the best N-of-1 trials is done by a family physician who takes care of the same patients for over 30-50 years of their career. However, the current managed care and insurance business models dictate changes to a person's family physician at any time based on insurance contracts. Therefore, N-of-1 individualized medicine is almost impossible. The power of the family physician observing and taking care of the same patient over a prolonged period, the true power of N-of-1 doctor-patient relationship, is replaced by mega databases of statistical analysis of people as groups, not individuals, by our government and insurance companies.

> **From my point of view, one of the best N-of-1 trials is done by a family physician who takes care of the same patients for over 30-50 years of their career.**

The American Academy of Anti-Aging (A4M) organization has been a leader in hormone replacement therapies and regenerative medicine. It has also been branching into many other related fields including, to my surprise, Energy Medicine. I had the opportunity to give a lecture on "Parasites and Energy Medicine" in a small room at their conference some years ago. The large auditorium was reserved mainly for hormone replacement therapy lectures.

In my lecture, I told the audience that regular "de-worming" with common parasite medications plus routine dental care, without root canals, implants, or mercury amalgams, might be the best anti-aging program you can have. Even better than hormone replacements, stem cell therapy, or trying to modify telomeres.

Using the word "de-worming" is based on one of my patients who is a horse breeder. She finds it interesting that I am prescribing her "horse" medications, for example, ivermectin and praziquantel, for her unexplainable medical symptoms. She is giving these same parasite medications to her horses. We started talking about horses and their life span.

In the old days, according to her, the average life span of horses was around twenty plus years. Now, with modern veterinary dental care and routine de-worming two to four times a year, horses can easily live over 40 years. That is doubling the life span simply by regular de-worming and routine dental care!

In that American Academy of Anti-Aging conference, most of the audience took my statement, that the best anti-aging program might be routine de-worming and dental care, with chuckles and skepticism. I gave a similar lecture at the Medical Week Conference in Baden-Baden, Germany and received similar responses.

At that Medical Week Conference, I met one of the founders of the A4M organization. I told him about my hypothesis, based on the truly unscientific anti-aging program of routine de-worming and dental care, that we may extend the human life span, from an average of 75-80 years to 120-150 years, if the horse breeder's story is true. He was interested and wanted evidence and data to back up my statement, not just a tall, fairy tale story.

This is my unscientific basis of an anti-aging, longevity program. It is based on my clinical observation, just like one horse breeder's experience extending the life span of horses and pondering the power of N-of-1. I have seen many patients recover from serious illness after multiple rounds of parasite/fungal medications and dental care, beating the odds of survival from poor prognoses and extending many years of quality life. If any readers have any experience of extending the life span of horses (and humans) based on using parasite medications and dental care, let me hear about it. That will be the power of "N-of- 2." Imagine yourself as a racehorse and choose your parasite medications and your dentist wisely.

> **Imagine yourself as a racehorse and choose your parasite medications and your dentist wisely.**

Conclusion: Knowledge for Healing Comes from Within

The Acupuncture meridian system has been known for thousands of years. Yet we don't fully understand how the complexity of meridians interacts in our physical body, emotions, spiritual level, and life force. Before RNA, DNA and organs manifested at the time of conception, there was an energy field, a Life Force: you may call it Chi, Prana, or Universal-Empty-Quantum-Energy Field. The meridians are one of the energy fields we can measure based on Electro-acupuncture according to Dr. Voll (EAV) or simplified, acupuncture meridian assessment (AMA).

My goal in this book is to present a medical acupuncture-related clinical case series based on my observations as an Internal Medicine physician. I am not an acupuncturist. My understanding of acupuncture meridians is limited, but I hope this book will stir interest and help the patients, physicians, and dentists who want to explore a simple, practical guide to complex medical problems.

When you get bogged down with too much information but face a confusing medical scenario, ask your integrative physician, biological dentist, acupuncturist, or EAV-AMA practitioner to use this book to guide you based on my writing on the Medical Acupuncture series.

Ask them which meridians, how many, and to what degree they help reveal your dominant problems. Go beyond the teaching of the traditional Pulse Diagnosis. Challenge the old belief system as much as Göbekli Tepe will challenge the entire academic archaeology and ancient history that we know. Don't bury the evidence of ancient, authentic, acupuncture intelligence.

> **Don't bury the evidence of ancient, authentic, acupuncture intelligence.**

My first two books, *Accidental Cure: Extraordinary Medicine for Extraordinary Patients* and *AcciDental Blow Up in Medicine: Battle Plan for Your Life*, provide a foundation for you to connect the dots beyond current medical teaching. This third book, *Accidental Cure 3*, is a practical guide for exploring the dawning/ancient era of mysterious, unknown AI.

AI becomes Acupuncture Intelligence, Ancient Intelligence, Alien Intelligence, Authentic Intelligence, Applied Intelligence. Real AI is here for a cure. It is not an accidental cure. AI is you.

It is time to crack the code. You have control over the domain of your whole body. Knowledge for healing comes from within.

Part 11

Everything You Want to Know About Acupuncture Meridian Assessment

Chapter 15 Frequently Asked Questions

By Atel Hemat, Dr. med., Cologne, Germany

Introduction

In this chapter, I will answer some of the questions that may arise before or during a treatment following Dr. Yu's approach. I will draw upon Dr. Yu's books and what I have learned from the multiple seminars I attended with Dr. Yu in St. Louis and in Europe, as well as our private conversations. I have begun organizing AMA Training seminars for him/with him in Europe.

These FAQs are organized into five sections: 1. General Questions, 2. Parasite Treatment, 3. Dental Treatment, 4. Allergy-Immunology Meridian Disturbance: Mycotoxins, Toxic Metals, Environmental Toxins, 5. Accompanying Treatments, and 6. FAQs for Practitioners.

1. General Questions

Q1: What does AMA stand for?

A: AMA stands for **Acupuncture Meridian Assessment**, developed by Simon Yu, MD, based on Dr. Reinhard Voll's Electroacupuncture system. Unlike traditional acupuncture, AMA does not involve needles. Instead, a blunt metal probe is applied to a system of 40 acupuncture points on your hands and feet to identify meridian imbalances in your system. Meridians run throughout your body like thin invisible energetic cables connecting different organs, tissues, joints and sensory organs with each other. The device tests the local resistivity at these points, with a normal range of 45-55 on the scale.

Readings below 45 indicate degenerative issues and chronic inflammation (signaled by a lower pitched sound), while readings above 55 suggest acute infection and inflammation (signaled by a higher pitched sound). Despite the probe being blunt, testing some points might be more uncomfortable than others. Dr. Yu encapsulates the essence of AMA as follows: "Acupuncture Meridian Assessment can reveal unique biofeedback information about a patient's energy patterns based on ancient knowledge of acupuncture and meridian flow of the body."

Q2: The AMA did not show my heavy metal issues/dental issues/parasite issues!

A: AMA is not an inventory method that lists all issues you might be dealing with. It reveals what is predominantly an issue at the time of evaluation. Your body, in its wisdom, will prioritize the issues that need attention first. For instance, I recall a patient whose initial AMA only showed a dental issue that needed to be addressed first. After the extraction of the infected root canal, the second AMA revealed a parasite and heavy metal burden, which was then addressed. Some bodies can't handle multitasking well (simultaneous dental, parasite, antifungal, chelation treatment), and these patients will benefit from a step-by-step approach. Think of it like peeling an onion: each layer removed reveals what needs to be addressed next.

Q3: How should I prepare for the AMA?

A: Prior to your AMA, ensure you are well-hydrated and avoid applying any lotion or cream to your skin, as this can interfere with the evaluation. Remove all jewelry and electronic devices (cellphones, smartwatches, etc.) before the examination. Implanted devices like ICDs and pacemakers are not an issue and will not be disturbed by the AMA reading.

Q4: What is Dr. Yu's advanced interrogation?

A: If the initial AMA reading shows no significant abnormalities or if there is a noticeable discrepancy between the patient's complaints and the AMA reading, your practitioner might use "advanced interrogation techniques." These techniques, which include acupuncture needles, lasers, or reading a few lines from a holy book, challenge your body to reveal hidden issues. Advanced interrogation unmasks what lies beneath.

Q5: Why are medications put in the tray of the device?

A: The metal tray is connected to the AMA device. Placing any medication or supplement into it puts your body in contact with the contents of the tray. This enables the practitioner to identify the ideal combination of medications to restore balance across all your meridians.

Q6: I was asked for a panoramic X-ray (Panorex) of my teeth, but I don't have any dental issues.

A: Dr. Yu's approach, most famous for the treatment of parasitic infections and for the use of antiparasitic medication for extraordinary patients, also places significant emphasis on oral health. A Panorex is required to rule out obvious issues that might include root canals, cavitations, infected implants, and mandibular joint issues (TMJ). A Panorex assists the practitioner in pinpointing hidden dental issues during the AMA. It is used to mark suspicious regions with low or high readings in the AMA, so that the dentist can confirm.

Dr. Yu's practice is equipped with a Panorex device, underscoring the importance of oral health in his concept. He may be the only non-dentist in the US equipped with a Panorex device. Some patients say, "My holistic dentist has treated all my cavitations and removed all root canals." However, AMA often reveals that hidden dental infections may still be present and require attention. An X-ray is essential for every patient to ensure thorough evaluation.

Q7: I was tested by an EAV specialist in the past and he could not find dental, parasite, or fungal issues. In which way is AMA according to Dr. Yu different?

A: Dr. Yu's method is unique in many ways:

- He simplified the complicated German approach involving measuring up to 500 points down to measuring up to 40 points.

- He has developed "advanced interrogation methods" that allow him to dig deep under the surface of disguise and compensation to unveil otherwise hidden dental, parasite, fungal issues.

- He mainly uses prescription medication to treat parasite and fungal infections, whereas classical EAV relies on plant-based remedies or homeopathic remedies.

Dr. Yu observed that antiparasitic and antifungal medications often have pleiotropic effects: they not only target the conditions they were designed to treat but can also address seemingly unrelated issues, helping to resolve long-standing chronic diseases. Additionally, many prescription medications can be repurposed as effective anti-cancer or antiviral treatments.

Q8: I was told I need three rounds of parasite medication. What does that mean?

A: Your treatment plan is individually tailored to your needs based on AMA. Typically, one round lasts 7 to 14 days, followed by a pause of 1 to 3 weeks. This is then followed by a second or third round in the same manner. This is a general rule; some patients might need 2 weeks of antiparasitic medication, then 2 weeks of antifungals. More serious diseases might need 6 months of continuous treatment with antiparasitics and antifungals.

Q9: How will I be able to tell what made me healthy, when I was taking antiparasitic medication, antifungal medication, chelation agents, supplements, and had dental work done?

A: Your body is a complex system, and it is often challenging to attribute the cause of a disease to a single factor. Our brains tend to simplify things by attributing our suffering to a single life event (for instance, a trip to Thailand that caused diarrhea). However, our bodies are more complex. Multiple factors weaken our immune system over time and make our terrain more susceptible to infections by parasites, bacteria, viruses, or fungi. The journey to better health thus requires various interventions. If you regain your health, it's because your immune system has regained its balance and your detox systems work more efficiently.

Q10: Which stressors can disturb my biological terrain and make me sick?

A: The most common stressors include Poor Diet and Nutrition, Lack of Adequate High-Quality Water, Psychological Stress and Negative Emotions, Medical Therapy and Medications, Environmental Poisoning and Heavy Metal Toxicity, Hidden Dental Problems, Parasites and New Emerging Infections, Allergies, Inactivity (lack of motion), Vaccinations, Structural Imbalance, Lack of Natural Sunlight and Cosmic Rays, Electromagnetic Pollution, Genetically Modified Organisms, and Scars. For details on each potential stressor, see: Simon Yu, *Accidental Cure: Extraordinary Medicine for Extraordinary Patients* (2010), page 42.

Q11: I know viruses and bacteria come after parasites in the order of treatment, but I have several positive tests for EBV and Borrelia species. Should I treat those first?

A: Dr. Yu's AMA provides a roadmap and a prioritized list of issues to address. Parasite medication is remarkably powerful, capable of balancing all meridians except for the Dental and Allergy-Immunology points. I have frequently observed that, following a thorough parasite cleanse lasting 6-9 months — alongside dental work such as root canal removal and treatment of dominant cavitations — lab tests for conditions like acute EBV reactivation, Borrelia (Lyme disease), Babesia, and Bartonella often return to normal. Parasites serve as hosts for these viruses and bacteria, making treatment of parasites the top priority if detected through AMA. Don't be misled by lab tests — parasites and dental issues are often the root cause.

Q12: Symptoms I have been suffering from for 30 years did not disappear after 3 months of parasite cleanse, is that normal?

A: Long-lasting symptoms and diseases will not disappear overnight, be patient, let yourself be reevaluated, the second AMA might show that you need crucial dental work or another combination of parasite or antifungal medication.

Q13: I am feeling pretty healthy, but my AMA showed several meridian disturbances, I don't see that it correlates with my absence of any symptoms.

A: AMA being an energetic testing method can pick up on issues prior to their clinical appearance. During my stay in Dr. Yu's clinic, I remember seeing a patient that revisited Dr. Yu after 3 years.

The first AMA, when the patient was feeling fine, was showing low readings on both "nervous degeneration meridians" and one dental meridian. Dr. Yu had recommended parasite cleansing and some dental work. The patient, feeling healthy at the time, opted for a plant-based parasite cleanse and did not address his dental issues. Three years later, when I saw the patient during the second visit, he was suffering from Multiple Sclerosis.

I recall a patient who came to see me for chronic asthma. Out of 40 meridians, 15 were imbalanced, with a significant issue in the left dental meridian. She had only one root canal, tooth number 14, which was not directly connected to her primary concern (lungs/asthma) but rather to the stomach, breast, and spleen meridian. Interestingly, her left breast point measured low in the AMA. She assured me there were no nodules or tumors in her breast and that she performed regular self-examinations.

Using the pinpoint method (also taught in kinesiology) we found that touching tooth number 14 balanced both the left dental meridian and the breast point. I recommended that she remove the root canal-treated tooth and have breast thermography. However, the patient decided to postpone treatment to seek a second opinion.

Five months after the AMA evaluation, she discovered a nodule in her breast and was diagnosed with ductal carcinoma in situ. Despite this, she remained hesitant to remove the affected tooth or start the antiparasitic medication.

The examples above are not meant to scare you but to inform you. AMA, like thermography and other energetic testing methods, can detect disturbances long before they are identifiable through lab work or radiological tests. Think of AMA as a valuable prevention tool — after all, energy shifts occur before chemical or structural changes manifest.

Q14: I've undergone six months of IV and oral antibiotics for Lyme disease, yet I continue to experience relapses. I identify as a Lyme survivor. What could be causing these persistent relapses?

A: Aggressive usage of antibiotics for Lyme may weaken your terrain and cause fungal invasion. If you think Lyme, think dental: have an AMA practitioner check for hidden dental and parasite infection as a root cause for your Lyme. Once hidden dental, parasite and fungal/mold issues have been resolved, Lyme might just accidentally disappear. Lyme can mimic almost every disease, as can a lot of parasites.

What makes you sure that it was mainly Lyme that caused your debilitating situation? Parasites are at the top of the food chain and include many known and unknown kinds, these parasites often bring additional uninvited guests: bacteria (including Lyme), fungi, and viruses. When parasites, dental and fungal/mold issues are taken care of, the other issues are often resolved.

Q15: I will travel from abroad to Dr. Yu or one of his students. If I do the parasite cleanse, antifungal treatment,

and dental work, can you guarantee that it will fix my issue?

A: There is no guarantee in medicine. "Medicine is a science of uncertainty and an art of probability." (Sir William Osler, Professor of Johns Hopkins Hospital). We also cannot give you a probability regarding the success rate: every case is unique. You are your own statistic.

Q16: I suffer from Chronic Fatigue Syndrome (CFS). During treatment, I suddenly felt free of brain fog and experienced a surge of energy—I can't remember the last time I felt that way. I even went for a jog but crashed afterward, and now I'm back to where I started. What went wrong?

A: CFS patients often suffer from secondary mitochondriopathy, where their mitochondria—damaged by various factors—are unable to produce sufficient ATP (the body's energy currency) to support normal daily activities. In severe cases, CFS can leave patients bedridden or capable of walking only a few meters before becoming exhausted for hours. Parasite medication can sometimes create "miracle"-like effects, resulting in a sudden burst of energy. However, this is only a glimpse of what the future could hold, not a permanent recovery. I always caution my patients that this energy surge is borrowed, not yet earned.

Regenerating mitochondria takes time and cannot be rushed. Many CFS patients are Type A personalities—perfectionists, pleasers, or individuals who push through pain. They often view their body as a machine that has betrayed them for months or years and feel compelled to "make up for lost time." This mindset often leads them to overdo it, such as going for a jog during their first burst of energy. When they crash afterward, they regret it but may repeat the same mistake when the next surge of energy comes.

The key is learning the technique of pacing and carefully managing newfound energy. I always advise my patients to spend no more than 10% of their gained energy and to resist the temptation to push further. Patience and adherence to this principle are critical for achieving sustained, long-term success.

2. Parasite Treatment

Q17: Can I drink alcohol during the parasite cleanse?

A: Alcohol is a liver toxin, so it's important to avoid anything that places additional strain on the liver. Stop alcohol consumption at least two weeks before starting your parasite cleanse and reintroduce it in moderation two weeks after completing the medications. This recommendation also applies to antifungal treatments.

Q18: I have elevated liver enzymes due to fatty liver degeneration; will I be able to tolerate the medication?

A: We have repeatedly seen that liver enzymes even normalized during antiparasitic treatment. If you want to be on the safe side, have your liver enzymes (Bilirubin, AST, ALT, ALP, GGT, Creatinine and white blood count checked before the treatment and during the last third of each round. The best preparation for the parasite cleanse is a gall-bladder-liver flush 1 week before the start of the first round and then one in each pause between the rounds.

Q19: My AMA results indicate that I need four different antiparasitic medications. Will my body be able to handle this treatment?

A: Yes, most patients do very well on parasite medication. The fact that multiple medications directed against parasites are better tolerated than single medication is what I call "Dr. Yu's Antiparasitic Medication Pseudo-Paradox." Patients with multiple sensitivities and intolerances tend to be very careful with medication, and they are right in doing so. Anything that can be avoided should be. Most of the oversensitive patients are well-informed and some of them already tried single parasite medication (e.g. ivermectin), they might recollect that the medication improved some symptoms but worsened others. They will describe that they had a so-called "Herxheimer" reaction. Online forums and Facebook groups might applaud them on the so-called "herxing" reaction as they consider it as symptoms caused by parasite die-off.

If a patient truly experiences a Herxheimer reaction after taking ivermectin, one might assume that combining multiple antiparasitic medications would result in an even stronger reaction. However, clinical experience shows the opposite: triple or quadruple antiparasitic treatments are generally better tolerated than single medications. Why would ivermectin alone cause stronger side effects or Herxheimer-like reactions, while combinations like ivermectin, pyrantel pamoate, and praziquantel (a common triple therapy) result in minimal or no side effects?

My Hypothesis: If a patient has a multi-parasite infection—for simplicity, let's label the parasites as A, B, and C—and AMA reveals the need for a triple-antiparasitic combination (medications 1, 2, and 3), taking only medication 1 would target parasite A exclusively. This leaves parasites B and C unaddressed, giving them less competition for resources in the host environment. Consequently, parasites B and C may thrive, potentially exacerbating symptoms and creating what is perceived as a Herxheimer reaction.

I call this phenomenon "Dr. Yu's Antiparasitic Medication Pseudo-Paradox." It suggests that treating with multiple medications simultaneously not only produces fewer side effects but also reduces the likelihood of a perceived Herxheimer reaction. This hypothesis casts doubt on the idea that single-medication treatments truly provoke a classic Herxheimer reaction. Instead, the reaction may be a result of unbalanced treatment that inadvertently allows other parasites to flourish.

Q20: I have visited an AMA practitioner, I got the medication and necessary supplements, but I am hesitant to start, is this even the right treatment for me?

A: Nobody can force you to take the medication. Nobody will guarantee that you will benefit from the medication. Many of my patients who are familiar with Dr. Yu's books and his approach using prescription medications travel from abroad, often from European countries, to seek treatment. These patients invest significant time and money—traveling to Germany, paying for their stay, and purchasing medications and supplements. Yet, some become hesitant to start the treatment.

Rationally, one might wonder: why would someone go to such lengths, only to avoid taking the prescribed medications? Hesitant patients often say things like, "The medication is sitting on the shelf, but when I look at it, I get scared," or "My gut feeling tells me it's not the right thing to do." But what if it isn't your gut feeling after all?

Research shows that parasites can influence the behavior and decision-making of their hosts—a scary but true phenomenon. In some cases, I encourage patients to critically reevaluate and "reprogram" their so-called gut feelings. For example, if a patient has three root canals and their gut instinct tells them these pose no health risks and should be left alone, I have to challenge that belief. Root canals often carry significant health risks and can be detrimental to overall health. In such cases, it's vital to distinguish between genuine intuition and decisions influenced by other, alien factors.

Q21: My parasite-related issues came back after I stopped the medication! What can I do?

A: There could be several reasons for this:

1. You might have been reinfected through the environment (pets, raw meat, sushi, exotic countries).

2. Your partner or other family members might be asymptomatic carriers of parasites. They might need treatment too. It's interesting to note that I've repeatedly seen several members of the same family requiring different antiparasitic medications for treatment. So, sharing your medication might work, or it might not.

3. You might need additional rounds of medication. Some patients will be fine after three rounds, but most need six or more rounds.

4. Do you have untreated dental issues? Small parasites like Dientamoeba fragilis love root canals and

cavitations and will escape the medication by hiding in these dental regions. Once the medication is stopped, procreation starts anew as they leave the safe cave (cavitation, root canal). Unresolved dental issues are among the most common causes for failed treatment.

Q22: How do I take parasite medications?

A: Yes, it is correct, if you are prescribed three or four different antiparasitic medications, they can be taken all at the same time. To facilitate and in order not to overcomplicate matters: take your parasite medication with a meal containing some natural fat source. Some parasite medications may have to be chewed (Pyrantel Pamoate tablets and Niclosamide for instance), most of the others come in capsules or tablets and must be swallowed. Some medication is taken twice daily, others three or four times daily, your practitioner will inform you about these details.

Q23: I saw long slimy worm-shaped structures in my stool, are these parasites? Is this a rope-worm?

A: It's difficult to tell, they may just be stuck food remnants mixed with mucus. You can only tell for sure if it is a parasite if it is still alive and moving when you inspect your stool. Don't obsess too much about finding parasites in your stool, some of them can only be seen with a microscope.

Q24: Will the AMA give me a detailed list of which parasites I am dealing with? My stool tests showed Blastocystis hominis and Giardia lamblia.

A: No, AMA does not test for presence of specific parasites, bacteria, or viruses. AMA detects meridian imbalances; in a second step the practitioner tries to balance out the meridians with different medications. Antiparasitic medication is amongst the medications that are tested (other medications that are tested to balance out meridians are antifungals, chelating agents, and binders for environmental toxins).

At the end of the examination, your practitioner might tell you that you need three antiparasitic drugs to balance out your meridians, so AMA will not test for specific parasites, but for a specific combination of antiparasitic medications. Don't focus too much on specific parasites, patients generally have a mixed parasite infection. The ones we can detect in stool samples (Dientamoeba fragilis, Blastocystis hominis, Giardia lambia etc.) are often only the tip of the iceberg. Don't rely too much on lab testing or stool testing, parasites are elusive and at the top of the food chain, they outsmart most testing methods, esp. laboratory testing, and often have a complex life cycle outside of the intestinal tract. There are many hundred known parasites that can affect humans and many unknown ones. How can you test for something that has not even yet a name?

Q25: If I am prescribed antiparasitic medication after my AMA, does that prove that I have a parasitic infection?

A: Technically it does not. It just shows that your meridian system will most probably benefit from the medication and will help your body in correcting imbalances. Antiparasitic medication is often pleiotropic which means that it can have multiple effects on different physiological systems and different infectious agents beyond its primary intended therapeutic action.

These additional effects can include anti-cancer properties (e.g. mebendazole, ivermectin, niclosamide etc.), antiviral (e.g. ivermectin, niclosamide etc.), antibacterial (e.g. tinidazole). Thus, if AMA shows that you need antiparasitic medication it might also be because your body will likely benefit from the antiviral effect or general immune-modulating effect of the medication.

Q26: Since I have been taking the antiparasitic medication, my asthma has been resolving, but now the long-gone anal itching is recurring, what can I do?

A: If deep-seated symptoms/diseases like asthma resolve and more superficially localized symptoms: mucosal (anal itching) or skin symptoms (eczema) for instance recur, this is a good sign of a healing reaction. Continue with the treatment. If symptoms that reoccur burden you, try Vitamin C 2000 mg every hour until you reach bowel intolerance (diarrhea), then continue with half the dosage every hour for 1 day.

Q27: I am hesitant, will antiparasitic medication harm my gut microbiome?

A: Interestingly, parasite medication might even have the opposite effect on your microbiome. Many antiparasitics have been shown to be beneficial for microbiomes. The biggest disruptor for the microbiome is a chronic parasite infection. While antibiotics may have a negative influence on the microbiome, antiparasitics may exert a very positive influence.

Q28: Is it possible that I have a parasite infection although I don't experience any diarrhea or abdominal pain?

A: While we often associate parasites with symptoms like diarrhea and cramps, this might not always be the case. Most chronic parasitic infections instead present with symptoms like bloating, flatulence, chronic constipation, multiple allergies, unexplained fatigue, or even parasitic relationships in their social life. Other patients with parasite infection might present with seemingly unrelated issues: a rare autoimmune disease, insomnia, teeth grinding, and many more.

Q29: I was prescribed ivermectin, praziquantel, and mebendazole. I already took them separately, but I did not notice any difference in my condition.

A: Dr. Yu's approach is unique in that he prescribes multiple medications in high doses simultaneously and for longer periods. The combined effect of these medications is significantly greater than taking each substance individually. It's a synergistic approach where the whole is more powerful than the sum of its parts. Think of it like baking a cake: the individual ingredients—flour, eggs, and milk—on their own cannot create a cake. However, when combined in the right proportions, they produce something entirely different.

Another critical aspect of Dr. Yu's method is the use of high dosages and, often, multiple treatment courses. Administering sublethal doses of antiparasitic medication can worsen the problem, as partially affected parasites may migrate deeper into the body, hiding in organs such as the pancreas. This highlights the importance of using the correct dosage and combination to ensure effective treatment.

Q30: I'd rather treat my parasite issues with natural/herbal remedies, is that possible?

A: Patients who are fairly healthy might be able to do a parasite cleanse with natural remedies, as their immune system is competent enough to handle parasite issues with mild support (natural/herbal remedies).

However, chronically ill patients have a compromised and burdened immune system. In these patients, follow-up AMA often reveals that subtherapeutic dosage of standard antiparasitic medication or use of natural/herbal antiparasitics only drives the parasites into deeper tissues, e.g., the pancreas meridian. This is always an alarming sign and needs fast action with antiparasitic medication. Remember, what does not kill a parasite, makes it stronger!

Q31: How can I make sure that I stay parasite free?

A: There will always be the possibility of reinfection with parasites. Nevertheless, there are several things you can do to reduce your risk of reinfection:

- Avoid raw fish and raw or bloody meat.
- Do a gallbladder-liver-flush once quarterly.
- Do preventative parasite cleansing with antiparasitic meds once a year. Avoid exotic travel for at least three years following your treatment.

I have repeatedly observed patients returning with parasite reinfections after holidays in regions such as South America, Southeast Asia, or Africa. Individuals who have previously experienced symptomatic parasite infections are more susceptible to reinfection during this period. It takes several years for the body to rebuild its defenses and restore its natural guard against reinfection.

As Dr. Yu explains, "The body begins to repair and correct itself when you remove underlying toxic conditions, such as heavy metals, hidden infections, and allergies." Building this resilience requires time, care, and avoiding unnecessary exposure to high-risk environments.

Q32: Since taking the antiparasitic medication I have been having diarrhea and abdominal cramps. What can I do?

A: Double the amount of the binder (e.g. activated charcoal) that you are already taking. If the symptoms persist, pause medication and contact your doctor.

Q33: Since taking the antiparasitic medication I have been developing body ache and a fever. What can I do?

A: Double the amount of the binder (e.g. activated charcoal) that you are already taking. Take Vitamin C 2000 mg every hour until you reach bowel intolerance (diarrhea), then continue with half the dosage every hour for 1 day. Contact your doctor if symptoms persist.

Q34: I suffer from severe histamine intolerance and/or MCAS (Mast Cell Activation Syndrome), that is why I am intolerant to many foods, medications and supplements. Will I be able to tolerate the medications?

A: Most patients with MCAS will tolerate the medications fine. MCAS in most cases is a secondary issue, it was caused by for instance chronic infections. Parasites and allergies/intolerances are causing similar reactions of the immune system. If you can treat the underlying cause, the histamine intolerance/MCAS might just vanish. Supportive treatment for patients with MCAS are antihistamines. You can increase your dosage during the antiparasite/antifungal cleanse.

Q35: I read that there is an ultimate "Dr. Simon Yu Antiparasite Protocol", is that correct?

A: No, despite what you might read on the internet, there is no standard antiparasitic protocol. As mentioned earlier, each case is individual: combination of medication, dosage per day, duration of cycle, and number of cycles. Please also note that the parasite cleanse is the easiest part of the treatment, but it might not be sufficient: you might need dental work, antifungal treatment, and chelation therapy. The individual nature of AMA is the reason why there are no online consultations; the first visit and measurement are done in the practice.

3. Dental Treatment

Q36: I have one root canal that was done 10 years ago. It does not hurt, nor does my dentist see any issue as far as the X-ray is concerned. I don't see how my asthma has anything to do with the root canal that is not bothering me at all. How come Dr. Yu said to extract it; my instinct tells me otherwise?!

A: Root canal treated teeth are essentially dead. They are killed by the treatment, killed by the dentist. Referring to a dead tooth as a "root canal" is a euphemism. If we call it what it is, plain and simple: a dead tooth, your instinct might tell you that having dead tissue in your body may not be healthy at all. In fact, the most important part of the treatment might be your dental work. We have seen numerous patients with unexplained diseases/issues that vanished with the removal of one dead tooth. Often, issues caused by a dead tooth start 10-15 years after the tooth was killed.

Q37: I was told that I have two cavitations in my wisdom tooth area (upper jaw left and right). I do not have any pain or swelling in that area, if it is an inflammation why do I feel nothing in the area?!

A cavitation is a cavity within a jawbone that previously held a tooth. It is the socket of an old tooth extraction site that has not filled in completely. That area can either show bacterial infection, or ischemic osteonecrosis (dead bone tissue due to lack of blood flow. Basically, cavitations can be compared to a cave inside the body where no blood vessels lead to. No blood vessels implies that our immune system is not able to reach that area properly. Bacteria, fungi, viruses, and parasites can enter these areas, hide there and reinfect your body repeatedly.

German dentist Fritz Kramer mapped the relationship between the teeth and organs/structures of the body in a Tooth-Organ Meridian Chart which is on Dr. Yu's website. The wisdom tooth area has a special place in the chart; as the wisdom tooth area shares the meridian with the following essential structures and organs: central and peripheral nervous system, energy production, small intestine, heart. That is why proper treatment of cavitations can resolve brain fog, neurological and psychological symptoms, trigeminal neuralgia, heart arrhythmia, chronic fatigue syndrome, small intestinal overgrowth, and many more. Dr. Yu sums up the importance of this area: "Whenever young people develop unexplainable medical symptoms, I immediately think of an old, infected wisdom tooth socket."

Q38: AMA showed several cavitations and infected teeth. Why can't I fix it all in one surgery?

A: Experience shows that surgeries in different quadrants (your mouth has four) at the same time make it more difficult for the body to heal. It is best if your practitioner – with the help of AMA - develops a roadmap that allows for a step-by-step approach. Moreover, AMA will give you a roadmap for prioritization. In the case of cavitations sometimes you might only need surgery for two out of four, as antiparasitic medications and other supportive treatments during your parasite cleanse might balance the other two cavitations.

Traditional dentists often deny the existence of cavitations and the notion that root canals are inherently burdensome to the body and eventually need removal. On the other hand, holistic dentists may sometimes over-diagnose cavitations or overlook infections in teeth that are vital. AMA can help identify hidden dental infections and provide a clear roadmap for addressing dental issues effectively. However, it is essential not to rush into dental procedures without first establishing a proper sequence of antiparasitic treatment, detoxification and nutritional support. This preparatory work ensures that your body is better equipped to handle dental interventions and promotes more effective and lasting outcomes.

Q39: What should I do to prepare myself for my dental surgery (root canal removal or cavitation)?

A: As stated earlier, the sequence of surgery should be determined by the AMA practitioner. Ideally, each quadrant should be addressed separately. New cavitations can develop if the area is not healing properly. To prepare your body for the healing process, I recommend:

- Ensuring optimal Vitamin D levels in the upper third of the reference range
- Taking Boron, Magnesium, Calcium, and consuming bone broth
- Ensuring good sleep and rest
- Performing soft lymph massage to prevent swelling
- Taking homeopathic Arnica 200C, 2-3 granules/drops twice daily for 2 days starting right after the surgery

Q40: I would like to have my Amalgam fillings removed. Can I just have my regular dentist remove them?

A: No, the removal of Amalgam fillings should be done by a specially trained dentist who is aware of the precautions that need to be taken in this context. We have seen many patients fall sick after improper removal of Amalgam fillings. For more on Mercury in Amalgam fillings, see Simon Yu, *Accidental Cure: Extraordinary Medicine for Extraordinary Patients* (2010), pages 67-83, and *AcciDental Blow Up in Medicine* (2019), pages 132-134.

In the US, visit "The Safe Mercury Amalgam Removal Technique (SMART)" thesmartchoice.com, at the International Academy of Oral Medicine and Toxicology's (IAOMT) website, iaomt.org, where qualified dentists are listed. There are additional listings and information at the International Academy of Biological and Dental Medicine's (IABDM) website, iabdm.org.

Q41: I was told that I need to remove a root canal to heal my gut issues and brain fog. I do not understand the connection?!

A: In recent years, we have gained more knowledge about the oral microbiome ("oralome") and its significant effects on the whole body and gut microbiome specifically. To put it simply: the gut starts in the mouth. Therefore, addressing oral issues is a crucial part of improving your microbiome. Bacteria and parasites residing in the mouth can be translocated to the gut, especially considering that you are swallowing 1-1.5 liters of saliva daily. Leaky gums can cause leaky gut and leaky brain.

Trying to fix your leaky gut without addressing your leaky gums is like trying to clean the oceans from plastic garbage without stopping the pollution of the rivers that carry the plastic into the oceans. On a side note, I suggest that we need to avoid euphemisms like "root canal" and instead call it what it is: "a dead tooth, killed by the dentist". Many patients don't even realize that a root canal treated tooth is always dead, that is how successful this euphemism is. Once more and more people realize what a root canal treated tooth is, more patients might be inclined to rid their body of this deadly burden.

Q42: My root canal was performed by an endodontist. He uses advanced technology, including a modern microscope and ozone, to disinfect the entire tooth thoroughly. Given these advanced techniques, will a root canal still pose a risk to the body?

A: Yes, it will, eventually. A root canal-treated tooth is still a dead tooth. To draw a comparison, whether a person is stabbed or euthanized, the result is the same: a lifeless body. Similarly, no matter how advanced the method used to treat the tooth, it remains dead. Sooner or later, it can lead to issues within the body. The more severe a patient's condition, the sooner they should address dental issues and consider removing root canals, following the recommendations of their AMA practitioner and dentist.

Q43: Can jaw infections from extracted teeth (e.g. dry socket, cavitation) cause mental disorders?

A: Yes, the trigeminal nerve (cranial nerve 5) is the thickest of the twelve cranial nerves and leads directly to the brainstem. Through this pathway, small parasites, Lyme-like bacteria, and viruses can directly impact the brain. The trigeminal nerve is influenced by the lymphatic jaw meridian (dental meridian). For further information I recommend: Patrick Störtebecker, *Dental Caries As a Cause of Nervous Disorders* (1982). The vagal nerve (CN 10) is mainly dominated by the gallbladder meridian; disturbances of the gallbladder meridian directly affect the brain (see chapter 5 of this book). The vagal and trigeminal nerve can play a dominant role in neurological disorders, AMA measures these two brain nerves with their surrogate meridians: gallbladder and dental.

Q44: At what point in therapy do you recommend extracting an infected tooth. You have said Lyme hides in teeth. Should I try to take down Lyme in the body first before extracting the tooth because we do not know what infection is in there?

A: Again, there is no general rule. AMA is an individualized approach; each case can be different. AMA will give you the road map for the right sequence of procedures. Patients who run against time (ALS, cancer) might be recommended to rush the extraction of infected teeth (if there are several, your AMA practitioner will specify the order). In other cases (CFS and fibromyalgia for instance) your practitioner might decide to start you on 1-2 cycles of parasite medication first and have you extract the infected tooth during the third cycle. Around the time of surgery, you might need additional medications like Azithromycin and/or Tinidazole to prevent parasites/bacteria/viruses that are released during surgery from negatively affecting your system.

Q45: My dentist says tooth #29 looks fine and is hesitant to remove a healthy tooth. However, if the AMA identified tooth #29 as an issue, do I need to have it removed?

A: AMA, when applied by an experienced practitioner, is more sensitive than the radiological findings that most dentists rely on. Bone destruction from an infected tooth may only become visible on X-rays after 20–30% of the bone has already been destroyed, whereas AMA can detect issues earlier. However, there's no guarantee that removing a specific tooth will improve your condition. The decision is ultimately yours. It may be helpful to consult with a dentist who works closely with your practitioner, as they are typically more confident in addressing dental issues that do not show obvious signs of infection.

Q46: My holistic dentist says that the CBCT (Cone Beam Computed Tomography) showed 4 cavitations in the wisdom tooth extraction areas. How do I proceed?

A: Whereas traditional dentists deny such a thing as a cavitation, holistic dentists often overtreat them. Not every cavitation needs to be addressed surgically. Your AMA practitioner can help guide you: the reading will show which area to address first. In case of cavitations in the upper jaw gravity is on your side and may help drain the inflammation/infection during a parasite or antifungal regime. Lower jaw cavitations might need a surgical solution. AMA will give us a road map and a priority list. Sometimes 2-3 cycles of parasite medications will help resolve smaller cavitations. Don't jump right into it, plan it carefully with your practitioner.

Q47: My holistic dentist would like to treat the cavitation by injecting ozone gas into the socket.

A: Ozone has strong antibacterial and antiviral properties. Nevertheless, we strongly advise against these kinds of injections as they might spread the infections/inflammation across the whole jaw, which might end in a nightmare.

Q48: I will remove my root canals. Shall I get full ceramic implants right away?

A: Although your dentist might recommend getting an implant immediately to prevent bone loss, it's worth reconsidering.

Even full ceramic implants, which are considered more biocompatible, can become infected and may eventually need to be removed.

The best option for addressing the gap left by an extracted tooth is a removable partial denture, or for front teeth, a Maryland bridge that is bonded to the adjacent teeth. While many patients prefer a traditional bridge, it typically requires the adjacent teeth to be contoured and reshaped to accommodate the crowns. This process removes a significant amount of tooth structure, potentially leading to the eventual death of those teeth. The least favorable solution would be a titanium implant, as intolerances and allergies to titanium are relatively common.

Full ceramic implants are a better alternative than titanium, but, as mentioned earlier, they can also fail over time. For patients with serious health conditions, it's often best to opt for leaving the gap and using a partial denture. This allows the immune system and the body's healing potential to focus entirely on managing the underlying health issue rather than dealing with foreign structures embedded in the jaw.

Q49: I have metal braces/retainer. Can that cause irritable bowel syndrome?

A: Metal orthodontic appliances can disrupt the oral microbiome and may contribute to health issues. Nickel corrosion can trigger type IV allergies, affecting the gut. Additionally, these appliances can generate galvanic currents, potentially interfering with the body's natural electromagnetic field. The presence of metal in the mouth can contribute to various diseases and symptoms.

4. Allergy-Immunology Meridian Disturbance: Mycotoxins, Toxic Metals, and Environmental Toxins

Q50: Why do I need antifungal treatment?

A: Many patients require antifungal treatment because fungal infections often occur alongside parasite and dental infections or result from mold exposure. Additionally, antifungals can help prevent fungal overgrowth caused by rounds of antibiotics and antiparasitic medications. To support the process, patients should also take binders to facilitate the removal of removing mycotoxins from the body.

Q51: Which mycotoxins are burdening my body the most?

A: Your practitioner can perform tests to identify mycotoxins: antibody tests to evaluate your immune system's response to mycotoxins or urine tests to detect the presence of mycotoxins or their by-products.

Q52: I moved out of the mold-infested building, but I am still suffering from mold-related Chronic Inflammatory Response Syndrome (CIRS).

A: The most critical step in antifungal treatment is eliminating exposure to mold and mycotoxins. However, moving out of a mold-infested building might not be enough, as many patients unknowingly carry mold spores on their clothing or furniture to their new home. Consult an experienced mold expert to address this thoroughly. Additionally, mold and fungus can grow within the body, so multiple courses of prescription antifungals may be necessary to eliminate lingering fungal infections. Depending on your mycotoxin report, your primary source of mycotoxins may also come from contaminated foods; such as coffee, peanuts, or grains. Once your body is compromised, avoiding exposure to mold and mycotoxins is critical to prevent symptom flare-ups.

Q53: I am fine with the parasite cleanse, but the antifungals seem too much to handle, can I skip those?

A: If your practitioner picked up mold or fungal infection as an issue on the Allergy-Immunology Meridian, the issue should be addressed. Mycotoxins are among the strongest known immune-suppressants and carcinogens. Aflatoxin B1 is an especially hepatotoxic carcinogen. Ochratoxins from contaminated coffee can reduce Lymphocytes, and Trichothecenes can interfere with cytokine production.

Q54: I was prescribed three antifungals: Fluconazole, Itraconazole, and Nystatin. How can I reduce side effects?

A: Your practitioner will usually recommend that you take binders (charcoal, cholestyramine etc.) and may ask you to increase mycotoxin release by using an infrared sauna regularly. However, sauna can also mobilize these infections, so follow the instructions of your practitioner.

Q55: I am a cancer patient and don't remember that I was tested for mycotoxins, what are the antifungals for in my case?

A: In cancer patients or patients with degenerative neurological diseases we sometimes prescribe antifungals together with antiparasitic medications to balance several meridians. Many antifungals have shown strong anti-cancer activity by stopping malignant tumors from metastasizing or by inhibiting angiogenesis.

Q56: How can I detox from environmental toxins?

A: Apart from minimizing exposure to environmental toxins, I highly recommend the regular use of infrared saunas, particularly far-infrared saunas. These can support detoxification by helping the body eliminate heavy metals and other environmental toxins through the skin. To prevent the reabsorption of mobilized toxins into the bloodstream via the enterohepatic circulation, take 2 grams of activated charcoal immediately after the sauna session. The following day, replenish lost minerals by using a high-quality, low heavy metal salt and a comprehensive mineral supplement. Additionally, regular gallbladder and liver flushing can further aid in the excretion of environmental toxins, supporting overall detoxification.

Q57: How can I detox from heavy metals?

A: Chelation therapy with the appropriate chelating agent (DMPS, DMSA, EDTA, DTPA, Deferoxamine will help you excrete heavy metals. Your practitioner might conduct a hair mineral analysis and chelation mobilizing test to check for heavy metal poisoning. Of course, the source of the toxicity must be identified and eliminated (e.g. amalgam fillings, gold fillings, lead in drinking water, pesticides, paint etc.).

5. Accompanying Treatments

Q58: Is it enough to take the parasite and antifungal medication to achieve a successful cleanse?

A: Your practitioner might decide that you need additional therapeutic treatments at home or in the practice. These might include avoiding intolerant foods (IgG4 allergy testing), coffee enemas, gallbladder-liver-flush, IV chelation therapy, IV nutritional therapy, hyperbaric oxygen therapy, ozone therapy (including EBOO: extracorporeal blood oxygenation and ozonation), Insulin Potentiation Therapy, and bioresonance therapy. Your practitioner will work with you to determine which of the above interventions may be most beneficial for your healing process.

Q59: I got all the parasite medication from the pharmacy. Am I ready to start?

A: AMA practitioners typically recommend or prescribe additional supportive treatments such as herbal remedies, homeopathic remedies, and detox support to enhance the effectiveness of the therapy and increase the chances of success.

Q60: I am constipated; can I still start the medication right away?

A: It is essential to ensure regular bowel movements before you start the treatment. Consider using coffee enemas to stimulate bile production or performing a gallbladder-liver flush to help get the bowels moving. Colon hydrotherapy may be necessary in some cases.

Q61: Which test is recommended for food intolerances?

A: A food intolerance test measures a specific subgroup of antibodies, called IgG4, which can cause delayed symptoms that manifest hours or even days after consuming trigger foods. The key is to avoid your intolerant foods for a specified period based on your test results. After that, the foods can often be gradually reintroduced into your diet.

Q62: I was recommended to undergo Insulin Potentiation Therapy (IPT), what does it entail?

A: IPT is used by Dr. Yu in different chronic conditions to potentiate the effect of different substances. He will use antiparasitics, antifungals, antivirals, antibiotics, and immune-boosting nutrients together with Insulin to increase the intake of these substances into cancer cells or inflamed cells. IPT can successfully be used in cancer patients but also in a variety of other diseases. Dr. Donato Garcia who invented IPT first used it in a patient with neurosyphilis. See Dr. Yu's article, "Insulin Potentiation Therapy (IPT) for All Chronic Disease: Can Old Cranky Physicians Try New Approaches?"

Q63: I tried parasite cleansing, partner treatment, stayed away from reinfection, but I just can't overcome my issues. What can I do?

A: If dental issues have been ruled out, a less common cause of relapses could be geopathic disturbances. Patients affected by this often have trouble sleeping, aversion to going to bed, restless sleep, or nightmares. If this applies to you, your resistance to therapy might be linked to your bed being situated above a geopathic disturbance. Consider repositioning your bed or consulting a dowser to address this issue.

Q64: My hair mineral analysis and urine test came back positive for different heavy metals. What are the indicated therapies?

A: Your practitioner will test the right chelating agent for your case and recommend a therapy plan that will consist of regular chelation IVs and supportive vitamins and nutrients. The most crucial step is to stop further exposure by safely removing amalgam fillings and identifying other potential sources, such as lead from old water pipes.

Q65: I don't have any psychological issues. I am not crazy. How come I was asked to see a psychologist?

A: Every disease has a psychological component that should be addressed with the help of trained professionals. Sometimes, resistance to healing isn't just physical. In some cases, a parasitic relationship, whether emotional or behavioral, may play a significant role. Patients may unconsciously resist taking antiparasitic medication or cling to toxic relationships. True healing comes from within. While your practitioner is there to guide you, you are ultimately responsible for your own recovery.

6. FAQs for Practitioners

Q66: I am a health practitioner, medical doctor, or dentist, and I would like to buy an EAV machine and use it to evaluate my patients. Where can I purchase the device?

A: Before investing in equipment, you should attend at least one hands-on training course with Dr. Yu in St. Louis. Dr. Yu offers both a basic course and an advanced course once a year. Learning how to use an EAV device is like learning how to play a violin. It requires several months of training. Don't give up too quickly.

While it might be difficult to diagnose and pinpoint dental issues in the beginning, very low readings of meridians will be easier to detect. You will develop the skill step by step. It requires determination, regular practice, and patience. As for purchasing the device, you may want to research online or contact manufacturers directly to find a reputable supplier.

Always ensure the device meets the necessary standards and regulations for your location.

Q67: What attitude/mind set should I ensure before the AMA evaluation?

A: Free your mind of too much empathy, intention, or expectation. Let the body tell you what is wrong. Emotions should not influence your AMA reading. Dr. Yu tries to ignore symptoms, diagnoses, or syndromes as much as possible, as these can be misleading. AMA is intended to look for underlying root causes.

Q68: How should I prepare for and start the AMA?

A: Ensure the patient is well-hydrated and instruct them to avoid applying lotions or creams to their skin, as these can interfere with AMA readings. Ask them to remove all jewelry and electronic devices before the session; implanted devices like ICDs and pacemakers will not affect the AMA reading.

Start with the hand-to-hand reading taught in the basic course. Readings should ideally be above 70/100 (preferably >80/100). If the reading is below 70, moisturize the patient's skin with water. If necessary, have them do squats or eat a hot meal to raise their energy levels.

Once the hand-to-hand-reading is high enough proceed with the dental control point on the thumb, this point will show you how much pressure you need to get a proper reading. In severe cases, such as advanced cancer or ALS, these measures may not suffice, and all readings will be lower than normal. In those cases, you can still start AMA but bear in mind that all readings will be lower than normal. You may have to improvise and adapt, if the patients average reading is 30-40 on the most points, but some are 10-20, rate the latter ones as the pathological ones. Go through the sequence of the control measurement points on each hand, and then on each foot; 40 in total. Make sure the patient switches the bar from one hand to the other with each hand and foot.

Q69: I have read about 12 meridians in Traditional Chinese Medicine, but Dr. Yu talks about more meridians.

A: In addition to the 12 meridians in Traditional Chinese Medicine (Lung, Large Intestine, Stomach, Spleen, Heart, Small Intestine, Bladder, Kidney, Pericardium, Triple Warmer, Gallbladder, and Liver), Dr. Voll from Germany introduced new so called vessels; the ones that play an important role in AMA are Lymphatic, Dental, Nervous System, Allergy-Immunology, Organ Degeneration, Pancreas, Joint, Connective Tissue, Skin, and Fat. To keep it simple we refer to all these as meridians too. Additional points that should always be measured:

- **Adrenal Point** on the Triple Warmer Meridian
- **Breast Point** on the Triple Warmer Meridian (women)
- **Prostate/Uterus Point** on the Bladder Meridian

Q70: My patient has a serious condition, but their AMA readings seem balanced. How should I proceed?

A: During the advanced course you will learn how to handle cases where the AMA reading, and the clinical picture, are in complete contrast. Through techniques invented by Dr. Yu named "Advanced Interrogation" or "Enhanced Interrogation" (Operation Open Sesame), you will be able to lift the curtain of compensation or delusion and see the real picture. Afterward, balance the meridians using appropriate medications.

Q71: I am using a Vistron or M2 from Kindling and noticed an indicator drop on some points?

A: Unlike traditional EAV, indicator drops are not critical in AMA. The primary goal is to balance the meridian using the correct combination of medications and supplements. AMA is simple, as long as you can balance out the meridian with the right combination of medication and supplements; that is sufficient.

Q72: The dental meridians showed very low readings, the patient has no root canals, how should I proceed?

A: Start by trying to balance the meridians with two to three wooden tongue depressors (stacked horizontally) and have the patient bite down gently. If this balances the meridians, the issue is likely TMJ or bite-related. Reevaluate after several rounds of parasite treatment to see if the TMJ/bite issue resolves. If it persists, refer the patient to a TMJ/bite specialist. If the tongue depressors don't help, try antibiotics (e.g. Clindamycin, Tinidazole, Doxycycline). If these balance the meridians, deep cavitations may be the problem. Use the pinpoint method from Dr. Yu's advanced course to localize the issue. Note: TMJ/bite issues and cavitations can coexist.

Q73: How should I handle patients who overwhelm me with questions?

A: To manage patient expectations, provide them with this list of FAQs. This helps answer their questions and allows them to determine if you are the right practitioner for them. Encourage patients to read Dr. Yu's books and articles on his website before their visit to familiarize themselves with his approach. After the appointment, provide detailed written instructions to clarify recommendations. For extensive follow-up questions, consider charging for your time.

Q74: The Dental and Allergy-Immunology Meridians could not be balanced with the antiparasitic medications, what is the next step?

A: These meridians often represent separate medical issues:

- **Dental Meridian:** This is the most complex. Use advanced AMA techniques to identify infections, inflammation, or TMJ/bite issues.
- **Allergy-Immunology Meridian:** Imbalances can stem from:
    - Food and airborne allergies/intolerances
    - Fungal infections/mycotoxins (test with Fluconazole, Itraconazole, Nystatin)
    - Toxic metals (test chelating agents like DMPS, EDTA, DMSA)
    - Environmental toxins (test with binders)
    - EMFs

Q75: Dental, Heart, and Small Intestine Meridians are low. What does this indicate?

A: Until proven otherwise, this often points to cavitations in silent, often painless, wisdom teeth extraction sites.

Q76: I'm struggling to balance certain meridians. Any tips?

A: Use these guidelines:

- **Large and Small Intestine Meridians:** Try antiparasitics (e.g., Ivermectin, Pyrantel Pamoate, Albendazole), antifungals (e.g., Nystatin), or Tinidazole/ Nitazoxanide for diarrhea.

- **Gallbladder, Liver, Spleen, Pancreas Meridians:** Use Praziquantel.
- **Stomach/Spleen Meridians:** Tinidazole, Doxycycline, or Azithromycin
- **Breast Point on Triple Warmer Meridian:** Treat dental infections and try Tinidazole.
- **Kidney Meridian:** Use chelating agents, parasite medications, or treat dental issues.
- **Bladder/Uterus/Prostate Meridians:** Use Tinidazole, Praziquantel, or Ivermectin.
- **Allergy Immunology:** Try EDTA/DMPS/DMSA or Fluconazole, Itraconazole, Nystatin.
- **Cancer Patients:** All of the above.

Q77: How can I improve my reliability and reproducibility of my AMA readings?

A: Master the method by following Dr. Yu's techniques exactly for at least one year. Avoid making changes until you've thoroughly mastered the process. It took Dr. Yu over two decades to develop AMA to its current level. It would be unwise to assume you can improve or modify the method after attending just two courses. Mastery requires extensive practice and experience with patients. To maintain and enhance your skills, regularly attend AMA courses.

Q78: My patient has obvious dental issues but is not willing to address them as he is convinced that they are unrelated to his issues.

A: Dental work is often the most challenging yet effective part of treatment. Patients sometimes sabotage their progress by avoiding necessary dental interventions, often unconsciously deciding not to heal. Approach these situations with patience and guidance.

References

Simon Yu, *Accidental Cure: Extraordinary Measures for Extraordinary Patients* (2010)

Simon Yu, *AcciDental Blow Up in Medicine: Battle Plan for Your Life* (2019)

Additional Sources:

Dawn Ewing, *Let the TOOTH Be Known* (2010)

George Meinig, *Root Canal Cover Up* (2008)

Patrick Störtebecker, *Dental Caries As a Cause of Nervous Disorders* (1982)

Thank you to Dr. Atel Hemat for preparing these FAQs.

Appendix:
Patient Resources on my Website

Here are the Patient Resources listed on my website:

Introductory Articles: Principal Causes of Illness

- Five Principal Causes of Illness - Heavy Metals and More
- Food Allergies - Often Overlooked Contributors to Chronic Illness
- Dental - The Root Cause of Chronic Illness
- Diet, Nutrition, Weight Loss and Longevity
- Parasites - Often Hidden and Undiagnosed
- Planet Earth, Human Ecology and Environmental Illness

Tooth-Organ Meridian Chart

View this very important Tooth-Organ Meridian Chart to understand the Tooth/Body Connection, and why a biological dentist or oral surgeon referral may be part of your "battle plan" to regain your health.

Patient Instructions and Resources

- Detox Recommendations based on Mosaic Diagnostics test results
- Gallbladder-Liver Flush Program
- Oil Pulling Therapy
- Parasite Remedies: Guidelines for Taking Medications
- Referral List of Biological Dentists

Most Common Parasite Medications I use

Here is a list of the most common parasite medications I use, with typical dosages and duration (for 150-180 lb. person):

- **Ivermectin** 12mg 3-4 x/day with **pyrantel pamoate** 725 mg 3-4 x/day for 10-30 days
- **Tinidazole** 2000 mg at bedtime or 500 mg 3-4 x/day up to 30 days, or **nitazoxanide** (**Alinia**) 500 mg 2-3 x/day for 3-10 days
- **Albendazole** 200-400 mg 4 x/day for skin problems or **mebendazole** 100-200 mg 4 x/day for 2-4 weeks
- **Praziquantel** 600 mg 4 x/day for 2-4 weeks
- **Levamisole** 50 mg 3-4 x/day
- **Niclosamide** 500 mg 3-4 x/day

For more information, see Chapter 12, "Parasite Medication Guidelines: for Physicians, Medical Hackers and Braves," in my book, *Accidental Blow Up in Medicine*, pp. 279-303.

Basic Biohacking Resources

See Chapter 13, "For Patients: Self-Help Strategies and Resources," of *AcciDental Blow Up in Medicine*, for basic biohacking resources, pp. 304-325.

They include One Hundred Dollar Cure for Braves, Skeptics and El Cheapo, Ten Dollar Cure When One Hundred Dollar Cure Fails, Additional Therapies to Consider, Detox Recommendations Based on Mosaic Diagnostics Test Results, Gallbladder/Liver Flush Instructions, Folk Remedy from Russia: Oil Therapy by Dr. Karach, Self-Help Resources on the Web, and How to Find a Biological Dentist.

Helpful Links and Resources:

Integrative Medicine

American College for Advancement in Medicine
> The voice for integrative medicine; offers conferences and education. https://www.acam.org

International College of Integrative Physicians
> Translating science into clinical practice; conferences, education and newsletter. https://www.icimed.com

Townsend Letter
> The Examiner of Alternative Medicine; newsletter, archives and blog. https://www.townsendletter.com

Biological Dentists

Referral List of Biological Dentists
> Here is Dr. Yu's Referral List of Biological Dentists in the St. Louis and beyond. https://preventionandhealing.com/resources/#helpful_links

International Academy of Oral Medicine and Toxicology
> Conferences, research, and a list of biological dentists in the US and worldwide. https://iaomt.org

International Academy of Biological Dentistry and Medicine
> Conferences, information, and a list of biological dentists and allied professionals. https://iabdm.org

Holistic Dental Association
> Promotes whole body approach to dental care, has list of holistic dentists. https://holisticdental.org

The SMART Choice

Learn about the Safe Mercury Amalgam Removal Technique (SMART), and how to find a SMART-certified dentist. https://thesmartchoice.com/

Dental Amalgam Mercury Solutions (DAMS)

Additional information and a free information packet are available from Dental Amalgam Mercury Solutions (DAMS), 1041 Grand Ave #317, St Paul MN 55105, 651-644-4572. https://www.amalgam.org/

Self-Help Websites

Know the Cause

Doug Kaufmann's site with videos, blog, information and resources on the role of fungi, mold and mycotoxins in chronic diseases. https://knowthecause.com

Better Health Guy

Blog and podcasts by Scott Forsgren, FDN-P, HHP who researches many approaches for overcoming chronic health issues. https://www.betterhealthguy.com

Debug Your Health

Website by Susan Luschas, PhD on what she learned about diagnosing and treating Lyme, coinfections, parasites, and more. https://www.debugyourhealth.com

Praxis2Practice

Carolyn Winsor has a range of helpful information and courses on Acupuncture and EAV, bioresonance, and biological medicine. https://praxis2practice.com. To order publications, go to Occidental Institute Research Foundation. https://oirf.com

About the Author

Dr. Simon Yu, MD

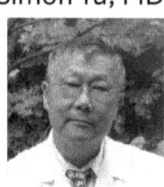

Dr. Simon Yu combines internal medicine with integrative medicine at Prevention and Healing, Inc., which he founded in 1996. Dr. Yu received his B.S. degree from Washington University and did postgraduate research in diabetes at Washington University Medical Center. He earned a Master of Science degree through a joint program at Washington University Medical Center and University of Missouri-St. Louis, where he conducted research on immunology. He graduated from the School of Medicine at the University of Missouri in 1984 and completed residency training at St. Mary's Health Center in St. Louis.

Dr. Yu worked as a regional medical director at a large health maintenance organization (HMO) medical group in Missouri for 10 years. He also served as a medical officer in the US Army Reserve for 25 years, further expanding his experience. Dr. Yu experienced first-hand the limitations of Western medicine's and HMO health systems' medication-management approach to patients with cancer and chronic diseases. He began studying integrative and complementary medicine over two decades ago. He took 300 hours of acupuncture training in a program at Stanford University School of Medicine.

Dr. Yu is certified by the American Board of Internal Medicine and is a member of the American College of Physicians. He serves on the advisory board of the International College of

Integrative Medicine (ICIM) and is active in many integrative medical organizations.

Dr. Yu lectures across the United States and around the world and has studied Biological Medicine extensively in Europe. Here are some of the experiences that shaped his career.

Dr. Yu attended Dr. Douglas Cook, DDS's "Conference on Energy in Medicine and Dentistry" in Chicago in 1996. Another medical doctor who attended the conference, Dr. Tom Stone, MD, succinctly stated what Dr. Yu felt was his reason for attending: *"To find out how dentists are killing my patients."*

Until this event, Dr. Yu did not realize the magnitude of the relationship between the oral cavity's pathology and patient health. At the conference, Dr. Cook introduced participants to computerized electrodermal screening (CEDS). Skeptical at first, Dr. Yu took a second CEDS course before realizing that the EAV (electroacupuncture according to Voll) tool provides medical doctors or dentists with a valuable method for evaluating connections between the teeth and the body.

Dr. Yu began to acquire and test modern, updated digital machines, and developed Acupuncture Meridian Assessment (AMA) to guide detection and treatment of root causes of diseases. Using AMA, he learned how energy meridians and energy fields can transform medical practice, enabling patients to move beyond lifelong medication of symptoms to restoring health.

In 2001, Dr. Yu's work as an Army Reserve medical officer took him on a mission to Bolivia where he treated 10,000 Andes Indians with parasite medications. He saw this not only resolved parasite problems, but many reported it helped them overcome a range of additional health problems

Dr. Yu wondered how many of his US patients might be helped by detection and treatment of parasites. He learned to search for evidence of parasite problems using AMA and saw many of his patients with chronic and unexplained medical conditions respond favorably to antiparasitic medications. Parasite problems are often linked with fungal problems, and he learned to treat these as well.

Dr. Yu's knowledge has been enriched through learning about German Biological Medicine and attending many annual Medical Week events and presentations in Baden-Baden, Germany over the years. Dr. Yu has been honored to give many presentations in connection with Medical Week and offer international AMA seminars, and to bring international medical innovative leaders to the United States.

Dr. Yu offers Special Training on Acupuncture Meridian Assessment (AMA) for doctors, dentists and prescribing health professionals. He writes a monthly newsletter, has over 250 articles on his website, and selected videos on his YouTube channel, www.youtube.com/preventionandhealing.[60] He thanks his colleagues who together are shaping the practice and science of medicine and dentistry to learn about and use energy medicine to detect and guide treatment of underlying problems and restore health and vitality.

Endnotes

[1] Bruce H. Lipton, *The Biology of Belief: Unleashing the Power of Consciousness, Matter & Miracles*, 10th anniversary edition. 2nd edition. (Carlsbad, California: Hay House, 2016).

[2] Douglas L. Cook, *Rescued By My Dentist: New Solutions to a Health Crisis* (BC, Canada: Trafford Publishing, 2009).

[3] Simon Yu, "Resources: Charts, Causes & Guides," *Prevention & Healing Inc.*, https://preventionandhealing.com/resources.

[4] Norman Doidge, *The Brain That Changes Itself: Stories of Personal Triumph from the Frontiers of Brain Science* (New York: Viking, 2007).

[5] H. Van Gelder, *The Process of Healing: A Field Theory Approach* (R. Martin Outsound, 1989).

[6] Per M Hellström, "This Year's Nobel Prize to Gastroenterology: Robin Warren and Barry Marshall Awarded for Their Discovery of Helicobacter Pylori as Pathogen in the Gastrointestinal Tract," *World Journal of Gastroenterology: WJG* 12, no. 19 (May 21, 2006): 3126, https://www.ncbi.nlm.nih.gov/pmc/articles/PMC4124396/.

[7] Carolyn Winsor, "Occidental Institute Research Foundation," *Publications/Courses and Manuals,* https://oirf.com

[8] Carolyn Winsor, "Praxis 2 Practice – Aus Der Praxis To Your Practice," *Praxis 2 Practice,* https://praxis2practice.com.

[9] "CDC - DPDx - Schistosomiasis Infection," last modified June 7, 2024, https://www.cdc.gov/dpdx/schistosomiasis/index.html.

[10] OIRF, *op cit*.

[11] Ilza Veith, ed., *The Yellow Emperor's Classic of Internal Medicine*, New ed. (Berkeley: University of California Press, 2016).

[12] Patrick Störtebecker, *Dental Caries as a Cause of Nervous Disorders: Epilepsy, Schizophrenia, Multiple Sclerosis, Brain Cancer; Additional Notes on Myasthenia Gravis, High Blood Pressure* (Orlando, Fla: Bio-Probe, 1986).

[13] Aigerim Mashekova et al., "Early Detection of the Breast Cancer Using Infrared Technology – A Comprehensive Review," *Thermal Science and Engineering Progress* 27 (2022): 101142, https://doi.org/10.1016/j.tsep.2021.101142.

[14] Y. R. Parisky et al., "Efficacy of Computerized Infrared Imaging Analysis to Evaluate Mammographically Suspicious Lesions," *American Journal of Roentgenology* 180, no. 1 (2003): 263–269, https://doi.org/10.2214/ajr.180.1.1800263.

[15] OIRF, *op cit*.

[16] Samantha J. Merwin et al., "Organophosphate Neurotoxicity to the Voluntary Motor System on the Trail of Environment-Caused Amyotrophic Lateral Sclerosis: The Known, the Misknown, and the Unknown," *Archives of Toxicology* 91, no. 8 (August 2017): 2939–2952, https://doi.org/10.1007/s00204-016-1926-1.

[17] Patrick Störtebecker, *op. cit.*

[18] Thomas Seyfried, *Cancer as a Metabolic Disease: On the Origin, Management, and Prevention of Cancer*, 1 edition. (Hoboken, N.J: Wiley, 2012).

[19] Jane McLelland, *How to Starve Cancer: ...And Then Kill It With Ferroptosis* (England: Agenor Publishing, 2021).

[20] S Fadhil Ali Malaa et al., "Assessment of Entamoeba Gingivalis and Trichomonas Tenax in Patients with Chronic Diseases and Its Correlation with Some Risk Factors," *Archives of Razi Institute* 77, no. 1 (February 28, 2022): 87–93, https://doi.org/10.22092/ARI.2021.356549.1868.

[21] Frederick T. Guilford and Simon Yu, "Antiparasitic and Antifungal Medications for Targeting Cancer Cells Literature Review and Case Studies," *Alternative Therapies in Health and Medicine* 25, no. 4 (July 2019): 26–31, https://pubmed.ncbi.nlm.nih.gov/31202208/.

[22] *Ibid.*

[23] *Ibid.*

[24] Donald B. Giddon, Donald R. Moeller, and Curtis K. Deutsch, "Use of a Modified Mandibular Splint to Reduce Nocturnal Symptoms in Persons With Post-Traumatic Stress Disorder," *International Dental Journal* 71, no. 2 (2021): 167–171, https://doi.org/10.1111/idj.12619.

[25] Felix Liao, *Six-Foot Tiger, Three-Foot Cage: Take Charge of Your Health by Taking Charge of Your Mouth: Holistic Mouth Solutions for Sleep Apnea, Deficient Jaws, and Related Complications* (Carlsbad, CA: Crescendo Publishing, 2017).

[26] Seyfried, *op. cit.*

[27] For a list of Dr. Ko's publications see her website, Young Hee Ko, "KoDiscovery | 3-BP | Young Hee Ko | Metabolic Cancer Therapy," *KoDiscovery*, https://www.kodiscovery.org.

[28] *Ibid.*

[29] Katrin Hoffmeyer et al., "Wnt/β-Catenin Signaling Regulates Telomerase in Stem Cells and Cancer Cells," *Science* 336, no. 6088 (June 22, 2012): 1549–1554, https://doi.org/10.1126/science.1218370.

[30] Joe Tippins, https://mycancerstory.rocks/the-blog/.

[31] Simon Yu, Parasite, Fungal, Dental Infections and Cancer: Unconventional Diagnostic Therapies (2024): YouTube. https://www.youtube.com/watch?v=6S3qKGV39jc

[32] Natalie C. Silmon de Monerri and Kami Kim, "Pathogens Hijack the Epigenome: A New Twist on Host-Pathogen Interactions," *The American Journal of Pathology* 184, no. 4 (April 2014): 897–911. https://doi.org/10.1016/j.ajpath.2013.12.022.

[33] Bobak Robert Mozayeni et al., "Rheumatological Presentation of Bartonella Koehlerae and Bartonella Henselae Bacteremias: A Case Report," *Medicine* 97, no. 17 (2018): e0465, https://doi.org/10.1097/MD.0000000000010465.

[34] Uwe Pleyer et al., "Toxoplasmosis in Germany: Epidemiology, Diagnosis, Risk Factors, and Treatment," *Deutsches Ärzteblatt international* (June 21, 2019), https://doi.org/10.3238/arztebl.2019.0435.

[35] Joseph Adrian L Buensalido, et al., "Rhinovirus (RV) Infection (Common Cold): Practice Essentials, Background, Pathophysiology" (February 6, 2025), https://emedicine.medscape.com/article/227820-overview.

[36] Leon Caly et al., "The FDA-Approved Drug Ivermectin Inhibits the Replication of SARS-CoV-2 in Vitro," *Antiviral*

Research 178 (June 2020): 104787. 104787, https://doi.org/10.1016/j.antiviral.2020.104787.

[37] Juliana Cepelowicz Rajter et al., "Use of Ivermectin Is Associated With Lower Mortality in Hospitalized Patients With Coronavirus Disease 2019," *Chest* 159, no. 1 (2021): 85–92, https://doi.org/10.1016/j.chest.2020.10.009.

[38] Vika Guloyan et al., "Glutathione Supplementation as an Adjunctive Therapy in COVID-19," *Antioxidants (Basel, Switzerland)* 9, no. 10 (September 25, 2020): 914, https://doi.org/10.3390/antiox9100914.

[39] David Weinberger, "The Machine That Would Predict the Future," *Scientific American*, last modified December 1, 2011, https://www.scientificamerican.com/article/the-machine-that-would-predict.

[40] *Ibid.*

[41] Prevention and Healing, Simon Yu, M.D., *Dr Simon Yu MD 2018: Parasite Medications Targeting Cancer Cells* (2018), https://www.youtube.com/watch?v=pr-prRfV5_8.

[42] Hanns Hippius and Gabriele Neundörfer, "The Discovery of Alzheimer's Disease," *Dialogues in Clinical Neuroscience* 5, no. 1 (March 2003): 101–108. https://doi.org/10.31887/DCNS.2003.5.1/hhippius.

[43] Mayo Clinic Staff, "The Role of Genes in Your Alzheimer's Risk." *Mayo Clinic*, https://www.mayoclinic.org/diseases-conditions/alzheimers-disease/in-depth/alzheimers-genes/art-20046552.

[44] Patrick Störtebecker, *op. cit.*

[45] Marijke De Couck et al., "The Role of the Vagus Nerve in Cancer Prognosis: A Systematic and a Comprehensive Review," *Journal of Oncology* 2018 (July 2, 2018): 1–11, https://doi.org/10.1155/2018/1236787.

[46] Dr. Med. Helmut Retzek, Holistic Medicine, Website. https://ganzemedizin.at/en/homepage-ganzemedizin-english/ .

[47] Ari Whitten, *The Ultimate Guide to Red Light Therapy* (Florida: Archangel Ink, 2018).

[48] F. Gonzalez-Lima and Allison Auchter, "Protection against Neurodegeneration with Low-Dose Methylene Blue and near-Infrared Light," *Frontiers in Cellular Neuroscience* 9 (May 12, 2015), https://doi.org/10.3389/fncel.2015.00179.

[49] Prashant R. Ginimuge and S. D. Jyothi, "Methylene Blue: Revisited," *Journal of Anaesthesiology, Clinical Pharmacology* 26, no. 4 (October 2010): 517–520. https://pmc.ncbi.nlm.nih.gov/articles/PMC3087269.

[50] "The Nobel Prize in Physiology or Medicine 1998." *NobelPrize.Org*, https://www.nobelprize.org/prizes/medicine/1998/summary.

[51] Mark Sloan, *The Ultimate Guide to Methylene Blue: Remarkable Hope for Depression, COVID, AIDS & Other Viruses, Alzheimer's, Autism, Cancer, Heart Disease, ... Targeting Mitochondrial Dysfunction* (Endalldisease Publishing, 2020).

[52] Thomas Butler, "The Jarisch–Herxheimer Reaction After Antibiotic Treatment of Spirochetal Infections: A Review of Recent Cases and Our Understanding of Pathogenesis," *The American Journal of Tropical Medicine and Hygiene* 96, no. 1 (January 11, 2017): 46–52, https://doi.org/10.4269/ajtmh.16-0434.

⁵³ Helmut Retzek, *For Dr. Simon Yu: Parasite Patient Testimonial*, 2021,
https://www.youtube.com/watch?v=zi7LXiCzSH4.

⁵⁴ Bruce H. Lipton, *The Biology of Belief: Unleashing the Power of Consciousness, Matter & Miracles*, 10th anniversary edition. 2nd edition. (Carlsbad, California: Hay House, 2016).

⁵⁵ "Drug Expiration Dates — Do They Mean Anything?," *Harvard Health*, last modified November 1, 2003,
https://www.health.harvard.edu/staying-healthy/drug-expiration-dates-do-they-mean-anything.

⁵⁶ Erik Vance, "Power of the Placebo," *Discover Magazine*, last modified July 19, 2014,
https://www.discovermagazine.com/power-of-the-placebo-3059.

⁵⁷ Jonathan Kipnis, "Immune System: The 'Seventh Sense,'" *Journal of Experimental Medicine* 215, no. 2 (February 5, 2018): 397–398,
https://doi.org/10.1084/jem.20172295.

⁵⁸ *Ibid*.

⁵⁹ Nicholas J. Schork, "Personalized Medicine: Time for One-Person Trials," *Nature* 520, no. 7549 (April 30, 2015): 609–611, https://doi.org/10.1038/520609a.

⁶⁰ Simon Yu, "Prevention and Healing, Simon Yu, MD," *YouTube Channel*, https://www.youtube.com/channel/UCSO7O3Xa5yxRDtv83r1c Zdg.

Bibliography

Becker, Robert, and Gary Selden. *The Body Electric: Electromagnetism And The Foundation Of Life.* 1 edition. New York: William Morrow Paperbacks, 1998.

Buensalido, Joseph Adrian L et al. "Rhinovirus (RV) Infection (Common Cold): Practice Essentials, Background, Pathophysiology" (February 6, 2025). https://emedicine.medscape.com/article/227820-overview.

Butler, Thomas. "The Jarisch–Herxheimer Reaction After Antibiotic Treatment of Spirochetal Infections: A Review of Recent Cases and Our Understanding of Pathogenesis." *The American Journal of Tropical Medicine and Hygiene* 96, no. 1 (January 11, 2017): 46–52. https://doi.org/10.4269/ajtmh.16-0434.

Caly, Leon et al. "The FDA-Approved Drug Ivermectin Inhibits the Replication of SARS-CoV-2 in Vitro." *Antiviral Research* 178 (June 2020): 104787. https://doi.org/10.1016/j.antiviral.2020.104787.

Cook, Douglas L. *Rescued By My Dentist: New Solutions to a Health Crisis.* BC, Canada: Trafford Publishing, 2009.

De Couck, Marijke et al. "The Role of the Vagus Nerve in Cancer Prognosis: A Systematic and a Comprehensive Review." *Journal of Oncology* 2018 (July 2, 2018): 1–11. https://doi.org/10.1155/2018/1236787.

Doidge, Norman. *The Brain That Changes Itself: Stories of Personal Triumph from the Frontiers of Brain Science.* New York: Viking, 2007.

Fadhil Ali Malaa, S et al. "Assessment of Entamoeba Gingivalis and Trichomonas Tenax in Patients with Chronic Diseases and Its Correlation with Some Risk Factors." *Archives of Razi Institute* 77, no. 1 (February 28, 2022): 87–93. https://doi.org/10.22092/ari.2021.356549.1868.

Gerber, Richard. *A Practical Guide to Vibrational Medicine: Energy Healing and Spiritual Transformation.* New ed. edition. New York; London: William Morrow Paperbacks, 2001.

Giddon, Donald B., Donald R. Moeller, and Curtis K. Deutsch. "Use of a Modified Mandibular Splint to Reduce Nocturnal Symptoms in Persons With Post-Traumatic Stress Disorder." *International Dental Journal* 71, no. 2 (2021): 167–171. https://doi.org/10.1111/idj.12619.

Ginimuge, Prashant R., and S. D. Jyothi. "Methylene Blue: Revisited." *Journal of Anaesthesiology, Clinical Pharmacology* 26, no. 4 (October 2010): 517–520. https://pmc.ncbi.nlm.nih.gov/articles/PMC3087269/.

Gonzalez-Lima, F., and Allison Auchter. "Protection against Neurodegeneration with Low-Dose Methylene Blue and near-Infrared Light." *Frontiers in Cellular Neuroscience* 9 (May 12, 2015). https://doi.org/10.3389/fncel.2015.00179.

Guilford, Frederick T., and Simon Yu. "Antiparasitic and Antifungal Medications for Targeting Cancer Cells Literature Review and Case Studies." *Alternative Therapies in Health and Medicine* 25, no. 4 (July 2019): 26–31. https://pubmed.ncbi.nlm.nih.gov/31202208.

Guloyan, Vika et al. "Glutathione Supplementation as an Adjunctive Therapy in COVID-19." *Antioxidants (Basel, Switzerland)* 9, no. 10 (September 25, 2020): 914. https://doi.org/10.3390/antiox9100914.

Harvard Health. "Drug Expiration Dates — Do They Mean Anything?" *Harvard Health.* Last modified November 1, 2003. https://www.health.harvard.edu/staying-healthy/drug-expiration-dates-do-they-mean-anything.

Hellström, Per M. "This Year's Nobel Prize to Gastroenterology: Robin Warren and Barry Marshall Awarded for Their Discovery of Helicobacter Pylori as Pathogen in the Gastrointestinal Tract." *World Journal of Gastroenterology:*

WJG 12, no. 19 (May 21, 2006): 3126. https://www.ncbi.nlm.nih.gov/pmc/articles/PMC4124396.

Hippius, Hanns, and Gabriele Neundörfer. "The Discovery of Alzheimer's Disease." *Dialogues in Clinical Neuroscience* 5, no. 1 (March 2003): 101–108. https://doi.org/10.31887/DCNS.2003.5.1/hhippius.

Hoffmeyer, Katrin et al. "Wnt/β-Catenin Signaling Regulates Telomerase in Stem Cells and Cancer Cells." *Science* 336, no. 6088 (June 22, 2012): 1549–1554. https://doi.org/10.1126/science.1218370.

Kipnis, Jonathan. "Immune System: The 'Seventh Sense.'" *Journal of Experimental Medicine* 215, no. 2 (February 5, 2018): 397–398. https://doi.org/10.1084/jem.20172295.

Ko, Young Hee, "KoDiscovery | 3-BP | Young Hee Ko | Metabolic Cancer Therapy." Website. *KoDiscovery*, https://www.kodiscovery.org.

Liao, Felix. Six-Foot Tiger, Three-Foot Cage: Take Charge of Your Health by Taking Charge of Your Mouth: Holistic Mouth Solutions for Sleep Apnea, Deficient Jaws, and Related Complications. Carlsbad, CA: Crescendo Publishing, 2017.

Lipton, Bruce H. *The Biology of Belief: Unleashing the Power of Consciousness, Matter & Miracles*. 10th anniversary edition. 2nd edition. Carlsbad, California: Hay House, 2016.

Mashekova, Aigerim et al. "Early Detection of the Breast Cancer Using Infrared Technology – A Comprehensive Review." *Thermal Science and Engineering Progress* 27 (2022): 101142. https://doi.org/10.1016/j.tsep.2021.101142.

Mayo Clinic Staff. "The Role of Genes in Your Alzheimer's Risk." *Mayo Clinic*. https://www.mayoclinic.org/diseases-conditions/alzheimers-disease/in-depth/alzheimers-genes/art-20046552.

McLelland, Jane. *How to Starve Cancer: ...And Then Kill It With Ferroptosis*. England: Agenor Publishing, 2021.

Carolyn McMakin, The Resonance Effect: How Frequency Specific Microcurrent Is Changing Medicine, 1 edition. Berkeley, California: North Atlantic Books, 2017.

Merwin, Samantha J. et al., "Organophosphate Neurotoxicity to the Voluntary Motor System on the Trail of Environment-Caused Amyotrophic Lateral Sclerosis: The Known, the Misknown, and the Unknown." *Archives of Toxicology* 91, no. 8 (August 2017): 2939–2952. https://doi.org/10.1007/s00204-016-1926-1.

Mozayeni, Bobak Robert et al. "Rheumatological Presentation of Bartonella Koehlerae and Bartonella Henselae Bacteremias: A Case Report." *Medicine* 97, no. 17 (2018): e0465. https://doi.org/10.1097/md.0000000000010465.

Oschman, James L. *Energy Medicine: The Scientific Basis*. 2nd edition. Edinburgh: Churchill Livingstone, 2015.

Parisky, Y. R., et al. "Efficacy of Computerized Infrared Imaging Analysis to Evaluate Mammographically Suspicious Lesions." *American Journal of Roentgenology* 180, no. 1 (2003): 263–269. https://doi.org/10.2214/ajr.180.1.1800263.

Pleyer, Uwe et al. "Toxoplasmosis in Germany: Epidemiology, Diagnosis, Risk Factors, and Treatment." *Deutsches Ärzteblatt international* (June 21, 2019). https://pmc.ncbi.nlm.nih.gov/articles/PMC6706837.

Rajter, Juliana Cepelowicz et al. "Use of Ivermectin Is Associated With Lower Mortality in Hospitalized Patients With Coronavirus Disease 2019." *Chest* 159, no. 1 (2021): 85–92. https://doi.org/10.1016/j.chest.2020.10.009.

Retzek, Helmut. "Holistic Medicine." Website. https://ganzemedizin.at/en/homepage-ganzemedizin-english/.

Retzek, Helmut. *For Dr. Simon Yu: Parasite Patient Testimonial*, 2021. https://www.youtube.com/watch?v=zi7LXiCzSH4.

Schork, Nicholas J. "Personalized Medicine: Time for One-Person Trials." *Nature* 520, no. 7549 (April 30, 2015): 609–611. https://doi.org/10.1038/520609a.

Seyfried, Thomas. *Cancer as a Metabolic Disease: On the Origin, Management, and Prevention of Cancer*. 1 edition. Hoboken, N.J: Wiley, 2012.

Silmon de Monerri, Natalie C., and Kami Kim. "Pathogens Hijack the Epigenome: A New Twist on Host-Pathogen Interactions." *The American Journal of Pathology* 184, no. 4 (April 2014): 897–911. https://doi.org/10.1016/j.ajpath.2013.12.022.

Sloan, Mark. *The Ultimate Guide to Methylene Blue: Remarkable Hope for Depression, COVID, AIDS & Other Viruses, Alzheimer's, Autism, Cancer, Heart Disease, ... Targeting Mitochondrial Dysfunction*. Endalldisease Publishing, 2020.

Störtebecker, Patrick. *Dental Caries as a Cause of Nervous Disorders: Epilepsy, Schizophrenia, Multiple Sclerosis, Brain Cancer; Additional Notes on Myasthenia Gravis, High Blood Pressure*. Orlando, Fla: Bio-Probe, 1986.

Swanson, Claude. *Life Force, the Scientific Basis: Volume 2 of the Synchronized Universe*. 2nd edition. Tucson, AZ: Poseidia Press, 2011.

Tennant, Jerry L. *Healing Is Voltage: The Handbook, 3rd Edition*. 3rd edition. CreateSpace Independent Publishing Platform, 2010.

"The Nobel Prize in Physiology or Medicine 1998." *NobelPrize.Org*. https://www.nobelprize.org/prizes/medicine/1998/summary/.

Van Gelder, H. *The Process of Healing: A Field Theory Approach*. R. Martin Outsound, 1989.

Vance, Erik. "Power of the Placebo." *Discover Magazine*. Last modified July 19, 2014. https://www.discovermagazine.com/power-of-the-placebo-3059.

Veith, Ilza, ed. *The Yellow Emperor's Classic of Internal Medicine*. New ed. Berkeley: University of California Press, 2016.

Weinberger, David. "The Machine That Would Predict the Future." *Scientific American*. Last modified December 1, 2011. https://www.scientificamerican.com/article/the-machine-that-would-predict/.

Whitten, Ari. *The Ultimate Guide to Red Light Therapy*. Florida: Archangel Ink, 2018.

Winsor, Carolyn. "Praxis 2 Practice – Aus Der Praxis To Your Practice." Website. https://praxis2practice.com.

Winsor, Carolyn. "Occidental Institute Research Foundation." Website. *Publications*. https://oirf.com.

Yu, Simon. *Accidental Blow Up in Medicine: Battle Plan for Your Life*. 1 edition. St. Louis, Mo.: Prevention and Healing, 2019.

Yu, Simon. *Accidental Cure: Extraordinary Medicine for Extraordinary Patients*. St. Louis, Mo.: Prevention and Healing, Inc., 2010

Yu, Simon. "Prevention & Healing." Website. https://preventionandhealing.com.

Yu, Simon. *Parasite Medications Targeting Cancer Cells*, Prevention and Healing, 2018. https://www.youtube.com/watch?v=pr-prRfV5_8.

Yu, Simon. *Parasite, Fungal, Dental Infections and Cancer: Unconventional Diagnostic Therapies*, 2024. https://www.youtube.com/watch?v=6S3qKGV39jc.

Yu, Simon. "Prevention and Healing," *YouTube Channel*. https://www.youtube.com/channel/UCSO7O3Xa5yxRDtv83r1cZdg.

Index

A

AcciDental Blow Up in Medicine: Battle Plan for Your Life, Simon Yu, 157, 325, 365
Accidental Cure: Extraordinary Medicine for Extraordinary Patients, Simon Yu, 325, 332, 349
Acid Reflux, 77–78
Addiction, 271
Adrenal Burnout, 167, 237, 239
Adrenal Point, 120, 361
Advanced interrogation, 59, 329–330, 361
Advanced respiratory distress syndrome (ARDS), 251
Airborne allergies/intolerances, 363
Airway, 52
Alien Intelligence, 325
All-cause mortality, 222
Allergy/immune system problems, 99
Allergy Immunology, 364
Allergy related symptoms, 300
Allopathic Test Substance, 43
ALS, diagnosis of, 141, 277
Alzheimer's disease, 162, 262–265
AMA with "Enhanced Interrogation", 239
AMA evaluation/readings/testing, 36, 200, 202
AMA Störtebecker Diagram, 115
AMA technical advancements, 42
AMA Wavelength, 282–283
Amalgams, 52
Amyotrophic lateral sclerosis (ALS), 63, 79, 141–145, 162, 168, 263, 275, 277, 293, 351, 360
Ancient Intelligence, 40, 193, 278, 310, 325
Ancient Romans, 67, 306
Anemia, 95, 124, 154, 223
Anger, 97
Angiostrongylus cantonensis, 264
Antibiotics:
  amoxicillin, 163, 178
  Augmentin, 163, 178
  azithromycin, 163, 178, 189
  clindamycin, 178
  doxycycline, 178, 189
  metronidazole, 195
  sulfadiazine, 235–236
  tinidazole, 178

Antifungals:
  fluconazole, 88–89
  itraconazole, 88
  nystatin, 73, 88–89
Antiparasitic Medication Pseudo-Paradox, 337–338
Antiparasitics, 78, 103, 166, 196, 300, 331
  albendazole, 189, 363
  anti-malarial drug, 286
  fenbendazole, 197–198, 305
  hydroxychloroquine, 285
  ivermectin, 306–307, 322, 337
  mebendazole, 200, 239, 341, 343
  niclosamide, 200, 340–341
  praziquantel, 239, 307, 322, 337, 343
  pyrantel pamoate, 307, 337, 340, 363
  pyrimethamine, 235–236
Antiviral, 43, 173, 200, 248, 252–253
Anxiety/depression, 59, 67
Arthralgia (pain), 135, 139, 154
Arthritic pain, 116
Artificial Intelligence (AI), 32, 40, 46, 69, 75, 80, 84, 255, 273, 278, 280–281, 291, 310, 325
Autism, 79, 87, 89–90, 215, 240–241, 287, 319

Autism and Autism Spectrum Disorder, 90
Autism Treatment Evaluation Checklist (ATEC), 89–90
Autoimmune:
  Disease, 112, 119–120, 122
  Problems, 211, 237
  Symptoms, 118, 120
Autonomic Nervous System, 86, 90–91, 110, 175
Autonomic Response Testing (ART), 13, 319
azithromycin, 163, 178, 189, 195, 246

B

Bacteria:
  Actinomyces, 160, 165
  Anaplasmosis, 225
  Bartonella, 225, 332
  Borrelia (Lyme disease), 225–227, 332
  Enterobacter, 160
  Haemophilus, 160
  Mycoplasma, 244, 264
  Prevotella, 103, 160
  Serratia, 160
  Staphylococcus, 160
Bacterial infections, 70, 78–79, 161, 163, 178, 231, 263
Balanced diet, 123
Becker, Robert O., 34
Bio-feedback therapy, 309
Biocybernetics, 33–34, 44–46, 282

Biohacking, 191–192, 195–196, 216
Biological Dentistry, 52
Biological Terrain, 35, 100, 104, 139, 164–165
Biologics, 138–141
The Biology of Belief, Bruce H. Lipton, 33, 295–297, 301
Biophotons, 33, 45, 283, 317
Biophysics, 33, 317
Biopsy, 112, 128–129, 136–137
Bioresonance, 261, 280, 357
Biotoxins, 94, 144, 165
Bipolar Disorder, 271
Bite, Breathing, Brainstem (BBB), 174
Bite-TMJ issues, 144
Blood:
  Chemistry, 192
  Pressure, 192
  Products, 140
The Body Electric: Electromagnetism and The Foundation of Life, Robert O. Becker, 34
Bonding Materials, 52
Boron, 246, 348
Borrelia spirochete infection, 225
Brain fog, 43, 89, 95, 99, 232, 266, 335, 347, 349
Brain-Gut Connection, 318
Brain-Gut-Immune Connection, 317, 319
Brain Neuromodulation, 262, 268–271
Brain Neuromodulation Therapy, 262, 268–273
Brainstem connections, 174
Breast:
  Cancer, 86, 98–99, 101
  Cancer treatment, 257
  Thermography, 136, 333
  Tissue, 165
Breastfeeding, 174, 176
Breathing exercise, 276
Bronchiectasis, 66, 252
Bronchoscopy, 148
Bruxism, 52, 95, 178
Bypass operation, 107

C

Caffeic Acid, 189
Calorie Restricted Diet, 148
Cancer:
  cells, 166, 170, 172–173, 183
  cells' development, 183–184
  mitochondria, 150, 183–184
  promoting immune activation, 43
Cancer as a Metabolic Disease, Thomas Seyfried, 150, 182
Candida, 162, 166
  Dimorphic, 166
Cardiovascular disease, 107, 110, 170, 291, 296
Cardiovascular problems,

109–110, 216–217
Cavitations, 52
Cellular degeneration, 134
Centers for Disease Control (CDC), 83, 92–94, 100, 249, 258, 289
Central nervous system, 77, 79, 90, 264
Cerebral learning disabilities, 271
Chakras, 282–283
Chemical:
  Exposures, 99, 185
  Poisoning, 286
Chemo/immunotherapy, 150
Chemotherapy, 63, 78, 99, 148, 160, 182, 206, 209, 212–213, 258, 292, 304
Chest pain, 74, 107–108, 110, 200, 216
Chronic Diarrhea, 82, 232
Chronic illness, 35, 43–44, 48, 164, 184–185, 290, 299, 320
Circulatory system, 86–87, 107–108
Clark, Hulda, 66
Cluster phenomenon, 145
CNS symptoms, 265
Coffee enemas, 357
Cognitive Enhancement, 287
Colon, 69, 257, 303, 357
  Cancer treatment, 257–258, 292
  Hydrotherapy, 357
Color Spectrum, 281–284

Composite Materials, 52
Connective/fibroid tissue, 134
Constipation, 87, 92, 95, 175, 342
Control Measurement Points (CMPs), 38–39, 361
  Foot Control Measurement Points, 39
  Hand Control Measurement Points, 38
Cook, Doug, 51
Coronary bypass, 257
COVID-19, 70, 76, 106, 140, 243–254, 262, 297, 299, 305
COVID, Seasonal Activity, 247
Cranial-Dental Vertebral Vein, 114
Creatinine, 123, 232, 336
CT scan, 147–148, 304
Cyber, 261
Cyprus, 269, 272–273, 275
Cyst/tumor, 95
Cytokines, 140, 183, 276, 318, 320
Cytomegalovirus, 160

D

Dementia, 162, 262–263, 266, 268
Dementia Spectrum Disorder, 263, 268
Dental Biopsy, DNA Connexions result of, 219

Dental Caries as a Cause of Nervous Disorders, Patrick Störtebecker, 114–115, 145, 350, 365
Dental DNA test, 54–55
Dental Infections, 62, 71, 74, 76
Dental Materials, 140, 144
Dental/Medical Complex Problems, 52
Dental meridian, 86, 91
Dental meridian disturbances, 108
Dental Pathogens, 162
Dental Problems, 108
Dental Procedures, 62, 123, 125, 127, 185, 300
Dental related infections, 195
Dental-related parasite problems, 236
Dental work, 130, 136–137, 140
Dental X-ray, 145, 148
Depression, 59, 67, 124, 163, 175, 222, 235, 271, 273, 287, 297, 308, 310, 313, 315
Dermatomyositis, 119
Detox/detoxification, 54, 73, 98
Diabetes, 51, 78, 107, 123–125, 127, 152, 201, 222, 252, 264, 291
Diabetes mellitus retinopathy, 222
Diarrhea, 82, 87–88, 92, 95, 121, 228, 232, 258, 331, 342, 344–345, 363
Digestion, 77, 79–84, 91, 96, 98, 106, 122, 175
Dizziness, 82, 235, 265
DNA:
    Connexions, 55, 102, 169, 180, 219
    Tests, 103
DNA Connexions, 55, 102, 169, 180, 219
Doctor-patient relationship, 314, 322
Dormant, 243–245
DPDx, 94
Drug therapy, 92, 120
Drugs, 68, 78, 87–88, 96, 104, 251–252, 264, 268, 314, 320–321, 341

E

EAV-AMA evaluation, 200
EBV reactivation, 332
Echinococcus spp., 264
Eczema, 67, 95, 138–139, 141, 201, 342
Effective anti-cancer, 330
Einstein, Albert, 174
Electroacupuncture
    According to Voll (EAV), 34, 40–43, 47, 59, 324, 330, 359, 362
Electrolyte imbalance, 124
Electromagnetic fields, 33
EMFs, 363

emotional changes/stress/trauma, 91, 97
Empty Sellar Syndrome, 82
Endocrine organs, 70, 76, 97, 106, 118, 122
Endotoxins, 292
Energy Medicine: The Scientific Basis, James L. Oschman, 34
Enhanced Interrogation Technique (EIT), 60, 62, 72–73, 238
Entamoeba histolytica, 165, 264
Environmental toxins, 60–61, 73–74, 78–79, 98, 144–145, 341, 354, 356, 363
Eosinophilia, 92, 95
Epigenetic(s), 215, 281, 292, 295–296
Epileptic seizures, 175, 265
Epstein-Barr Virus (EBV), 57, 332
Esophageal Reflux, 77, 82
Esophageal/stomach cancers, 77
"excessive mobility", 216
Extracorporeal blood oxygenation and ozonation (EBOO), 292–293, 357
Extracorporeal blood oxygenation and ozonation (EBOO), 292–293, 357
Extreme weakness, 124

F

Facial nerve (CN7), 99
Fake sugars, 139
Fat-soluble vitamins, 96
Fatigue, 335, 342, 347
FDA, 140–141, 198, 248, 252
Fear, 88
Fever of unknown origin (FUO), 67, 82–83, 85, 247–251
Folinic acid, 236
Food allergies, 87, 95, 139, 312
Food cravings, 95
Foot Control Measurement Points, 39
Frequency Specific Microcurrent (FSM), 271
Frequent infections, 124
Frequently Asked Questions (FAQs), 40, 327, 359, 362
Frontal lobe, 209
Fungal medications, 61, 73, 88–89, 104, 150–151, 160, 200, 250, 323
Fungi/Fungal infection:
   Candida, 162, 166
   Yeast, 139, 166

G

Gallbladder-liver-flush, 344, 357
Galvanic currents (the mouth battery), 52
Garcia, Donato Perez, 290, 292, 358

Gas/Bloating, 95
Gastrointestinal (GI), 66, 77, 80–81, 108–109, 116, 122, 167, 175, 193, 257
Genes, 46, 200, 215, 217, 231, 240
Glaucoma, 222
Glioblastoma Multiforme (GBM), 186, 205–208
Glossopharyngeal nerve (CN), 99, 226, 264–266, 300
Glucose/ketone ratio, 188, 190
Glutathione (GSH), 150, 246, 252–254
Gluten, 87, 139–140, 203
Glycolysis, 189
GMO food, 87
Guilford, Frederick T., 150, 170–173
Guilt, 127, 302, 311
Gut-brain connection, 55, 264
Gut-Immune connection, 118, 317, 319

H

Hair Tissue Mineral Analysis (HTMA), 61, 187–188, 190, 195
Hand Control Measurement Points, 38
Headache, 67, 79, 82, 90, 92, 95, 100, 116, 120, 237, 252, 265, 291, 297
Healing is Voltage: The Handbook, Jerry L. Tennant, 34
Heart:
 arrhythmia, 347
 attack, 88, 100, 107–110
 disease, 74, 172, 378
 health, 287
 meridian, 86, 99, 107, 112, 117
 rhythms, 74, 192
 transplant, 126, 257
Heart rate variability (HRV), 276
Heavy Metal Toxicity, 42, 83, 188, 228, 241, 259, 332
Heavy Metals, 52
Heisenberg and Schrodinger's quantum theory, 32
Hemat, Atel, 40, 253–254, 269, 327
Herxheimer reaction, 290, 337–338
Hesperidin, 189
Hidden dental infection, 35, 43, 45, 74, 78, 99, 216–220, 274, 315, 330, 348
Hidden Dental Problems, 51, 68, 126, 151, 225, 273–274, 301, 332
High Speed Drill, 52
Holistic biological dentists, 74
Homeopathic remedies, 330, 357
Hormone therapy, 129–130
Horowitz, Richard, 252, 254

How to Starve Cancer, Jane McLelland, 150
Human Genome Project, 33, 46, 240
Hyperbaric oxygen therapy (HBOT), 267, 357
Hyperbaric oxygen therapy (HBOT), 267, 357
Hypertension, 51, 70–71, 74, 76, 92, 107–110, 286, 291
Hyperventilation, 110
Hypoglossal nerve, 80
Hypothyroidism, 71

I

IBS/colitis, 95
IBS symptoms, 67
Immune deficiency, 95, 118, 120, 122
Immune Dysregulation, 44, 153, 156, 182
Immune suppression, 112, 118, 120
Immune System, 83, 99, 101, 104, 134, 139, 141, 155, 301, 310, 317–319, 331, 343, 345, 347, 353–354
Immunotherapy, 129, 148, 150, 182
Implants, 52
Infectious disease, 92, 172, 184, 200, 226, 249
Influenza, 247
Initial AMA Evaluation, 53, 200, 238
Insecurity, 235, 311

Insomnia, 59, 82, 116, 226, 232, 266, 271, 343
Insulin, 84, 130, 140, 145, 171, 200
Insulin potentiation therapy (IPT), 130, 145, 171, 206, 210
Insurance reimbursement, 120
Interstitial fibrosis of the lung, 119
Intestinal infection, 87
Intrauterine Device (IUDs), 116
Irritable Bowel Syndrome (IBS), 67, 82, 87–89, 95, 232, 252, 315, 353
Ischemic osteonecrosis, 346
IV chelation therapy, 267, 357
IV nutritional therapy, 357
IV UV/Ozone, 104, 206, 210

K

Ketogenic diet (KD), 151, 183–184, 186, 188
Kidney:
　disease, 355, 358–359
　Failure, 112, 123–124
　Meridian, 123–124, 126–127
　Problems, 217
　Transplant, 126, 257
Kipnis, Jonathan, 317
Klinghardt, Dietrich, 204, 319
Known and Unknown, Fear of the, 304

L

Lack of Adequate High-Quality Water, 331
Lambert-Eaton myasthenic syndrome (LEMS), 277
Lechner, Johann, 152, 156
Leg edema (swelling), 71, 124, 130, 200, 233, 235
Legal blindness, 222
Let the TOOTH Be Known, Dawn Ewing, 365
Lethargy/fatigue, 95
Leukemia, 199–202
  cause of, 199
Level Intravenous (IV), 63, 104, 171, 200, 267, 284
Life Force, The Scientific Basis: Volume 2 of the Synchronized Universe, Claude Swanson, 34
Lightheadedness, 74
Lipton, Bruce H., 33
Liver enzymes, 336
Liver fibrosis, 92
Living organisms, 33
Longevity, 182, 184, 187, 320, 323
Loss of appetite, 124
Low back pain, 82, 226
Lower wisdom teeth, 105, 111, 117, 122
Lumbago/low back pain, 82
Lung cancer, 70, 76, 148–150, 193, 212–213, 305
Lupus, 152–155, 246
Lyme, 234, 237, 243, 264, 266
  disease, 226–227
  DNA test, 103
  Long, 104
  Lyme-like bacteria, 350
  Panel, 167–168
Lymphadenitis, 233
Lymphatic, 51, 53, 89, 125, 148, 178, 223, 264, 350, 361
Lymphoma, 150, 154, 165, 199, 201

M

Macular Degeneration, 222–225, 265
Malaria, 92, 233, 235, 285
Man with Cancer, DNA Connexions for, 55
Mantle Cell Lymphoma, 203
Mast-cell activation, 237
MCAS (Mast Cell Activation Syndrome), 345
McMakin, Carolyn, 34, 271
Medical and Dental Disconnection (MAD), 48, 51, 53, 56–57, 131, 138, 149, 155, 237–238, 240
Medically unexplained symptoms (MUS), 71, 76, 93, 164
Meinig, George, 365
Melanoma, 139
Meningeal syndrome, 265

Mental Illness, 232, 236–237
Mercury, 83, 89, 114, 119, 121, 144, 155, 179, 201, 204, 210, 212–213, 228–229, 264, 267, 322, 349
Mercury fillings, 179, 204, 212
Meridians, classical:
   Bladder, 37, 39
   Gallbladder, 37
   Heart, 37–39
   Kidney, 37, 39
   Large Intestine, 37–38
   Liver, 37, 39
   Lung, 37–38
   Pericardium, 86–87
   Small Intestine, 37–38
   Spleen, 37, 39
   Stomach, 37, 39
   Triple Warmer, 37–38
Meridians, lesser known:
   Allergy/Immunology, 101, 109, 119, 134, 226
   Dental/Lymph, 54, 134
   Joint/Cartilage, 134–135
   Nerve Degeneration, 134, 141–144
   Skin, 134, 138–141
Metabolic dysfunction, 183
Metabolic Therapy, 182–184, 186, 189
Metabolism, 86, 96, 98, 105, 122, 127–128, 172, 179, 186, 231, 281, 285
Metal Allergies, 52

Metal orthodontic appliances, 353
Methylene Blue, 281, 284–287
Microbiome, 48, 100, 103, 139, 164, 179
Microcalcifications, 136
Microorganisms, 54–55, 114, 159, 265, 298
Migraine Headache, 67, 79, 90, 95, 141, 237, 252, 291, 297
Military Officers, case studies of, 81
Mind-Body Connection, 185
Miscommunication, 317
Mitochondria, 150, 183–184, 186, 190
   Damage, causes of, 184
   Dysfunction, 173
   Dysregulation, 181
Modern dentistry, 51, 145
Monoclonal antibody (mAb) products, 140
Morell, Franz, 33, 46, 283
MTHFR genes, 231
Multiple Risk Factors, 78, 264
Multiple sclerosis (MS), 66–67, 79, 99, 141, 144–145, 263, 265, 271, 291, 297, 333
Muscle/joint pain, 95
Myalgic Encephalomyelitis (CFS/ME), 98–99, 104, 192, 243

N

NAC, 253
National Center for Biotechnology Information (NCBI), 172
Nerve Degeneration (ND), 68, 100, 134, 141–142, 144
  Medical Acupuncture on, 141
Nerve Meridian Disorder, 142
Nervous Disorders, 114–115, 145, 350, 365
Nervous System:
  Autonomic, 86–87
  Central, 86
  Enteric, 86, 91
  Neurovegetative, 87
  Parasympathetic, 87
  Peripheral, 86
  Sympathetic, 87
Neurodegeneration, 263–264, 266
Neurodegenerative conditions, 79
Neurodegenerative Disease, 211, 240–241, 263, 265
Neuroinflammation, 43, 262–263, 266
Neurological:
  Diseases, 141, 147, 169, 190
  Disorder, 44, 53, 56, 145, 351
  and psychological symptoms, 347
  Symptoms, 43, 89, 116, 240
Neurological and psychological symptoms, 347
Neuromodulation, 86, 91, 261–262, 268–273, 275, 278, 313
Neuropathy, 156, 223, 237, 275
Neurovegetative activities, 87, 105, 108
  appetite, 87
  Concentration, 44, 85, 87
  Hormones, 84, 86–87
  Sleep, 82–83, 86–87
Night sweats, 95
Night waking/bed wetting, 95
Nightmares, 177, 358
NIH National Heart, Lung, and Blood Institute (NHLBI), 74
Nitric Oxide (NO), 183, 285–286
Non-Hodgkin's Lymphoma, 154
Non-Small Cell Lung Cancer, 148–150
Nutrition, 161, 164–167

O

Obesity, 51, 95, 264, 291
Occidental Institute Research Foundation (OIRF), 90, 99
On-and-off Atrial Fibrillation, 108
Optimizing health, 280

Oral circumcision, 161, 169
Organ Degeneration, 361
Oschman, James L., 34
Osler, William, 55, 161, 335
Ozone Dialysis Therapy, 292–293
Ozone therapy, 285, 357

P

Pain Reliever, 287
Palladium, 227–228, 230–232
Pancreatic cancer, 85–86, 93
Parasite medications, 53, 60, 66–71, 75, 83, 88–89, 93, 95–96, 267, 289, 297, 299, 340, 352, 364
Parasites:
   Angiostrongylus, 264
   Babesia, 332
   De-worming, 322–323
   E. gingivalis, 162–163
   Echinococcus, 264
   Entamoeba, 264, 266
   Infectious Relationships, 244–245
   Medications, 319, 322–324
   Metabolic Parasites, 150, 166, 184
   Multi-parasite infection, 337
   Parasite Infections, 71, 100–101, 139, 144, 154
   Parasitosis, 71, 223, 236, 300, 319
   Relationships, 244, 305, 342
   Schistosoma, 92, 96
   Taenia solium, 264
   Toxocara canis/cati, 264
   Toxoplasma, 264
   Treatment, 336
   Trichinella, 264
   Trypanosoma, 264
Parasites and Bruxism, 52
Parasympathetic, 87, 90, 105, 108, 276
Parkinson's disease, 79, 141, 144–145, 162, 200
Patient's AMA Evaluation, 36
Pelvic Vertebral Veins, 114
Periodontal Surgery, 161, 163, 169
PET scan, 148, 213
Phosphohexose isomerase (PHI), 170, 231
Placebo Effects, 297, 313–316
Pleomorphism of Bacteria and Protozoa, 52
Pneumocystis carinii, 235
Pneumonia, 66–67, 70, 245–246, 252, 297, 299
Poor Diet, 331
Popp, Albert, 45, 283
Positron emission tomography (PET), 148, 213, 314
Post-COVID syndrome (Long COVID), 56, 70, 75, 104, 110, 147, 242–243, 309
Post-Lyme Syndrome, 225–227, 243

Post-Treatment AMA Evaluation, 202
Postural orthostatic tachycardia syndrome (POTS), 237
A Practical Guide to Vibrational Medicine, Richard Gerber, 34
Practitioners, FAQs for, 327, 359
Praxis2Practice, 90
Prayer, 276
Price, Weston, 161
The Process of Healing, H. Van Gelder, 68
Proprioception, 52
Prostate Cancer, 128–131, 158, 196
Prostate Cancer Treatment, 196
Prostate-dental connection, 131
Prostate Specific Antigen (PSA), 112–113, 128–130
Protozoa, 52, 162, 166
    Babesia, 167
    Entamoeba, 164–167
    Toxoplasma, 235–236
    Trichomonas, 162
Protozoal parasites, 116, 160, 162, 164
PTSD, 313
Pulmonary arterial hypertension (PAH), 74
Pulmonary embolism, 74
Pulmonary Hypertension, 70–71, 74, 76, 286
pyrantel pamoate, 66–67, 73, 83, 89, 101, 109, 250, 307, 337, 340, 363
Pyrimethamine, 235–236

Q

Quantum Entanglement, 295–296, 298, 301

R

Random clinical trial (RCT), 144, 253
RANTES, 44, 152, 156
Real-time diagnostics, 46
Recirculatory Hemoperfusion (RHP), 293
Recurrent Tumor, MRI of, 209–210
Red Light therapy, 284–285, 287
Regulated upon activation, normal T-cell expressed and secreted, 156
Regulates blood glucose levels, 96
Regulates blood volume, 97
Rescued By My Dentist, Doug Cook, 51
The Resonance Effect, Carolyn McMakin, 34
Retzek, Helmut, 40–41, 157, 233, 246, 253, 269, 272, 275, 290
Rheumatic diseases, 156
Rheumatism, 135, 162–163,

234, 237
Rhinovirus, 247
Rocky Mountain Spotted Fever (RMSF), 226
Root Canal Cover Up, George Meinig, 365
Root Canals, 52
Routine dental care, 135, 322–323

S

Seeds of Deception and Corrupt Science, Jeffrey Smith, 215
Self-help, 272, 280
Severe Fatigue, 82, 100, 120, 226, 237
Sexual dysfunction, 95
Seyfried, Thomas, 150–151, 182
Shame, 311
Shortness of breath, 71, 74, 92, 94, 100, 234
Sickle cell disease, 74
Six-Foot Tiger, Three-Foot Cage: Take Charge of Your Health by Taking Charge of Your Mouth, Felix Liao, 177
Skin:
  diseases, 139
  Rashes, 139
Sleep:
  apnea, 82, 144, 174–175, 261
  Disruptions, 177
Patterns, 192
Social Parasites, 300, 305–306
Spontaneous Healing, 60, 104
Störtebecker, Patrick, 114–115, 145, 159, 265
Stress/anxiety disorder/management, 271
Structural Imbalance, 332
Submandibular Ganglion, 80
Swelling, 71, 124, 130, 200, 233, 235
Sympathetic, 87, 90, 99, 105, 108, 276, 320
Symptoms Associated with, 92, 229–230
  Lead, 228–230
  Mercury, 228–229

T

Tennant, Jerry L., 34
Testicular/ovarian plexus, 80
Textbook of Acupuncture, Felix Mann, 98
Thyroid, 53, 86, 98–99, 105, 108, 114, 134, 153, 165, 167, 169, 175, 266, 285, 302
Thyroid dysfunction, 98
Tippens, Joe, 193, 197, 305
Tiredness, 234–235
TMJ, 52
Tooth Injury, 112, 124
Tooth loss, 147, 162
Tooth-Organ Meridian Chart, 34, 40–43, 47, 59, 324, 330, 359, 362

Mandible-Lower, 48–50,
52, 69–70, 75–76, 111,
116–118, 122, 126, 132,
206, 347
Maxillary-Upper, 48–50,
52, 69–70, 116–118, 122,
126, 132, 206, 347
Toxic metals, 45, 61, 134,
228, 231, 327, 354, 363
Toxocara canis, 264
Toxocara cati, 264
Toxoplasmosis, 232–236
Toxoplasmosis questionnaire,
235
Toxoplasmosis Symptoms,
234
Traditional Chinese Medicine
(TCM), 34, 41, 46, 70, 76,
111, 282, 302, 361
Traditional Chinese Medicine
(TCM), 282, 302, 361
Transcranial Direct Current
Stimulation (tDCS),
269–273
Transcutaneous Auricular
Vagus Nerve Stimulation
(taVNS), 270–272
Trichinella, 264
Trigeminal nerve, 55, 90,
142, 144–145, 176–177,
261, 264–266, 277,
350–351
Trigeminal nerve-brainstem,
145
Triple-antiparasitic
combination, 337

Trypanosoma, 264
Type 1 diabetes, 152

U

*The Ultimate Guide to
Methylene Blue*, Mark
Sloan, 286–287
*The Ultimate Guide to Red
Light Therapy*, Ari
Whitten, 284, 287
Universal Ancestors,
evolutionary tree of, 244
Unresolved Emotions, 70, 302
Upper wisdom teeth, 105,
111, 117, 122
Ursolic Acid, 189
UV light laser color therapies
(UVLrx), 284

V

Vaccination, 140, 243, 257,
332
Vague GI problems, 108
Vagus nerve, 55, 80, 90, 142,
144, 177, 261, 264–266,
270, 275–276, 313,
318–319
Vagus nerve stimulation
(VNS), 270, 275, 313
Vagus parasympathetic
nervous system, 276
Vertigo, 110
Veterans, 292, 300
Vitamin supplements, 222
Vitamins, 69, 96, 203, 221,
314, 358

Voll Electroacupuncture Desk Reference Manual, 90, 99
Voll, Reinhold, 41, 51, 134, 138, 141, 196
Voltage-gated calcium channel (VGCC), 277

W

Wave-particle theory, 32
Weight loss/gain, 95
White blood cell count (WBC), 166, 199–200, 228, 336
Wnt signaling pathways, 191–194, 196
World War II, 285
World Without Cancer, Edward Griffin, 197

X

X-rays, 43–44, 108, 157, 208, 216, 351

Y

Yoga exercise, 276
Yu, Simon, 33, 35, 37, 39, 41–43, 45, 47, 49, 51, 53, 275, 277, 279, 281, 283, 285, 325, 363, 365

www.ingramcontent.com/pod-product-compliance
Lightning Source LLC
Chambersburg PA
CBHW060449030426
42337CB00015B/1529